Dental Implantology and Prostheses

Contributors

Charles A. Babbush, D.D.S., M.Sc.D., D.A.B.
Senior Visiting Oral Surgeon,
Mount Sinai Hospital;
Assistant Clinical Professor,
Case Western Reserve University School of Dentistry,
Cleveland, Ohio

Roy L. Bodine, D.D.S., F.A.C.D., D.A.B.
Clinical Professor, Advanced Prosthodontics,
University of Southern California School of Dentistry,
Los Angeles, California

Edwin S. Mehlman, D.D.S., F.I.C.D.
Assistant Clinical Professor of Endodontics,
Harvard School of Dental Medicine,
Staff Associate, Forsyth Dental Center
Boston, Massachusetts

Raymond J. Melrose, D.D.S.
Associate Professor,
Department of Pathology,
University of Southern California
School of Dentistry
Los Angeles, California

Myron Nevins, D.D.S., D.A.B.
Associate Clinical Professor of Periodontics,
Boston University School of Graduate Dentistry;
Boston, Massachusetts

Dental Implantology and Prostheses

Morton L. Perel, D.D.S., M.SC.D.

Assistant Clinical Professor
Department of Fixed Prosthodontics
Boston University School of Graduate Dentistry
Boston, Massachusetts
Assistant Dental Surgeon
Active Staff
Division of Dentistry
Department of Surgery
The Miriam Hospital
Providence, Rhode Island

605 Illustrations Including 37 in Color

J. B. Lippincott Company

Philadelphia • Toronto

ISBN 0-397-50347-4

Library of Congress Catalog Card Number 76-2596
Printed in the United States of America

1 3 5 6 4 2

Library of Congress Cataloging in Publication Data

Perel, Morton L
Dental implantology and prostheses.

Bibliography: p.
Includes index.
1. Implant dentures. I. Title. [DNLM: 1. Dental implantation. WU550 P437d]
RK667.I45P47 617.6'9 76-2596
ISBN 0-397-50347-4

This book is dedicated to the memory of Dr. Aaron Gershkoff (1915–1973). He was a compassionate and warm human being, a courageous pioneer in the field of dental implantology, a dear friend, and a genuine inspiration.

Preface

This textbook provides the essential facts of current clinical dental implantology, its practicability lying in the ability of the dental practitioner to attain an additional dimension of treatment by applying prescribed techniques in clinically feasible situations. Attention to detail in implant procedures and in related dental specialties is essential.

This book is not a historical review of dental implantology. Rather, it focuses on the types of implants that have withstood the tests of time. Instead of stressing a widened view encompassing implants of questionable design and technique, the emphasis is placed on dental implants that have served as *abutments* for both fixed and removable prostheses. This book is not merely a documentation of examples of successful dental implants, but is a purposefully sequential analysis of the making of a dental implant. The reader is given a step-by-step teaching discourse that (a) is attentive to the requirements of the patient, (b) illustrates the demands placed on the knowledge and skills of the dentist, and (c) is frank and honest, encouraging both the patient and the dentist to seek multispecialty counsel and treatment.

Animal and human histologic studies are included for three reasons. First, every clinician should be familiar with the histologic evidence that supports as well as disputes certain aspects of a practiced technique. Second, the nature and direction of research activities to date should lend direction to future investigations, even if they be tangential in approach. Third, it is as important for the researcher to be familiar with what is clinically expected from the dental implant as it is for the clinician to realize the basic limitations of dental implants, so that the development of materials and designs can be clinically sound.

The illustrations literally speak for themselves. Because concern for the supportive and surrounding hard and soft tissues is paramount, color photographs are selectively presented, in order to guide the reader in an appreciation for the colors and textures of the periodontal or peri-implant tissues. A standard of soft-tissue quality is set forth in the first chapter of this textbook. The total impact of its characteristics can only be appreciated by the student of implantology by extending his visual sense to its optimal capacity.

Techniques are placed within a framework of treatment planning. The viability of dental implants lies within case selection at one end of the spectrum and proper sequential treatment by other dental specialists at the other. For example, osteoporotic conditions generally are not amenable to implant procedures; and periodontal health must be fully restored *before* the impressions are taken for the final fixed prosthetic appliance.

The reader will follow proven techniques and learn to apply them properly. At no time should the hard and soft tissues, nor the prosthetic appliance of choice, be forgotten. As in any other dental specialty, the stomatognathic system as a functional, comfortable entity must be uppermost in the practitioner's mind.

Morton L. Perel, D.D.S., M.Sc.D

Acknowledgments

I extend my gratitude to Dr. David J. Baraban, Dr. Fredrick I. Muroff, Dr. Zoltan "Ben" Nyeste, Dr. Glenn Sutton, and Dr. Leo Talkov, for their guidance and their personal and professional concerns.

I appreciate also the help of Dr. Henry Goldman, Dean; Dr. Morris Rubin, Assistant Dean for Graduate Studies; and Dr. Herbert Schilder, Assistant Dean of Continuing Education; Boston University School of Graduate Dentistry, Boston, Massachusetts. Dr. Goldman and Dr. Rubin have had the foresight to include the teaching of basic precepts of oral implantology to graduate students in a sound academic environment. Dr. Schilder has fostered the implementation of postgraduate courses for dental practitioners through lectures and seminars with a multidisciplinary approach to dental implantology.

The cooperation and good will of my talented contributors to this textbook are appreciated: Dr. Charles A. Babbush, Dr. Roy L. Bodine, Dr. Edwin S. Mehlman, Dr. Raymond J. Melrose and Dr. Myron Nevins. Dr. Bodine wishes to acknowledge the following persons who have helped him in his histologic studies and analyses: Dr. Dale E. Grenoble, Assistant Professor of Dental Materials, School of Dentistry, University of Southern California, Los Angeles, California; and Dr. Clive I. Mohammed, Former Dean, School of Dentistry, University of Detroit, Detroit, Michigan. Dr. Nevins would like to acknowledge the contributions made to his chapter by Dr. Gerald M. Kramer, Professor and Chairman of the Department of Periodontics; and by Dr. Howard M. Skurow, Assistant Clinical Professor, Department of Prosthetics; Boston University School of Graduate Dentistry, Boston, Massachusetts.

Dr. Edward Listengart's assistance in oral surgery has been of real value. He has exposed complete arches for bone impressions and subperiosteal implant insertions.

Dr. Jeffrey Shapiro, Dr. Paul Segal, Dr. Daniel DeCesare, and Dr. Marvin Rosenberg, periodontists, have collaborated with me on combined treatment for various cases included in this volume.

Special thanks go to Mrs. Lois A. Gottlieb for her untiring and skillful typing and organizing of all phases of this manuscript. Her dedication and concern will always be appreciated.

Mr. Edward Hail has combined his artistic skills with a diligent study of oral implantology in order to render some of the fine drawings included herein. Mrs. Tina Powers is thanked for her responsible and proficient clinical assistance.

Ms. Marlene Levov has shown a remarkable talent as the copy editor of this text, and her study of the subject matter has reflected a rare dedication to her profession.

Mr. J. Stuart Freeman, Jr.'s advice, encouragement, and editorial counsel have reflected the positive attitude of a knowledgeable dental editor.

I wish to thank my father, Isadore Perel, and my mother, Estelle Perel, for their continuous interest and encouragement in all my professional endeavors.

I especially wish to thank my wonderful wife, Jane, whose love and understanding have sustained my own sense of purpose.

Contents

1 Implants in Perspective— An Introduction

THE PROSTHETIC ROLE OF DENTAL IMPLANTS

The dental implant should be viewed as part of the armamentarium available for a system of replacement. Lutz has advocated that fixed prostheses, removable prostheses, and implants be grouped under the heading of tertiary prevention.

Taxonomy of Preventive Dentistry

Primary Prevention
(Pre-pathosis)
1. Fluoride therapy, systemic or topical
2. Diet control
3. Plaque control
4. Sealants
5. Preventive orthodontics
6. Pulp protection
7. Tissue protection
8. Mouth guards, etc.

Secondary Prevention
(Intervention)
1. Restorative dentistry
2. Periodontics
3. Endodontics
4. Orthodontics
5. Oral surgery (most types)
6. Tissue biopsy

Tertiary Prevention
(Replacement)
1. Fixed prostheses
2. Removable prostheses
3. *Implants*

(Modified from Lutz, B. L.: Preventive dentistry: proposal for definition of terms. J. D. Educ., *37*:24-26, 1973)

A part or all of the dentition may be lost, so that the resultant dysfunction and disability are irreversible without the aid of replacement. Health maintenance in general may require the use of dental implants; dental implants may prevent people who are unable to masticate properly from deteriorating physically or psychologically.

Dental Disease, Dysfunction, or Disability Continuum

	Pathosis begins		*Loss of parts*	
Primary prevention	↓	Secondary prevention	↓	Tertiary prevention

(Modified from Lutz, B. L.: Preventive dentistry: proposal for definition of terms. J. D. Educ., *37*:24-26, 1973)

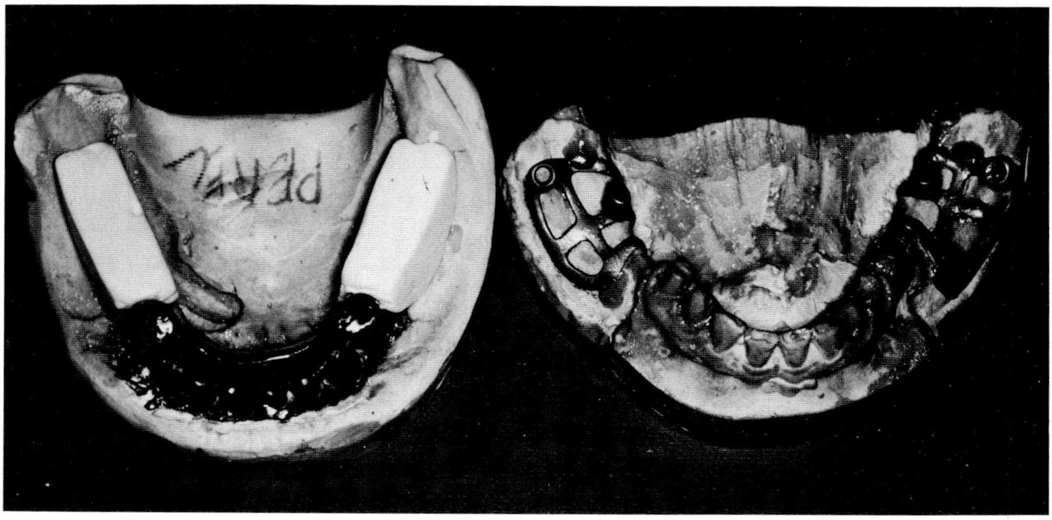

Fig. 1-1. Two cases with similar bilateral mandibular posterior edentulous areas. The combined anterior fixed segment *(left)* and posterior removable prosthesis is the treatment of choice. Bilateral subperiosteal implants *(right),* in conjunction with a fixed prosthetic superstructure, are used when the patient cannot tolerate a removable prosthetic appliance.

The oral implant then establishes itself in the continuum of oral disease treatment. In fact, the use of implants may be the last resort available in the rehabilitation of the dental cripple.

IMPLANTS WITHIN THE FRAMEWORK OF TOTAL DENTISTRY

Implants are not to be considered as equally acceptable alternatives to other forms of dental treatment. Rather, they are to be used only when other forms of treatment do not suffice in restoring the mouth to its function as a healthy, comfortable, masticatory organ. If the ridges of an edentulous arch are capable of supporting a removable complete denture, then this is the form of prosthesis that should be undertaken. Only if such prostheses are not tolerable by the patient should implantology be considered as a form of treatment. Also, the bilateral, free-end precision or semiprecision, removable mandibular denture is not to be supplanted by bilateral implants; however, if lingual bars or removable prostheses are not comfortable for the patient, then such implants may be offered as prosthodontic alternatives (Fig. 1-1). Implant dentistry does not supplant good total dentistry. To the contrary, the successful use of clinically acceptable dental implants is based on the sum total of the time, effort, skill, and knowledge that are basic to the performance of sound periodontal-prosthetic practices (Figs. 1-2 to 1-5). Any implant must be properly selected, properly designed, and properly inserted. But the implant is only the "means." The "end" is the prosthetic appliance that the implant must support in function, in comfort, and in a sound environment. Therefore, knowledge of implant procedures is but the beginning. Adherence to sound principles of periodontics and fixed and removable prosthodontics, along with an acceptable approach to occlusion, are necessary adjuncts in every aspect of oral implantology (Figs. 1-6 to 1-8).

Only the most knowledgeable and skill-

Chapter 1

Implants in Perspective—An Introduction

Plates 1–1—1–6

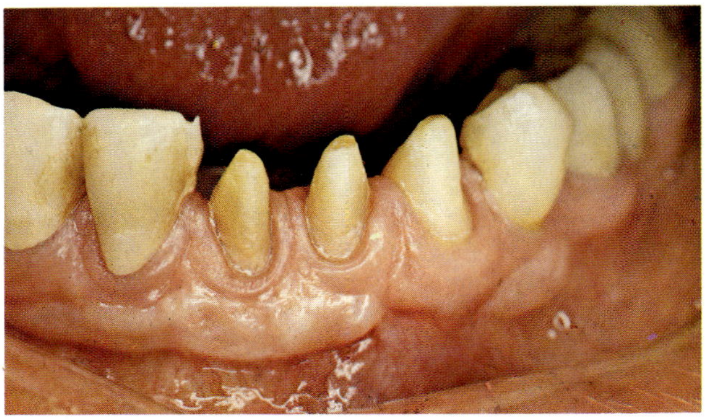
Plate 1–1. See Figure 1–2.

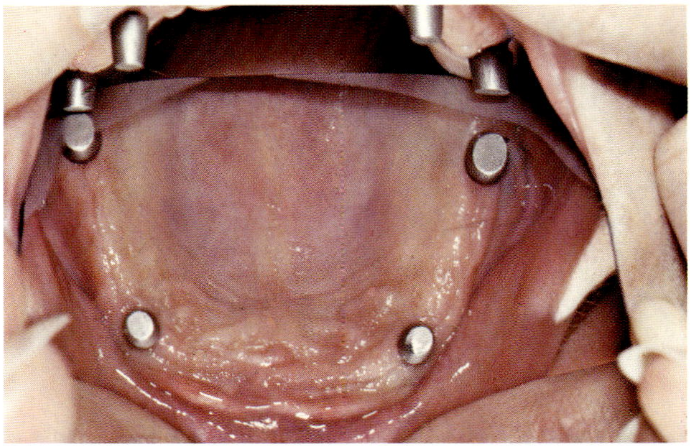
Plate 1–2. See Figure 1–3.

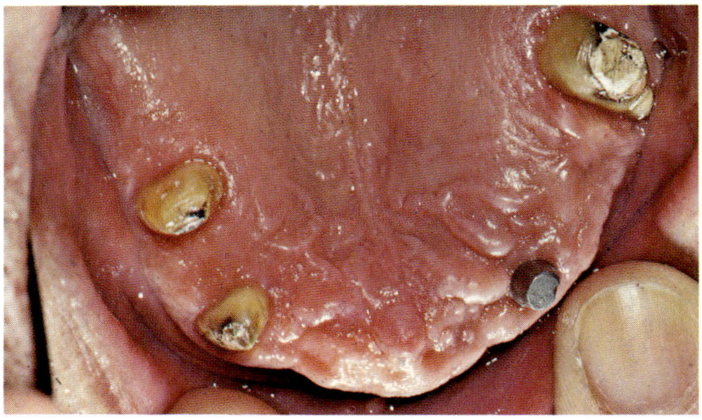
Plate 1–3. See Figure 1–4.

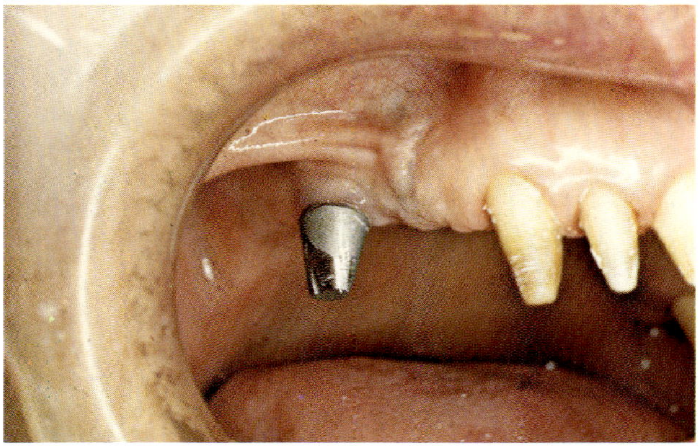
Plate 1–4. See Figure 1–5.

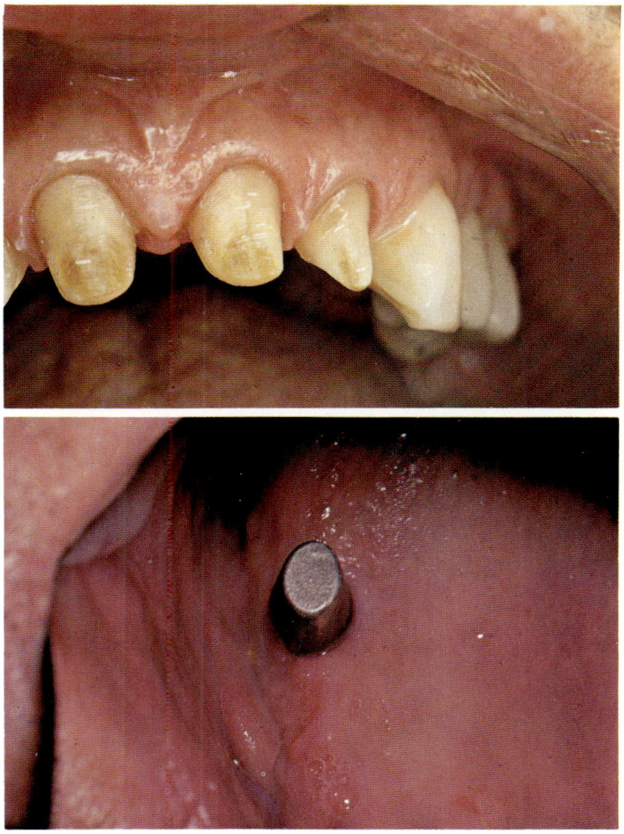

Plate 1–5. See Figure 1–13.

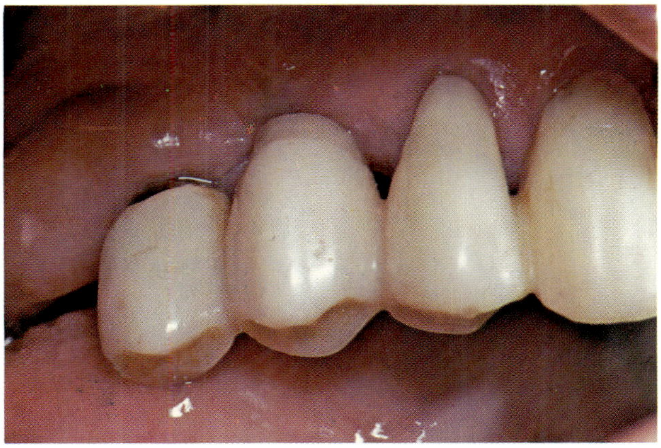

Plate 1–6. See Figure 1–16.

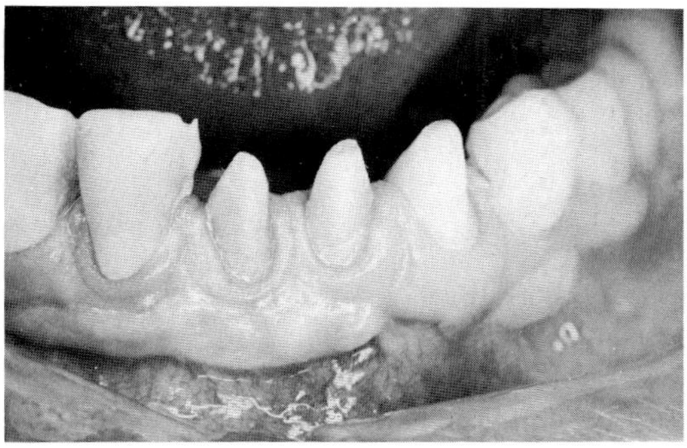

Fig. 1-2. Temporary acrylic-resin splint has been severed between the two central incisor teeth. A sound periodontal environment has been created with the aid of free gingival grafts. The restorative concern for the maintenance of a sound periodontium is exemplified by the topography, consistency, color, and cleanliness of the soft tissues. These periodontal and restorative standards are basic to all sound dental procedures. (See Plate 1-1.)

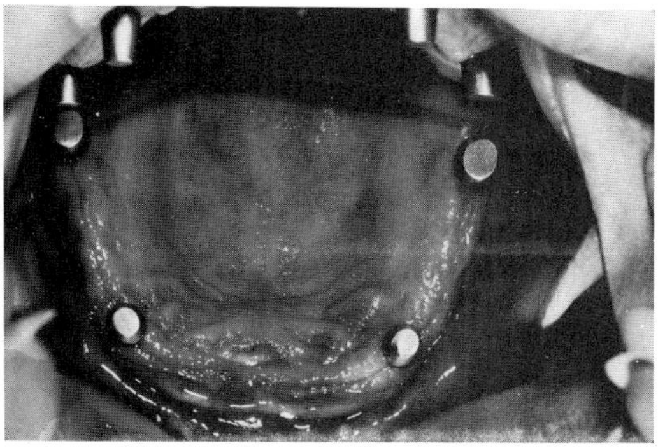

Fig. 1-3. Mirror view of the maxilla bearing a complete subperiosteal implant. The soft-tissue environment was maintained by means of a temporary removable appliance for 1 year prior to the fabrication of a permanent prosthesis. (See Plate 1-2.)

ful dentists—not those who are least capable of even executing the procedures of a three-unit fixed bridge—should be involved in implant procedures. If a team approach is to be used in executing the surgical and restorative phases of dental implants, a comprehension of one another's procedures is necessary. Communication and understanding of the interrelated disciplines is as necessary as the prosthodontist being knowledgeable in periodontal therapy and vice versa. Implant procedures are not merely surgical.

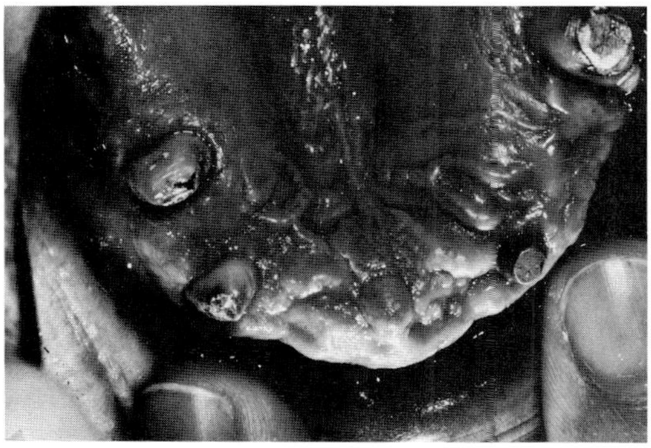

Fig. 1-4. Mirror view of the maxillary arch, showing an upper right cuspid, an upper right second bicuspid, an intermediary subperiosteal implant, and an upper left first molar which has been sectioned by the removal of the distobuccal root. Total treatment of this arch in preparation for a fixed prosthesis involved endodontics, periodontics, and implantology. The intermediary step that has allowed for the maintenance of the soft tissues consisted of an acrylic-resin provisional splint. (See Plate 1-3.)

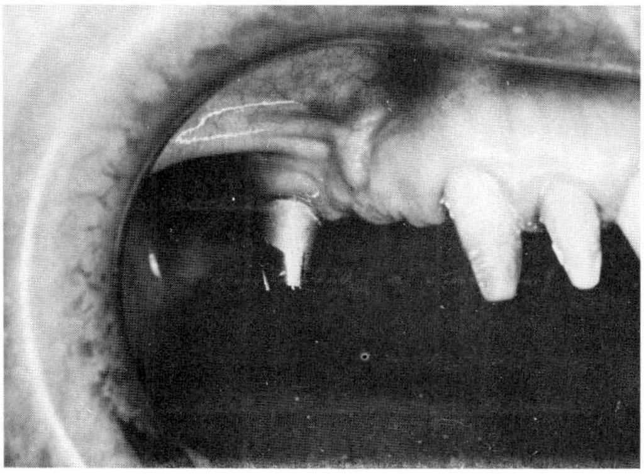

Fig. 1-5. An upper right unilateral subperiosteal implant in the area of the first molar. The implant was inserted after provisional splinting and periodontal treatment had been completed. Then, at the time of implant insertion, the provisional acrylic-resin splint was extended through two pontics to include the implant abutment post. This treatment precluded the use of a unilateral removable partial denture. (See Plate 1-4.)

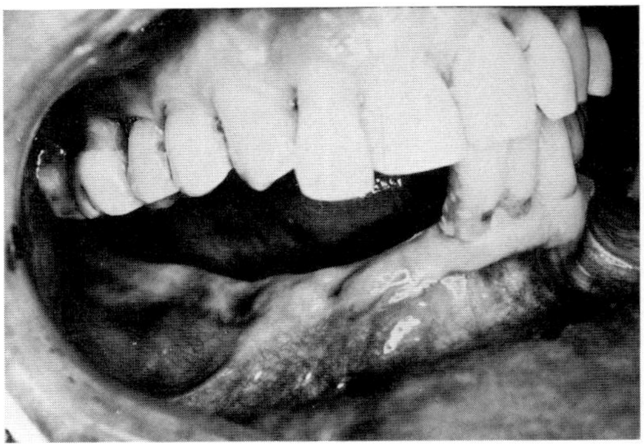

Fig. 1-6. At the examination, in conjunction with periodontal evaluation, the maxillary dentition was deemed to be hopelessly involved periodontally. The left mandibular remaining dentition was periodontally salvageable, with adequate supportive periodontium for a superimposed prosthesis. The resultant treatment plan was to fabricate a complete upper denture, and a complete lower fixed prosthesis with the supportive aid of implants.

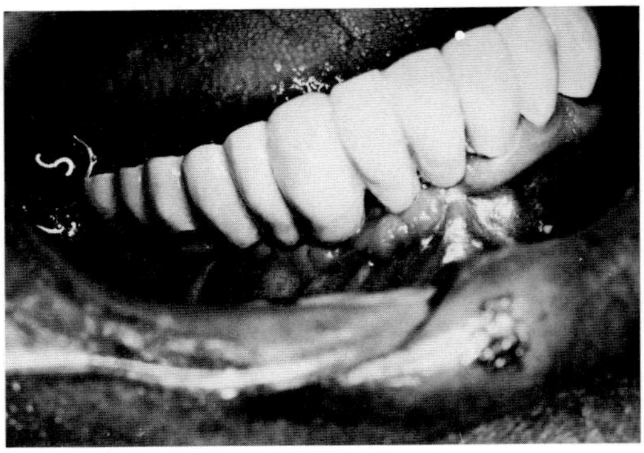

Fig. 1-7. The mandibular arch (see Fig. 1-6) has received a fixed acrylic-veneered prosthesis. This is supported by natural dentition on the left side extending through the lower left central incisor, by an endosseous blade-vent implant at the cuspid site, and by a terminal subperiosteal implant at the right molar area.

Implantology, periodontics, oral surgery, and occlusion must find their ultimate common denominator in the supportive role for a fixed or removable dental prosthesis:

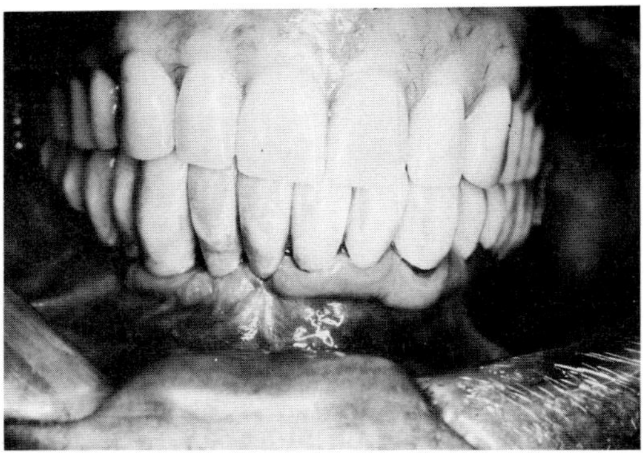

Fig. 1-8. Combined therapy allowed this patient to function comfortably with a complete upper removable prosthesis and a complete lower fixed prosthesis. The treatment included periodontics on the remaining mandibular natural dentition, implantology for the lower right edentulous ridge, and a conventional maxillary removable prosthesis opposing a modified mandibular fixed superstructure. The use of different types of implants for different osseous configurations within the same arch has allowed this patient to receive a comfortable fixed appliance rather than an extensive unilateral removable prosthesis (see Figs. 1-6 and 1-7).

The implant, through surgical procedures of insertion, serves as an abutment for a form of prosthetic tooth replacement.

The prosthetic teeth and their natural or implant abutments must be maintained in a healthy periodontal environment.

The stresses placed on the implant, and thus on the supportive bone through the articulated prosthesis, must be in harmony with properly distributed forces of occlusion.

The prosthesis must function comfortably and allow for the maintenance of the sound periodontal environment that was, at the outset, created for its supportive role.

TIME AND TIMING IN DENTAL IMPLANTOLOGY

Attention to detail is imperative. Skill in the execution of detailed procedures is imperative. Time is of no consequence, but timing may be very important. There are two types of timing to consider:

1. After extractions, the bone impression for a subperiosteal implant should not be considered for about 9 months. Although

empiric in its selection, this amount of time will safely allow for complete bone resolution in the healed areas. After the 9 months, an implant may be contraindicated because of poor bone topography; or, if an implant is indicated, arrangements may be made for the bone impression. This time serves as both a period of reevaluation for alternate treatment plans and as a period of healing, which allows for maximum predictability of osseous height and contour.

2. The second type of timing is sequential treatment. After the initial preparation, temporization is suggested before periodontal treatment. Periodontal therapy should be instituted before the insertion of any implants. After periodontal therapy, the healing period, *prior* to implant surgery, will usually vary from 6 to 10 weeks, according to the healing processes of the individual.

The amount of time that is required for any given implant prosthesis case should be based on the operator's ability to proceed with caution and skill, while unrelenting, detailed attention is being given to the sequential interplay of disciplines. Healing periods, proper temporization, sound attached gingiva, marginal adaptation, crown contours, vertical dimension, centric relation, and proper case selection—all of these factors focus on the eventual long-term success of any given dental implant. Shortcuts are incompatible with good dentistry and are surely to be rejected in dental implantology.

THE UNPREDICTABLE NATURE OF DENTAL IMPLANTS

In spite of the attention given to all of the aforementioned, there is and always will be an element of unpredictability in the field of oral implantology. It is mainly for this reason that the use of dental implants should be regarded as a last physical and/or psychological approach to sound dentistry. The lack of predictability is based essentially on the fact that we are working within both a closed system and an open system, both of which are subjected to the stresses of functional and nonfunctional forces. The success of sound nonsurgical endodontics is based on proper access cavity, proper instrumentation for the shaping of the root-canal system, and proper obturation. These all function within a closed system. Periodontics, on the other hand, has as one of its basic aims the treatment of the hard and soft oral tissues to conserve and maintain sound attachment apparatuses within an open field of treatment.

Closed Systems and Open Systems

The implant frame sits in a closed system, and its post sits in an open system, with the connecting neck acting as the link for a rather unnatural interplay between the oral cavity and the supportive bone. Aside from this intrusion of one system upon the other, there is a lack of a shock-absorber system in dental implants. There is no periodontal ligament to cushion and to dissipate the forces of mastication that are placed on the supporting bone. There is a membranous soft-tissue pad between the implant and the supportive bone that is referred to as "an implant periodontal membrane," or a peri-implant membrane (see Chaps. 6 and 8, on histology); however, the relative effectiveness of such a system can only be related to the success of the implants that such membranes surround. The abilities of these membranous soft-tissue pads to dissipate forces is based on sound conjecture, and their variance under different stressful circumstances has yet to determined.

Also, because of the lack of a true periodontal ligament, there is a lack of a neurophysiologic proprioceptive device to relay the fact that certain forces may be injurious. *The least determinable factor for the dentist to predict* is whether the supportive bone for any given implant will or will not

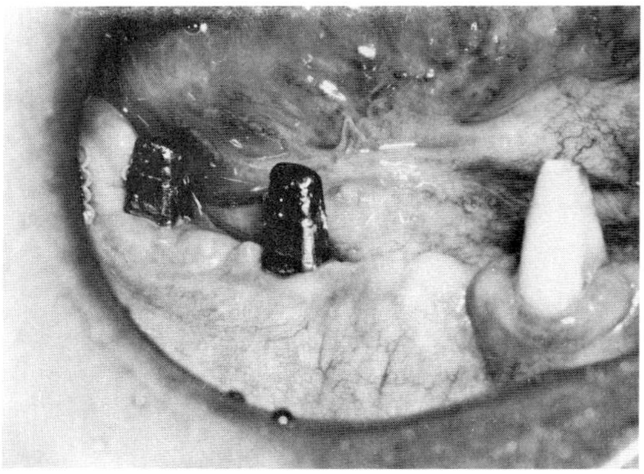

Fig. 1-9. An endosseous blade-vent implant with two posts has been inserted in the patient's lower right posterior mandibular edentulous ridge area. The posts are in alignment with the previously prepared lower right cuspid. The height of the residual ridge as compared to that of the supportive structures of the natural tooth indicates the presence of a substantial amount of remaining alveolar bone. It is for this reason that an endosseous implant was chosen rather than a supra-osseous implant. The firm, attached soft tissue through which the implant posts extrude is comparable to the gingival cuff that surrounds the cuspid.

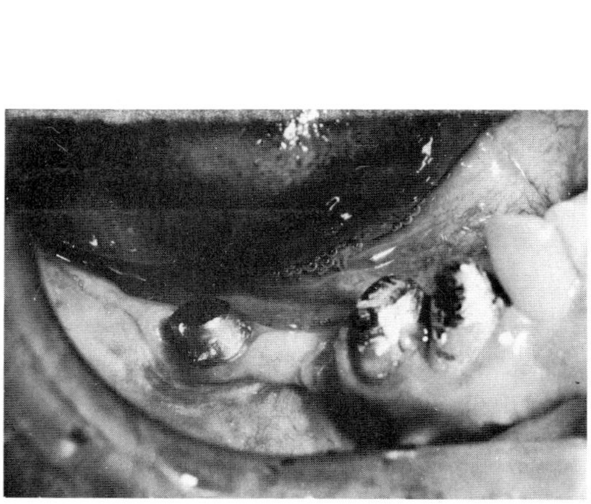

Fig. 1-10. A subperiosteal implant replaces the patient's lost natural lower right mandibular molar. The lower right cuspid and first bicuspid have been endodontically treated because of carious pulp exposures, and cast posts and cores have been inserted. A subperiosteal implant was selected because of severe ridge atrophy, wherein no alveolar bone remained. In this case, optimum use was made of the natural attachment apparatus by employing endodontic treatment and restorative intra-radicular procedures. The man-made attachment apparatus was the subperiosteal implant.

resorb under the stresses that can be brought to bear by the forces of mastication of any particular patient. What may constitute good supportive bone in one individual may not suffice in another individual. The subjection of sound bone to various components of force may yield unknown results under even "ideal" predetermined examination analysis.

In view of this complex relationship of closed systems, open systems, forces, materials, and prosthetic superstructures, certain questions which arise thereof have yet to be answered. It should not be forgotten, however, that there are many unanswered questions that have arisen in other aspects of dentistry, as well, over the decades. Prime examples are the debate as to what constitute the correct components of occlusion, and the debate over the employment of articulators in prosthetic and restorative dentistry. Nevertheless, despite such unanswered questions, these fields of dentistry are carried forth with excellent service to patients by conscientious dentists. Meanwhile, the dialogue on the subject of occlusion continues, as does occlusal and articulator clinical research. Likewise, the complexities involved in oral implantology do not preclude the sensible and sound use of dental implants in indicated clinical situations, while sound basic and clinical implant research are simultaneously being carried forth.

There is no room for dogmatism in dental implantology. Much as an endodontist may employ gutta-percha in certain situations and silver cones in other situations, so must the oral implantologist have both subperiosteal and blade-vent implants as part of his armamentarium (Figs. 1-9, 1-10). Those who have taken a single short course on one phase of implant techniques are ill-prepared to return to their offices and perform this single procedure because they do not have the background to evaluate and make a choice between subperiosteal and blade-vent implants.

Above all, implant dentistry does not

preclude good total dentistry. To the contrary, implant dentistry is dependent on the ability of the practitioner to analyze, plan, and skillfully carry through those phases of dentistry that predate modern oral implant techniques.

RATIONALE OF CLINICAL IMPLANTOLOGY

Implant dentistry has a type of symbiotic relation to other disciplines of dentistry. The implant technique of choice is based on a combined anatomic and surgical approach. A knowledgeable and skillful approach to either the subperiosteal or the endosseous blade implants should render a patient a successful implant. The implant, however, is strictly a means to an end. Its placement in the oral cavity is useless unless it can function comfortably. Herein lies the symbiotic relation. The implant of choice must support, in part or of itself, a removable or fixed prosthetic appliance (Figs. 1-11, 1-12). The superstructure prosthetic appliance of choice must be harmonious with the rest of the oral cavity. The superstructure must also provide an environment in which the implant on which it rests is subjected to the least number of stresses, and in which it is readily maintainable by both the patient and the dentist. There is, thus, an inseparable bond among the supporting bone, the surrounding soft tissue, the implant base, the implant neck and abutment, and the superimposed prosthesis. All principles that are inherent in the sophisticated approach to periodontal-prosthetic treatment are always present in the treatment planning, insertion, and follow-through of any oral implant.

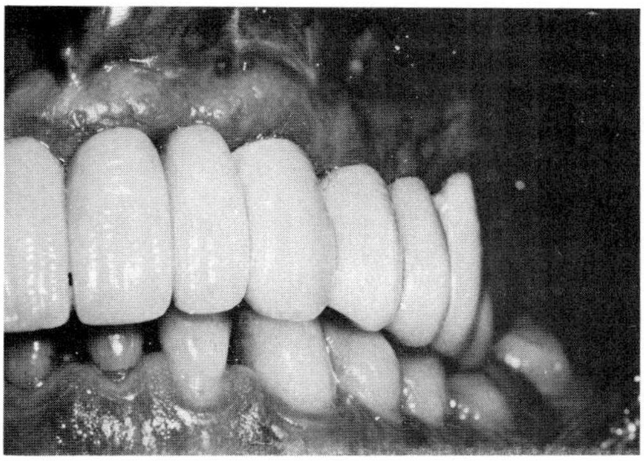

Fig. 1-11. An upper-arch, porcelain-fused-to-gold, fixed prosthesis is supported in part by an intermediary subperiosteal implant at the patient's upper left cuspid site. The passive superimposition of the soft tissues is accomplished by using modified ridge-lap pontics and adequate major embrasures. As in all fixed superstructures that are superimposed on any implant, the margins of the crown retainer are supragingival.

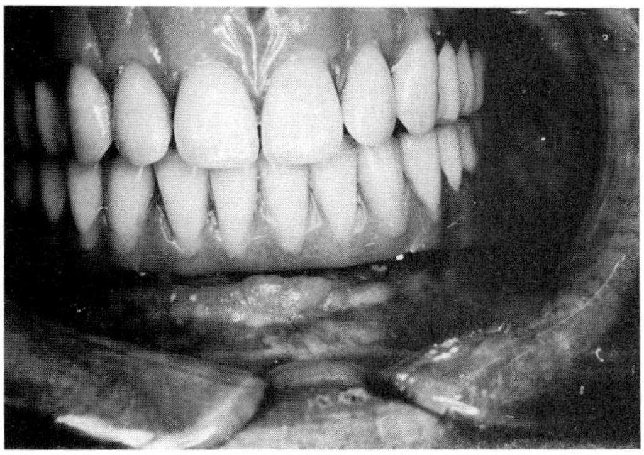

Fig. 1-12. A conventional complete maxillary denture is opposed by a complete lower denture that is supported by a complete subperiosteal mandibular implant. The flanges of the maxillary denture are part of the retentive structure, whereas the lower denture is completely supported by the implant posts. Here, as in the fixed prosthesis case, the implant posts are not completely covered by the prosthetic superstructure. This avoids impingement on the surrounding soft tissues, so that there is no compression of these tissues between the superstructure and the implant frame.

Man-Made Attachment Apparatus—A Concept

The very basis of sound restorative dentistry is the integrity of its foundation. The foundation to which we refer is the attachment apparatus of the individual tooth. This consists of the alveolar bone, the ce-

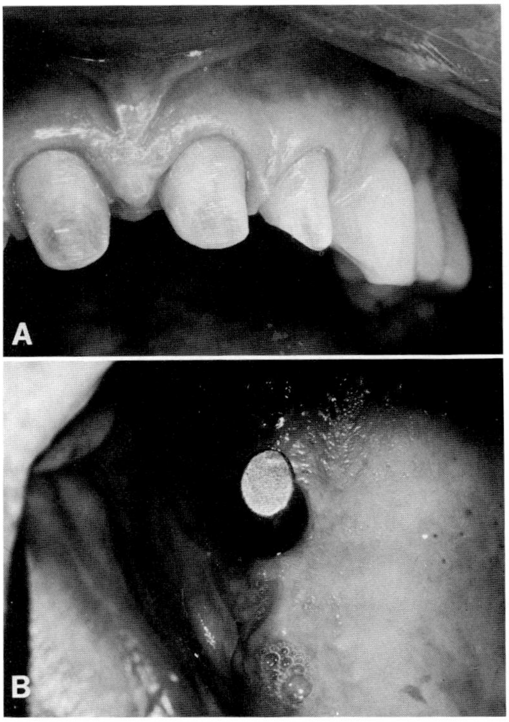

Fig. 1-13. A distinct similarity exists between the soft tissues surrounding prepared natural abutment teeth *(A)* and implant abutment teeth *(B)*. In both cases, there are parabolic curves of firm attached tissue that circumvent the immediate area from which the retainer portion extrudes. Likewise, the lack in bulk of either preparation allows for the accommodation of a cast retainer that can be adequately contoured so as not to impinge on these tissues that are basic to the supportive foundation. (See Plate 1-5.)

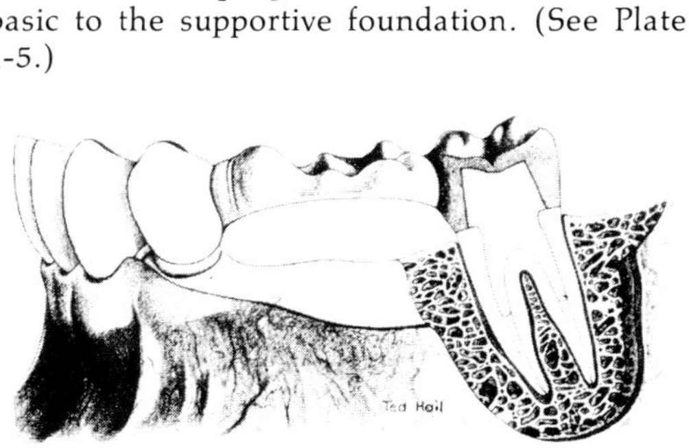

Fig. 1-15. A molar root has been made sound and useful by endodontic treatment within an adequate amount of healthy attachment apparatus. Subsequently, a post and core help to support a retainer that functions as a distal abutment for a fixed prosthesis. Such thorough treatment avoids the unnecessary extraction of a root and, thus, the unnecessary use of either a removable prosthesis or an implant abutment.

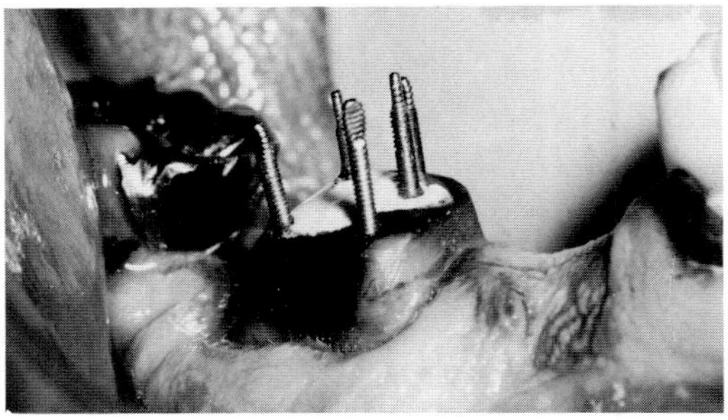

Fig. 1-14. A lower right first molar has been endodontically and periodontally treated. Thus, an adequate amount of sound attachment apparatus, in conjunction with pins and Adaptic* build-up, makes this tooth useful as an abutment.

mentum, and the intervening periodontal ligament. The amount, the soundness, and the configuration of the attachment apparatus around any given root determine to a large extent the fitness of that tooth to serve as an abutment for a fixed or removable prosthesis. Periodontal treatment may be instituted in any given situation to create and sustain a sound attachment apparatus (Fig. 1-13). Endodontics is also employed to this end, under different circumstances. Roots can be salvaged because conservative root-canal therapy can work within a closed system. Thus, even if the crown of a tooth has been mutilated by rampant decay, endodontics has enabled the attachment apparatus to be saved (Fig. 1-14). Subsequently, restorative techniques employing posts and cores and crown retainers make use of this sound foundation (Fig. 1-15).

Likewise, dental implants may be referred to as man-made attachment apparatuses. These implants are the foundations upon which retainers and prostheses are built (Figs. 1-16, 1-17). This does not imply that the histologic sections of an implant and a natural tooth are similar in appearance (see Chaps. 6 and 8, on histology). The term "man-made attachment ap-

*Johnson and Johnson Dental Products Co., East Windsor, New Jersey.

paratus" is simply used to enable the reader to understand the place of the implant in the continuum of dentistry.

We can then understand the appropriateness of creating as broad a base as is possible for the subperiosteal implant. This enlarges the area of man-made attachment apparatus. When speaking of blade implants, the same holds true. There are certain blade implant designs that are truly built-in failures. They may be doomed to fail merely by their inadequate bases—inadequate in depth and/or in length. As broad an area as possible, both mesiodistally and occlusogingivally, must be attained if the implant is to have a chance to succeed. In this context it is important to bear in mind that whether the implant is subperiosteal, blade, vitreous carbon, or an endodontic extension, the *concept* of man-made attachment apparatus is common to them all.

Reasons for Implant Failures

Scholastic prejudices notwithstanding, the right implant type is to be placed in the appropriate implant site (Fig. 1-18). The rules to date are mainly based on clinical empiricisms. Such empiricisms have been based on the results of successes and failures, and on histologic evidence. It is as important to evaluate the reasons for success at it is to evaluate the causes of failure.

Implant failures may, to some extent, be due to the surgical approach and insertion of the subperiosteal or endosseous designs; however, it is the abuse of the implants that appears to be the greatest cause of failures. The abuses may be:

1. Improper implant selection for the type of bone available
2. The extrusion of the implant neck through a soft mucosal area rather than through an attached gingiva-type of soft tissue
3. The inadequate design of the base of the implant which is to support the prosthesis of choice

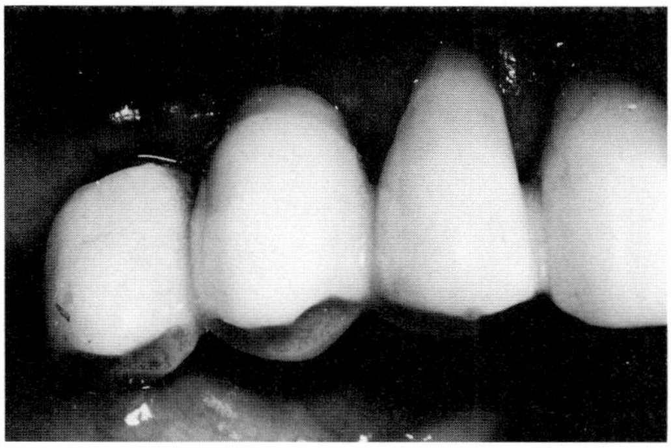

Fig. 1-16. Mirror view of an upper temporary acrylic-resin prosthesis that is part of a complete-arch periodontal prosthesis. The distal abutment is a subperiosteal implant. Principles that include marginal placement, tooth contours, and embrasure architecture are carried through the temporary appliance in order to better maintain the surrounding soft tissues. (See Plate 1-6.)

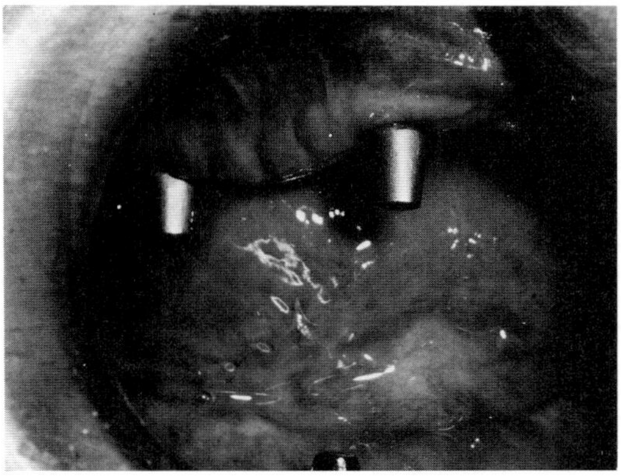

Fig. 1-17. The right segment of this complete upper subperiosteal implant exemplifies the nature of the supportive posts. Throughout the impression and try-in procedures, the implant posts and necks, and the surrounding attached gingival tissues have been kept impeccably clean by home care that had been allowed for by proper superstructure design.

4. The improper placement of the implant of choice in relation to the opposing dentition
5. The improper placement of the implant of choice relative to the remaining dentition in the same arch or with respect to other implants within the same arch

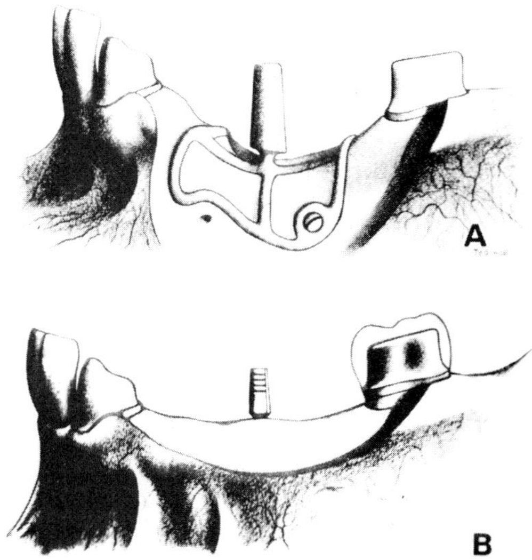

Fig. 1-18. A comparison is made of two different implant sites in two similar prosthetic situations. The long span from second molar to cuspid on the same side may preclude the use of a fixed bridge. In both situations, an intermediary implant may be used for the superimposition of a fixed appliance. In one case *(A)*, there is severe bone resorption of the edentulous ridge, so that only cortical bone remains. Such bone loss would indicate the use of subperiosteal implant. In the other case *(B)*, it is obvious that a substantial amount of alveolar bone remainds within an edentulous ridge that has very little resorption. This is the type of bone that would call for the use of an intra-osseous implant, such as a blade-vent endosseous implant.

6. The placement of implants in patients with such debilitating problems as advanced diabetes or alcoholism
7. The placement of implants in patients who are known to have a history of clenching or of bruxism
8. The disregard for the impeccable and intricate design of the superstructure
9. The lack of adherence to accepted principles of periodontal prosthesis
10. The disregard of a sound occlusal approach
11. The lack of consideration for the essential intermediary phase of temporization
12. The lack of impeccable oral hygiene allowed for, explained to, and carried out by the patient.

Naturally, there are those cases that will fail in spite of adherence to all sound principles. Some unpredictable factors are worth reiterating succinctly. The weak link in the chain is the passage of the neck of an implant through the soft tissue. This may allow the causative factors of infection to pass through the soft tissue, despite the best-intended home-care attention and the best tissue adaptation. Also, there may be a resorption of bone surrounding or subjacent to the implant of choice. Assuming that the bony environment was correct for the implant that was selected, resorption of bone usually is caused by unforeseen stresses that are exerted by the patient in occlusion. Implant failures also may occur in some patients simply because their bone —regardless of good implant design—will not tolerate and accept the forces of normal function. Obviously, success is based on case selection augmented by a skill and knowledge of implantology, prosthodontics, and periodontics. The nebulous characteristic referred to as "clinical judgment" is of overriding importance.

The Choices—Subperiosteal Implant, Endosseous Implant, or No Implant

The subperiosteal implant, the endosseous blade implant, and the endodontic implant have proved to be of value in different prosthetic cases—even in combination within the same arch of the same patient. To rely only on the blade implant or only on the subperiosteal implant is to limit one's scope and may foster the placement of the wrong implant in the right place. The condition and topography of any residual ridge area should dictate the selection of implant types. Time has proven that the subperiosteal implant, the blade implant, and the endodontic implant can be a part of the armamentarium of the prosthodontist. On the other hand, the mere existence of a space in any arch does not indicate that an implant should be inserted therein. In the same manner as the operator must choose between a removable prosthesis and a fixed prosthesis, so must he consider whether a patient might best be served in any given instance with a removable appliance rather than an oral implant.

Interestingly, the use of implants began because of the influence of the orally debilitated person. The complete-arch implant was considered first—prior to the presently used terminal and intermediary implants. It was those patients who could not tolerate a complete denture who sought and indirectly fostered the use of the complete implant. These patients usually presented with severe ridge resorption, which precluded the retention of any complete denture; or the patients were psychologically unprepared for and not receptive to any complete denture. It was because of their inability to tolerate dentures and, consequently, their inability to chew properly, that the patients became debilitated to some extent or other. Weight loss, frailty, and age do not eliminate the potential use of the implant technique. To the contrary, when such implants were inserted with their removable superstructures, the patients returned to a more comfortable ingestion of food through better mastication.

It was after such successful implantations that considerations were given to the possible replacement of the bilateral free-end saddle mandibular removable denture with two terminal subperiosteal implants. Other implant designs have passed through the dental scene with varying degrees of success and failure. But subsequent to the successes of the subperiosteal implant, none entered the armamentarium more auspiciously than the endosseous blade implant. To date, the subperiosteal and blade implant designs are clinically useful and very successful when properly used. Unfortunately, the very nature of the single-appointment blade insertion has opened the door to many abuses. All things being equal, if there is a choice in any given instance, the subperiosteal implant would still be the implant of choice as regards the prosthodontist. As previously alluded to, this does *not* preclude the use of the blade implant; its indications will become apparent in a discussion of treatment planning.

BIBLIOGRAPHY

Applegate, O. C.: Conditions which may influence the choice of partial or complete denture service. J. Pros. Dent., *7:*182-196, 1957.

———: Essentials of Removable Partial Denture Prosthesis. ed. 3. Philadelphia, W. B. Saunders, 1965.

Atwood, D. A.: The reduction of residual ridges, a major oral disease entity. J. Pros. Dent., *26:*266-279, 1971.

Avant, W. E.: Fulcrum and retention lines in planning removable partial dentures. J. Pros. Dent., *25:*162-166, 1971.

———: A study of some factors associated with denture retention. J. Pros. Dent., *29:*383-389, 1973.

Bar-oz, I.: Implantology today: an evaluation of literature and personal experience. Israel J. D. Med., *18:*39-45, 1969.

Bell, F. A., and Dobson, D. P.: Vestibuloplasty and floor-of-mouth revision with application of a split-thickness skin graft. North Carolina D. J., *57:*14-16, 1974.

Beresin, V. E., and Schiesser, F. J.: The Neutral Zone in Complete Dentures. St. Louis, C. V. Mosby, 1973.

Bodine, R. L.: Implant dentures: prosthodontic—favorable. J. Pros. Dent., *10:*1132-1142, 1960.

Boero, W., and Forbes, W. G.: Considerations in design of removable prosthetic devices with no posterior abutments. J. Pros. Dent., *28:*253-263, 1972.

Boucher, C. O.: Implant dentures: prosthodontic—unfavorable. J. Pros. Dent., *10:*1143-1148, 1960.

Boucher, L. J.: Injected Silastic in ridge extension procedures. J. Pros. Dent., *14:*460-464, 1964.

Boyne, P. J., and Cooksey, D. E.: Use of cartilage and bone implants in restoration of edentulous ridges. J.A.D.A., *71:*1426-1435, 1965.

Calagna, L. J.: A comprehensive treatment rationale combining prosthodontics and periodontics. J. Pros. Dent., *30:*781-788, 1973.

Campbell, R. L.: A comparative study of the resorption of the alveolar ridges in denture-wearers and non-denture-wearers. J.A.D.A., *60:*143-153, 1960.

Clarke, E. G. C., Hickman, J., Collins, D. H., and Scales, J. T.: Discussion on metals and synthetic materials in relation to tissues. Proc. Roy. Soc. Med., *46:*641-652, 1953.

Fenton, A. H.: Bone resorption and prosthodontics. J. Pros. Dent., *29:*477-483, 1973.

Fields, H. Jr., and Campfield, R. W. Jr.: Removable partial prosthesis partially supported by an endosseous blade implant. J. Pros. Dent., *31:*273-278, 1974.

Fish, E. W.: Principles of Full Denture Prosthesis. ed. 6. London, Staples and Staples, 1964.

Fish, S. F.: Free-end saddle dentures. Brit. D.J., *128:*495-502, 1970.

Flander, S.: Periodontic, orthodontic and endodontic considerations in conjunction with implant dentistry. D. Clin. North America, *14:*137-143, 1970.

Gatewood, J. B.: Reconstruction of the alveolar ridge with silicone-dacron implants: a pilot study. J. Oral Surg., *26:*441-448, 1968.

Gershkoff, A.: The subperiosteal unilateral implant as a distal abutment and as a support to periodontally involved teeth. D. Clin. North America, *14:*95-102, 1970.

Gershkoff, A., and Goldberg, N. I.: Implant Dentures. Philadelphia, J. B. Lippincott, 1957.

Glickman, I.: The periodontal structures and removable partial denture prosthesis. J.A.D.A., *37:*311-316, 1948.

Hammer, W. B., Topazian, R. G., McKinney, R. V. Jr., and Hulbert, S. F.: Alveolar ridge augmentation with ceramics. J. D. Res., *52:*356-361, 1973.

Hartsook, E. I.: Food selection, dietary adequacy, and related dental problems of patients with dental prostheses. J. Pros. Dent., *32:*32-40, 1974.

Heartwell, C. W.: Complete denture failures related to improper interpretation and improper preparation of the anatomy of the mouth. D. Clin. North America, *16:*127-144, 1972.

Howe, G. L.: Surgical aids to full denture construction. *In* Morrant, G. A.: Modern Trends in Dental Surgery. vol. 1. London, Butterworth, 1963.

James, R. A.: Periodontal considerations in implant dentistry. J. Pros. Dent., *30:*202-209, 1973.

Jordan, G. L. Jr.: Dental implantations: a review of the literature. J. Michigan State D. A., *55:*243-247, 1973.

Kelsey, C. C.: Alveolar bone resorption under complete dentures. J. Pros. Dent., *25:*152-161, 1971.

Kresse, E. J.: Rehabilitating the edentulous with implantation. J. Implant Dent., *4:*32-36, 1957.

Krol, A. J.: Clasp design for extension base removable partial dentures. J. Pros. Dent., *29:*408-415, 1973.

Kruger, G. O.: Ridge extension: review of indications and techniques. J. Oral Surg., *16:*191-201, 1958.

Lacue, J. J., and Armbrecht, E. C.: An approach to atrophic ridges. D. Survey, *46:*29-33, 1970.

Leake, D. L., Kent, J. N., and LaVelle, W. E.: New method for alveolar ridge augmentation. J. California D. A., *1:*50-52, 1973.

L'Estrange, P. R.: The use of implants as an aid to prosthodontics. Australian D. J., *15:*371-376, 1970.

Leuck, M. H., and LaVelle, W. E.: Preservation of the mandibular ridge through root retention. J. Acad. Gen. Dent., *21:*29-32, 1973.

Lutz, B. L.: Preventive dentistry: proposal for definition of terms. J. D. Educ., *37:*24-26, 1973.

McCracken, W. L.: Partial Denture Construction. ed. 2. St. Louis, C. V. Mosby, 1964.

Marziani, L.: Dental implants and implant dentures, their theory, history and practice. Internat. D. J., *4:*459-481, 1954.

Miller, E. L.: Periodontics-prosthodontics: their interrelationship. Arkansas D. J., *41:*15-19, 1970.

Molinari, J. A.: The immunology of implants. Oral Implantol., *3:*160-174, 1973.

Natiella, J. R., Armitage, J. E., Green, G. W. Jr., and Meenaghan, M.: Current evaluation of dental implants. J.A.D.A., *84:*1358-1372, 1972.

Ogesen, R. B.: Construction of free-end saddle partial dentures. D. Digest, *74:*381-385, 1968.

Ortman, H. R.: Factors of bone resorption of the residual ridge. J. Pros. Dent., *12:*429-440, 1962.

Osburn, R. C.: Preservation of the alveolar ridge: a simplified technique for retaining teeth beneath removable appliances. J. Indiana State D. A., *53:*8-11, 1974.

Potter, R. B., Appleby, R. C., and Adams, C. D.: Removable partial denture design: a review and a challenge. J. Pros. Dent., *17:*63-68, 1967.

Propper, R. H.: Simplified ridge extension using free mucosal grafts. J. Oral Surg., *22:*469-474, 1964.

Prowler, J. R.: A skin-grafted ridge extension:

new approach to atrophic ridge management. J. Oral Surg., *23:*123-129, 1965.

Ruben, M. P.: Fixed prosthesis: aid to periodontal health. D. Survey, *47:*32-33 1971.

Schwartz, R.: Occlusion and the endosseous implant. Oral Implantol., *4:*205-215, 1973.

Smith, B. B.: Report of the Committee on Scientific Investigation of the American Academy of Restorative Dentistry. J. Pros. Dent., *29:*647-682, 1973 (note pp. 670 and 671).

Steffel, V. L.: Planning removable partial dentures. J. Pros. Dent., *12:*524-535, 1962.

Stephens, A. P.: The free-end saddle partial denture. J. Irish D. A., *17:*110-115, 1971.

Swenson, M. G., and Terkla, L. G.: Partial Dentures. St. Louis, C. V. Mosby, 1955.

Swoope, C. C.: Predicting denture success. J. Pros. Dent., *30:*860-865, 1973.

Tallgren, A.: Alveolar bone loss in denture wearers as related to facial morphology. Acta odont. scandinav., *28:*251-270, 1970.

———: The continuing reduction of the residual alveolar ridges in complete denture wearers: a mixed-longitudinal study covering 25 years. J. Pros. Dent., *27:*120-132, 1972.

Tuckfield, W. J.: Problems of the mandibular denture. J. Pros. Dent., *3:*8-28, 1953.

Wiesenbaugh, J. M., Saunders, L. A., and Simmons, A. H.: Alveolar ridge deficiency correction with osseous transplant and vestibuloplasty skin graft: report of case. J. Maryland State D. A., *13:*241-244, 1970.

Wlodzimierz, J.: The influence of wearing dentures on residual ridges: a comparative study. J. Pros. Dent., *24:*137-144, 1970.

Yeager, J. E., and Boyne, P. J.: Use of bone homografts and autogenous marrow in restoration of edentulous alveolar ridges. J. Oral Surg., *27:*185-189, 1969.

Yoshizumi, D. T.: An evaluation of factors pertinent to the success of complete denture service. J. Pros. Dent., *14:*866-878, 1964.

2 Case Selection, Case Presentation, and Categorization

CASE SELECTION: THE INVESTIGATION AND ANALYSIS

Case selection is a procedure that may be described as the placement of the patient before a one-man board of review. The practitioner's office standards and criteria should conform to the highest ethics of the dental profession, which exhibit concern for the welfare of the patient. A coordination of the answers to the following questions should indeed reveal that integrity in case selection would eliminate many potential dental implant candidates:

1. Why has the patient presented himself for oral implants?
2. What does a visual examination of the oral cavity reveal?
3. What does palpation of the potential implant site reveal?
4. What is the interpretation of the radiographs of the potential implant site?
5. What is the current status of the occlusion?
6. What is the current medical health status; and what is the health history?

Listening to the Patient

Many patients who seek the use of oral implants may be better served by other forms of restorative or prosthetic dentistry. The patient who has read a magazine article about implanting teeth, after having neglected his mouth for quite some time, should be educated as to the potentialities of other more conservative dental treatments that are presently available. On the other hand, if a patient has consistently pursued good dentistry and is physically or psychologically unable to cope with other forms of prosthetic dentistry, then a further evaluation as to the possible use of dental implants is warranted.

The key is to listen to the patient, and then, after thorough examination, inform him of those forms of dental treatment that would best serve his situation, with no bias toward the dental implant. Obviously, this first phase takes time. Implant consultations should be allowed at least one initial 1-hour appointment. Briefer sessions are a rarity; they occur only when a team effort has allowed for basic explanations and screening by another dentist.

The General Visual Examination

The visual examination of the oral cavity may reveal the necessity for other restorations, periodontal therapy, extractions of hopelessly involved teeth, and endodontic treatment. The visual examination may also reveal mobility patterns of any existing teeth. It is imperative that the opposing arch be treated, to establish a total, functional, stomatognathic unit.

Observation should also be made of the standard of home care that has been practiced by the patient. If the patient has been unwilling or unable to maintain sound oral hygiene procedures to date, then such a negative attitude may preclude the use of any dental implant. The phases of initial periodontal preparation provide an opportunity for the practitioner to reassess the patient's true interest in receiving and maintaining sophisticated dental treatment. It is also imperative that *both* the dentist and the patient be willing to work with supportive dental disciplines, so that the dental implant may ultimately function in a sound periodontal and occlusal environment (Fig. 2-1).

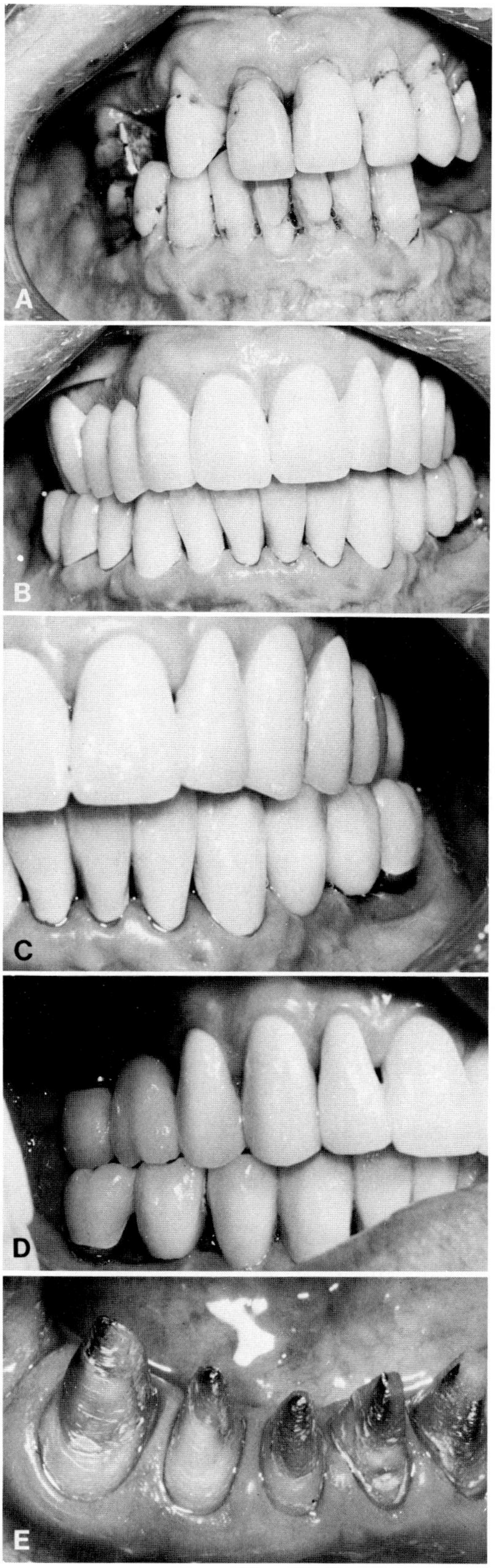

Fig. 2-1. A multidisciplinary approach over a span of $1^{1}/_{2}$ years has restored a mutilated stomatognathic system to an acceptable level of functional health. (*A*) illustrates the appearance of the mouth at the initial examination. (*B*) illustrates the final result that was obtained after a sequence of initial preparation, provisional splinting, periodontics, endodontics, unilateral left implants, and fixed prosthodontics. (*C*) and (*D*) reveal a direct view and a mirror view, respectively, of the upper and lower left posterior quadrants which received terminal implants. The upper arch received a subperiosteal unilateral implant, and the lower arch received a blade-vent unilateral implant. (*E*) illustrates a portion of the lower arch prior to the insertion of the final fixed prosthesis. Multiple endodontics was necessary, in conjunction with a customized acrylic-resin provisional prosthesis, to maintain the integrity of the periodontium.

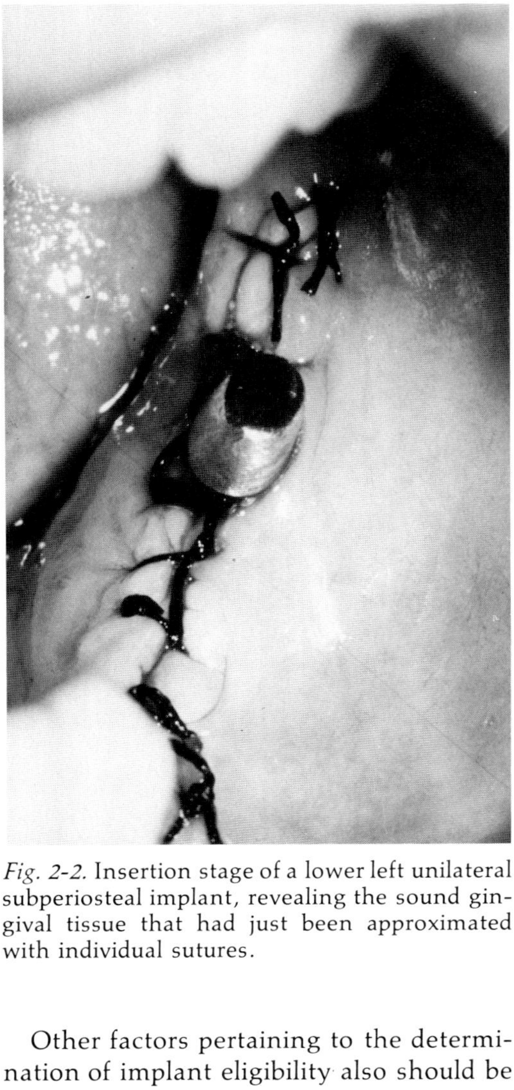

Fig. 2-2. Insertion stage of a lower left unilateral subperiosteal implant, revealing the sound gingival tissue that had just been approximated with individual sutures.

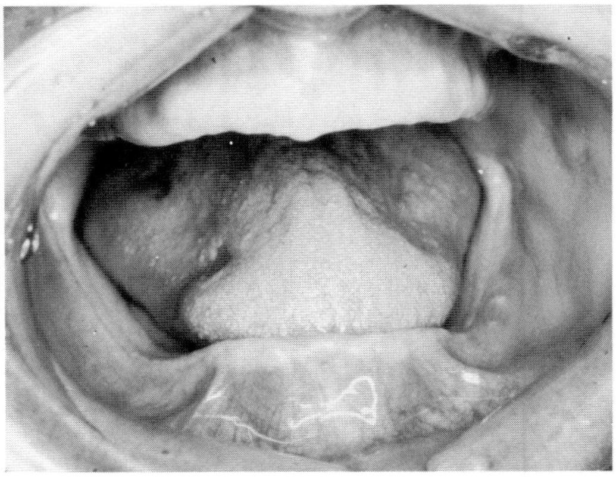

Fig. 2-3. Completely edentulous mouth requiring prosthetic restoration. The upper arch has an adequate amount of supportive bone and sound tissue for the use of a standard complete removable denture. The lower arch, which has denture sores in the lower left posterior quadrant, has posterior ridges that are confluent with the mucobuccal folds. Because of this patient's inability to support a complete lower removable denture comfortably, a complete mandibular subperiosteal implant, to support a removable prosthesis, was considered.

Other factors pertaining to the determination of implant eligibility also should be considered during the general visual examination. For example, in the partially edentulous mouth, the remaining dentition may exhibit severe occlusal and incisal wear. Such indications of bruxism and clenching would eliminate the patient from dental implant treatment. Also in the partially edentulous mouth, the implant may not be sufficient as the sole supportive structure for otherwise highly mobile teeth, and the implant may only share the mobility load when there are other sound teeth with which to share it.

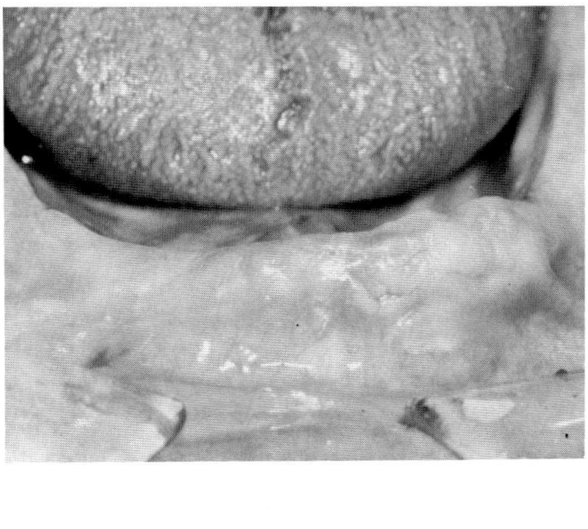

Fig. 2-4. Close-up view of the anterior segment of a completely edentulous lower arch. Although the posterior portions of this arch have no remaining alveolar bone and very flat supportive residual ridges, a small segment of the anterior ridge has irregular residual alveolar bone. If a complete implant were to be undertaken in this case, an alveolectomy would have to be performed in this anterior region, followed by a 9-month waiting period prior to implant consideration. Obviously, if such alveolar bone were to offer adequate support for a standard complete removable denture, then it would be improper to remove any part of the alveolus.

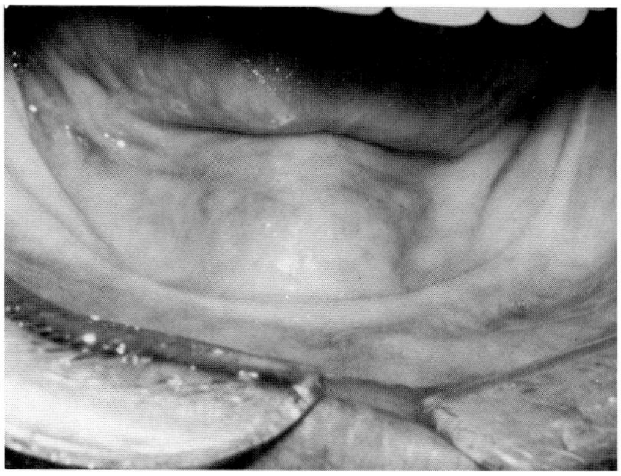

Fig. 2-5. This edentulous lower arch is a classic type of case that would require a complete subperiosteal implant to support a prosthetic appliance. In this case, there is no alveolar bone remaining, and the edentulous ridge is extremely flat. Radiographic examination of such a ridge usually reveals dense, compact bone below such healthy soft tissue. Although a complete removable denture cannot be tolerated comfortably by the patient, there is an adequate band of gingival tissue through which implant posts can extrude.

The Specific Visual Examination

The potential implant site should be examined visually for the following: (a) the topography of the residual ridge; (b) the amount and form of any attached firm tissue at the height of the residual ridge; and (c) the consistency and color of the soft tissue in the immediate vicinity (Figs. 2-2 to 2-5). It is as important to note the texture and consistency of the soft tissue over-

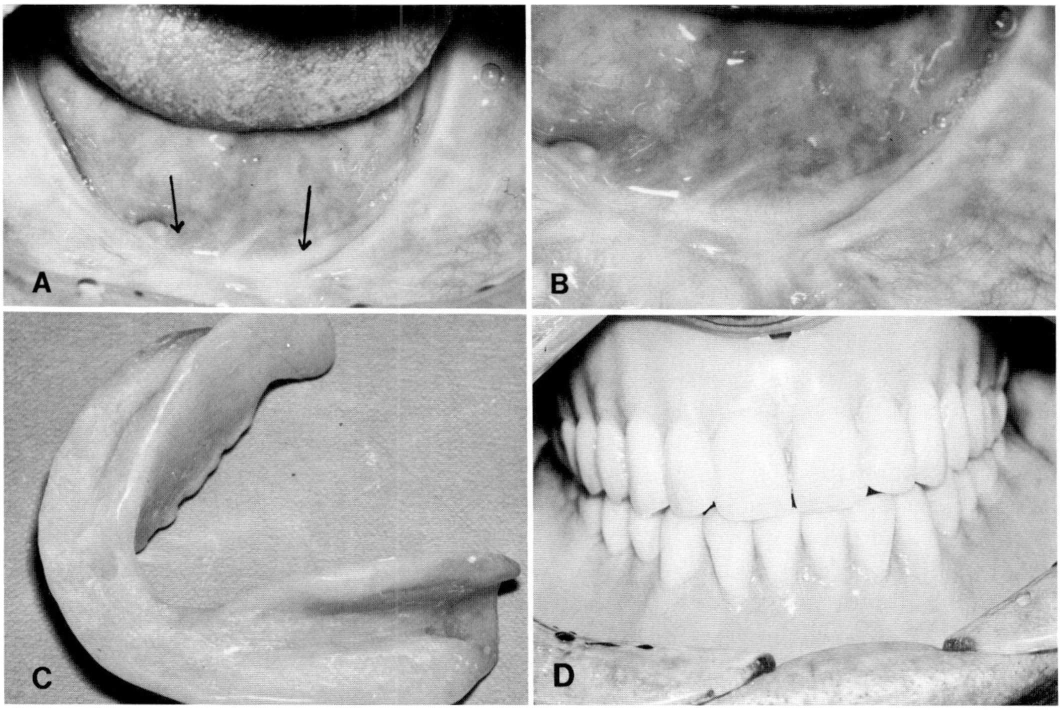

Fig. 2-6. Although this patient requested an implant prosthesis for the edentulous lower arch, a standard complete removable denture was used instead. Although (*A*) shows the extent of bone loss, with a flattened residual ridge that at times dips below the mucosal folds, (*B*) reveals a soft-tissue discrepancy in the anterior region. There is a lack of attached tissue, and a coalescence of the buccal mucosa with the sublingual mucosa at the height of the ridge. A positive health history precluded any grafting of tissue in this area. (*C*) and (*D*) demonstrate the extensive use of flanges in the fabrication of a standard complete removable denture for this patient. (Dentures fabricated by Dr. Charles Weitzner)

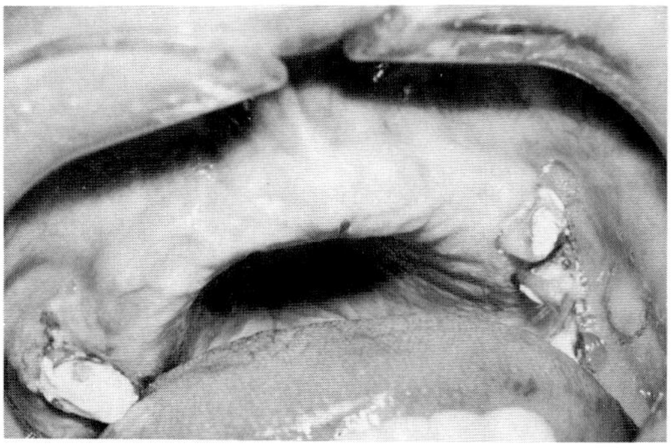

Fig. 2-7. Prior to periodontal treatment, the remaining roots of this maxillary arch have been treated endodontically. The upper right cuspid area has an adequate amount of attached gingiva through which an implant neck can extrude.

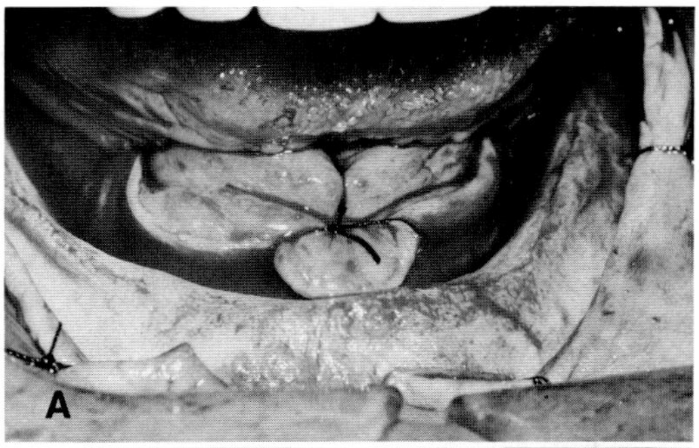

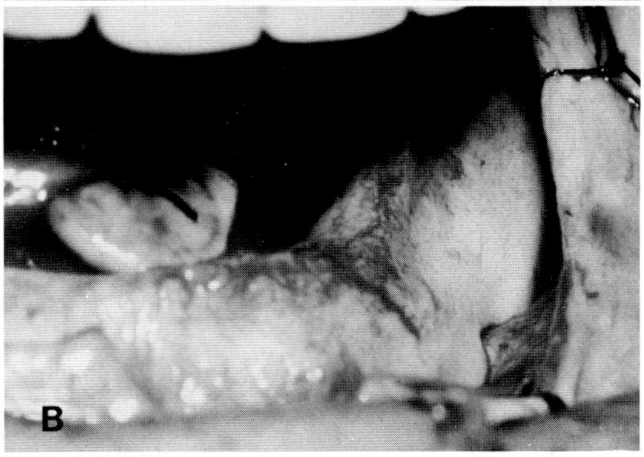

Fig. 2-8. Through visual examination, radiographs, and palpation, the implantologist should be able to anticipate the osseous topography that is to be exposed upon surgical entry. Palpation is especially useful, in order to anticipate overall contours (*A*) and specific contours such as the broad expanse of an external oblique ridge (*B*).

lying the residual ridge as it is to observe the bony configuration itself. All things being equal, if such tissue is only mucosal in nature, with no epithelium that resembles an attached gingiva-like tissue, then there are no adequate areas for the extrusion of the implant posts (Fig. 2-6).

Inasmuch as the apparent weak link in the implant chain is the connection of the oral cavity with the underlying bone, the soft-tissue cuff surrounding the implant neck is of special significance (Fig. 2-7). It is preferable that this tissue be firm and of gingival consistency, in order to form a snug mechanical collar. Often, there may be just a thin band of such tissue in a buccolingual dimension. This may indicate a lateral placement of the implant necks, despite a resultant inappropriate position regarding the opposing table. Otherwise, a free gingival graft may be donated to the implant site. Then, a waiting period of 6 to 10 weeks must precede any implant surgery.

The nature of the tissue in general that is superimposed on the residual ridge should be examined. If this tissue is friable, it may portend that the exposure of struts after insertion of a subperiosteal implant is inevitable. Just as periodontists see different consistencies in the healthy gingival tissues of different patients, so does the implantologist see varying soft-tissue conditions even among patients considered to be in good health.

Examination by Palpation

Palpation of the implant site between the forefinger and thumb helps to analyze the third dimension that is not seen in a two-dimensional radiograph. The broad expanse of an external oblique ridge, the labio-inferior thrust of an anterior symphyseal area, and the direction and amount of bony undercut in the mylohyoid ridge area are examples of such revelations found by palpation (Fig. 2-8). This exercise may aid in the selection of the appropriate type of site required for the insertion of the subperiosteal or the blade implant. If palpation indicates that the site is extremely narrow or has severe undercuts in

Morton L. Perel, B. Sc., D. D. S., M. Sc. D.

PRACTICE LIMITED TO PROSTHODONTICS

130 WATERMAN STREET
PROVIDENCE, RHODE ISLAND 02906
TEL.: 401-861-1343

October, 1973

Mrs. A.B.C.--CONSULTATION
Dr. Morton L. Perel--September, 1973.

UPPER ARCH

Complete upper reconstruction at present acrylic veneer full splint from UR 7 to UL 6 (cantilevered pontic).

LOWER ARCH

The present lower splint extends from LR 3 to LL 3. There are two cantilevered pontics at the distal of LR 3. The only additional abutments are LL 1 and LL 2. The lower right residual ridge is highly resorbed with a narrow band of attached tissue (2½ mm) on a rounded knife edge solid substructure. Although the buccal muscle attachments are quite high on the occlusal aspects of this ridge, there is no appreciable muscle pull nor flabbiness of soft tissues. The lingual aspect slopes at about a 60 degree angle for about 5 mm before there being any undercut.

The lower left residual ridge has had extractions within the past six weeks and healing has been superficially complete. This ridge is presently broad with a wide band of attached tissue (3 to 4 mm) with moderate resorption. The buccal soft tissues coalesce at about the same plane as the height of the ridge from a very broad external oblique ridge. The lingual aspect presents a distinct vertical drop of about 6 to 7 mm. There is no mobile tissue in the immediate vicinity of the height of the ridge.

Both ridges have the potential for the placement of an abutment at the sites of the lower first molars.

In order to accommodate a complete subperiosteal implant extractions of the remaining lower teeth would have to be performed in conjunction with an alveolectomy that would prepare the ridge for a subperiosteal frame. In the interim, the patient would have to wear a complete immediate lower denture for at least a period of nine months in order to afford complete resolution of the bone in the more recent extraction sites. Only after this mandatory waiting period would an implant be considered for the lower arch.

MLP:lag

Fig. 2-9. This example of an examination report is typical of the chair-side recordings made by a competent secretary. In this instance, the loss of the lower, periodontally hopeless, involved teeth was anticipated because of the severe bone loss. A negative health history, in conjunction with severe ridge resorption, allowed for consideration of an implant.

the buccolingual dimension, then a blade implant may be contraindicated.

It is important to touch and feel the edentulous arch in total. The depression of the soft mucosal tissues by the dentist's fingers can reveal much about the configuration of bone that potentially could bear a subperiosteal implant frame. This is a di-

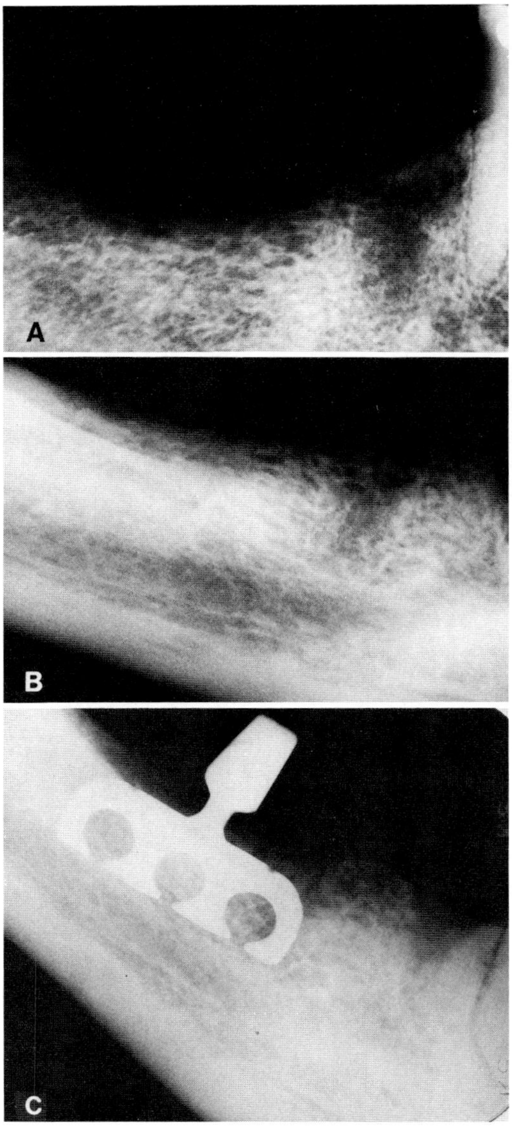

Fig. 2-10. These individual apical radiographs depict edentulous areas that may be amenable to intra-osseous implants. An appreciable amount of remaining alveolar bone negates the use of a supra-osseous implant. Such vital considerations as the inferior alveolar canal (*C*) limit the depth of placement of a blade-vent implant.

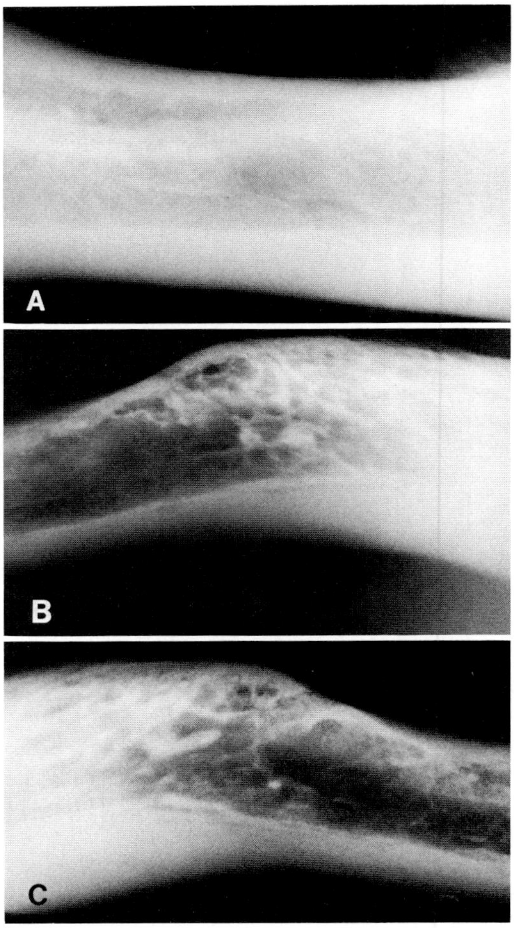

Fig. 2-11. These individual apical radiographs depict the type of bone that is suitable for the superimposition of a subperiosteal implant. In different cases, the posterior segment in the vicinity of the external oblique ridge (*A*), and the mandibular cuspid areas (*B*) and (*C*), have substantial bone resorption. The true density of the cortical plates can only be determined upon surgical exposure.

mension that cannot be achieved via any radiographic medium. Palpation can also lead to a mental image of the eventual subperiosteal implant framework design. For example, a severe and acute sublingual inclination at the mylohyoid ridge area may indicate that mechanical retention is attainable for the peripheral border or lingual fingers of a subperiosteal implant (Fig. 2-9).

The Radiographic Survey

There is no doubt that the use of a single panoramic radiograph *may* be useful. It may reveal areas that are of questionable

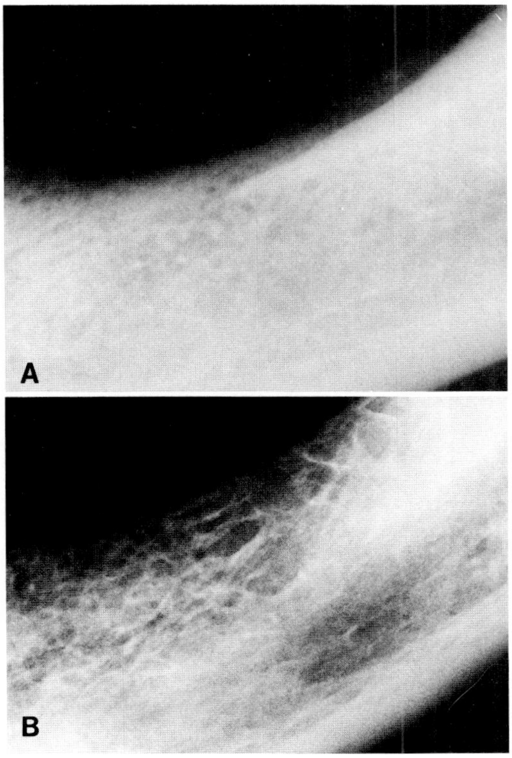

Fig. 2-12. These two apical radiographs show different left mandibular edentulous areas that may be suitable for intra-osseous implant insertion. If the unilateral edentulous area reveals remaining alveolar bone without a well-defined cortical plate, a subperiosteal implant is contraindicated. At times, it is necessary to surgically expose the osseous structure in preparation for *either* supra-osseous or intra-osseous implant procedures.

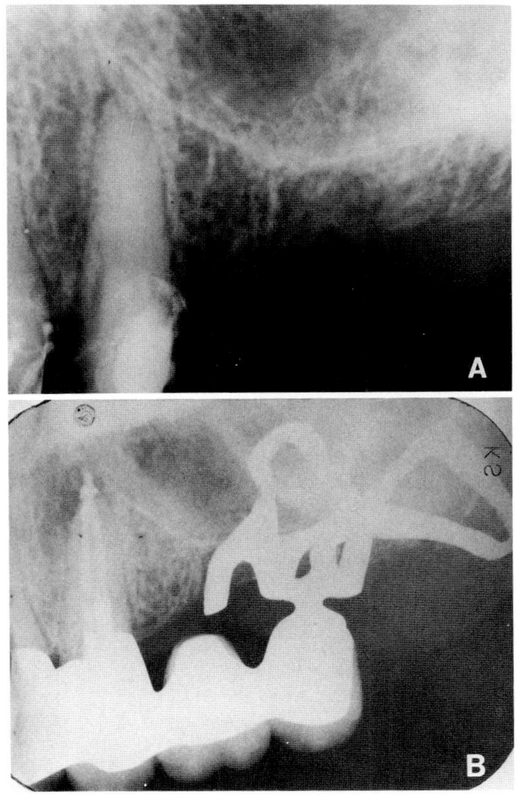

Fig. 2-13. The presence of a maxillary sinus may preclude the use of an intra-osseous implant (*A*). Despite the lack of a dense cortical plate in the maxilla, a unilateral subperiosteal implant has been used (*B*) (an exception to the rule). This implant serves as a terminal abutment for a fixed prosthesis, in conjunction with a mesial abutment tooth that has been treated endodontically.

status, and it may show the relative position of anatomic parts. Nevertheless, the serial view of the mandible or the maxilla through a series of individual apical radiographs is of greater value. Such a series can reduce the degree of distortion and also reveal bone structure with unparalleled clarity.

It is assumed that routine radiographic interpretations and observations are to be made. For example, retained roots, cystic formations, and anomalies in osseous configurations should all be attended to according to the normal routine of any complete mouth evaluation and subsequent treatment. Radiographic analysis alone, even postoperatively, however, is not an adequate means of implant evaluation.

One also should look for the density of bone at the height of the residual ridge, the density and configuration of the interstitial subcrestal bone, the relative anatomic pathways of the mandibular canal, the mental foramina, possible dehiscences, the positions of the maxillary sinuses, and the depth of the body of the mandible.

It is particularly important to note the density of bone at the height of the ridge of the mandible (Figs. 2-10, 2-11). It is

(Text continues on page 25.)

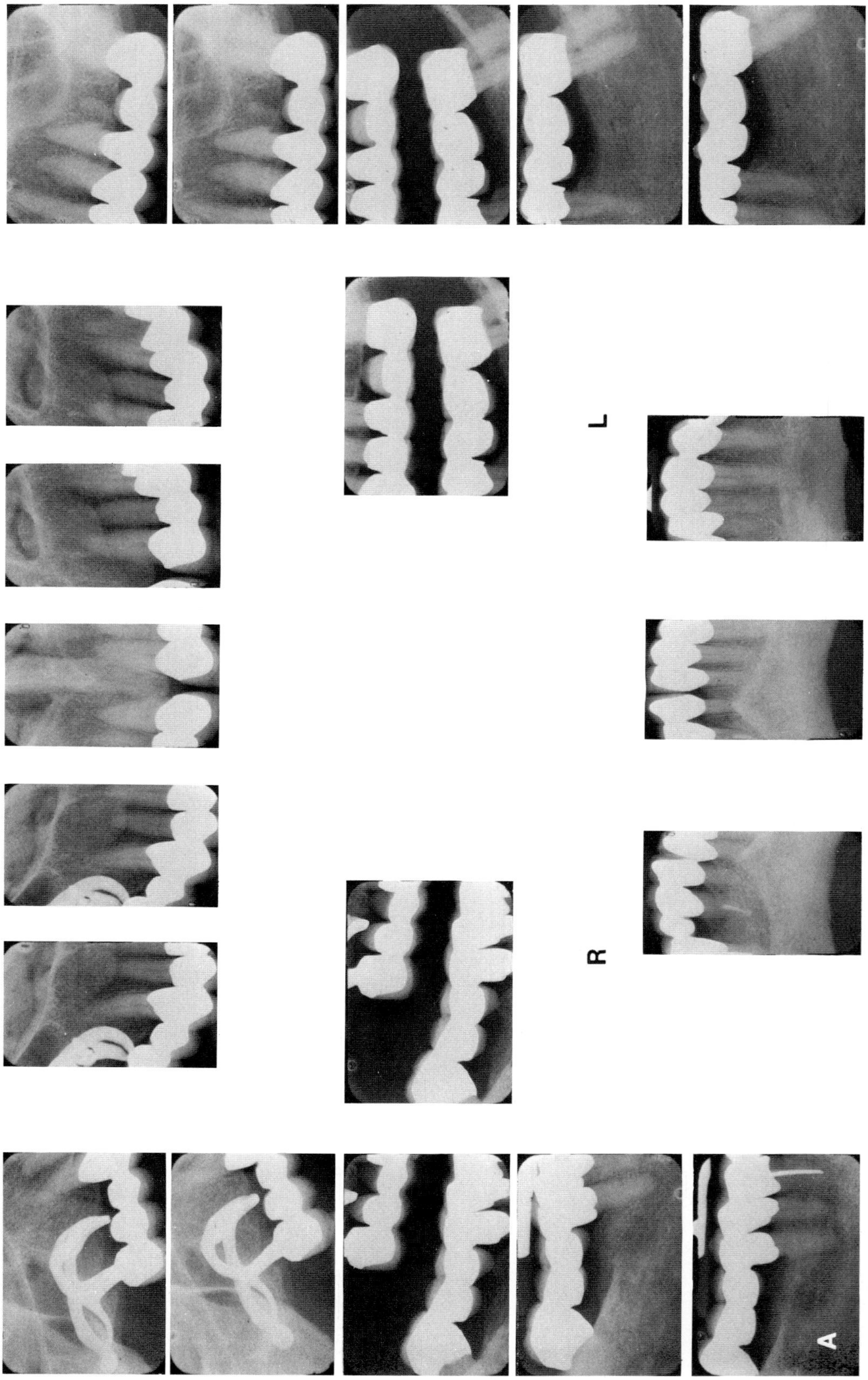
L
R
A

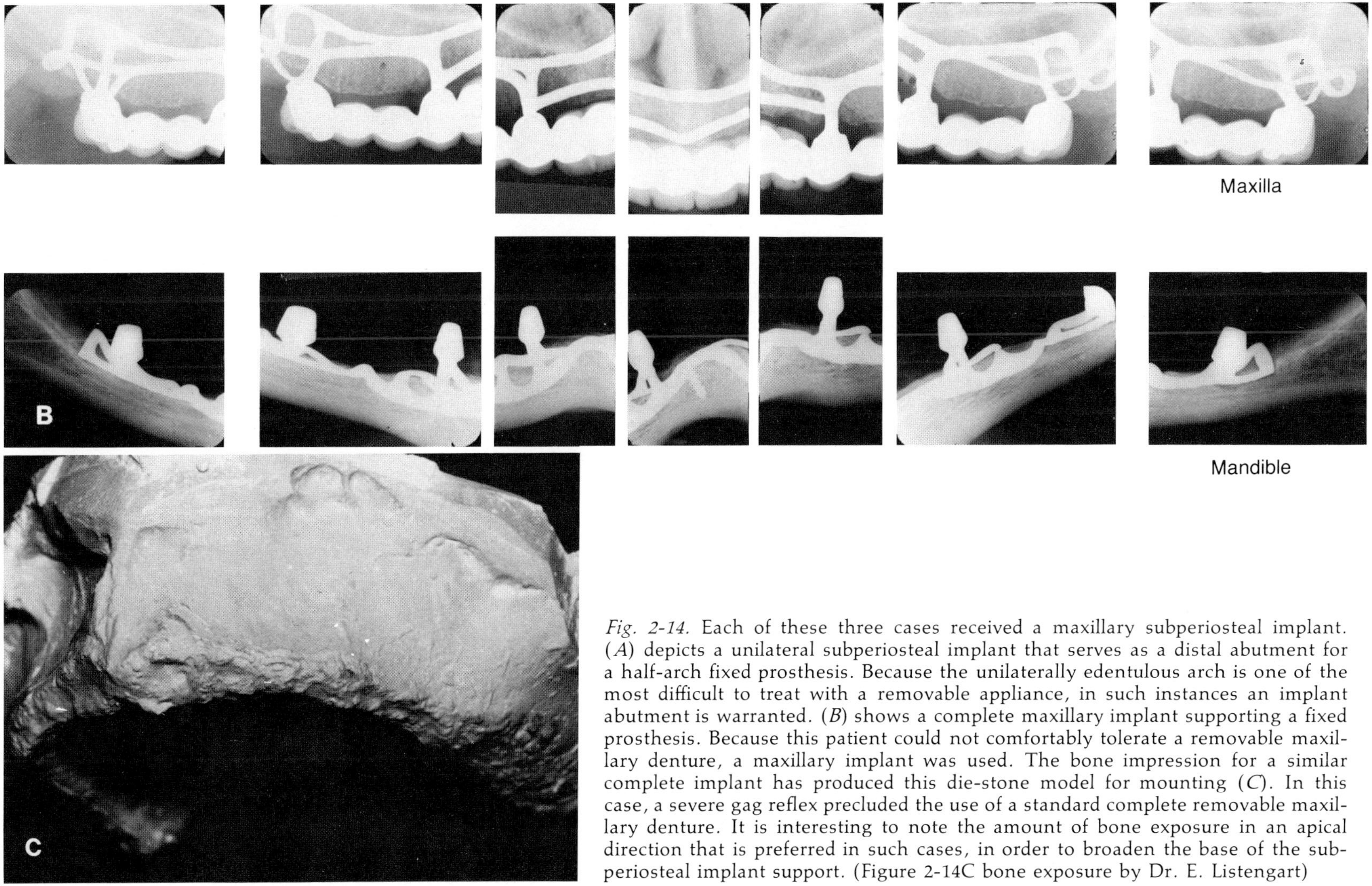

Fig. 2-14. Each of these three cases received a maxillary subperiosteal implant. (*A*) depicts a unilateral subperiosteal implant that serves as a distal abutment for a half-arch fixed prosthesis. Because the unilaterally edentulous arch is one of the most difficult to treat with a removable appliance, in such instances an implant abutment is warranted. (*B*) shows a complete maxillary implant supporting a fixed prosthesis. Because this patient could not comfortably tolerate a removable maxillary denture, a maxillary implant was used. The bone impression for a similar complete implant has produced this die-stone model for mounting (*C*). In this case, a severe gag reflex precluded the use of a standard complete removable maxillary denture. It is interesting to note the amount of bone exposure in an apical direction that is preferred in such cases, in order to broaden the base of the subperiosteal implant support. (Figure 2-14C bone exposure by Dr. E. Listengart)

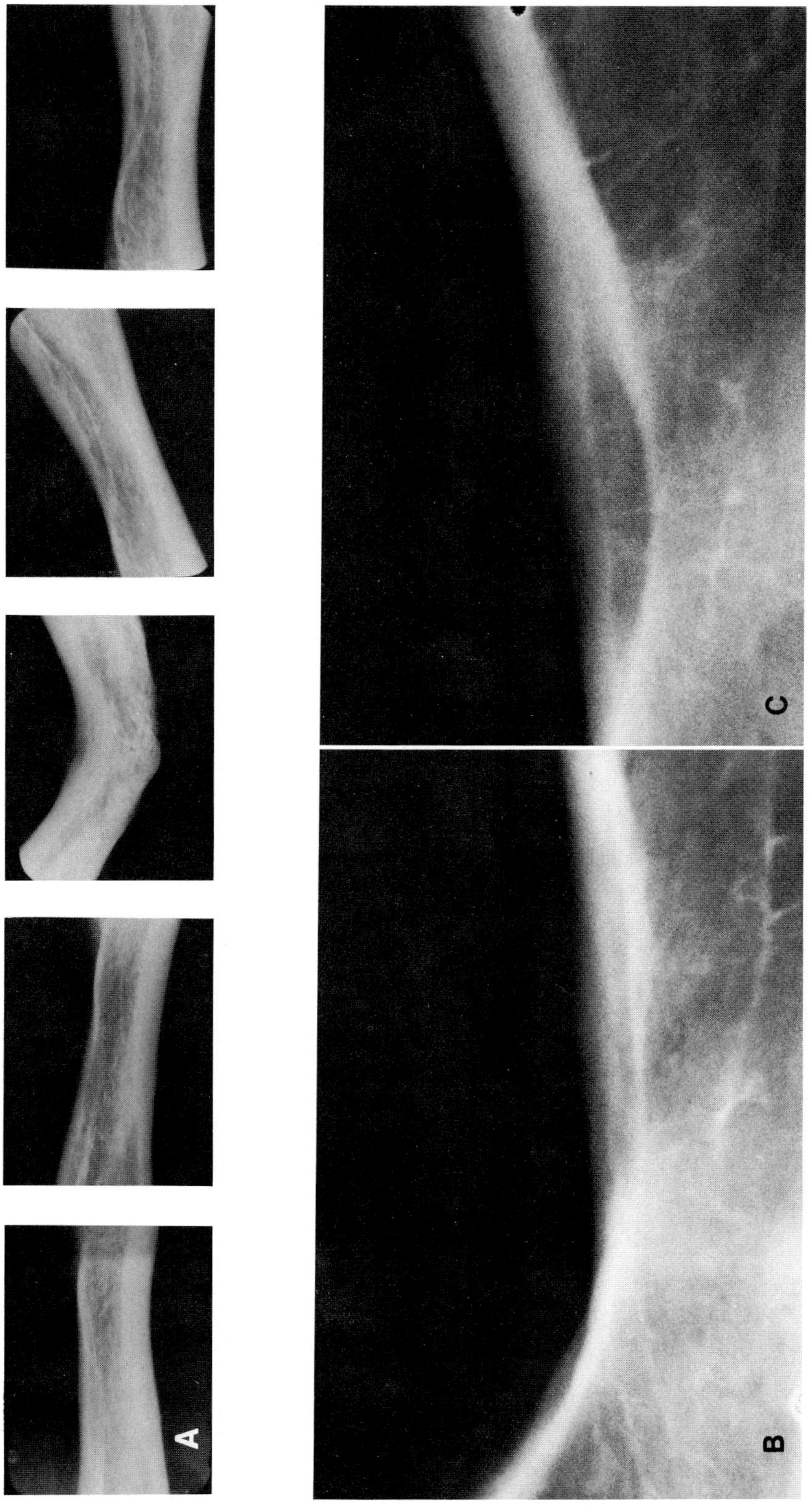

Fig. 2-15. A comparison of the multiple radiographs in (*A*) is made with each of the individual radiographs of (*B*) and (*C*). (*A*) depicts the typical, highly resorbed mandible that can serve as the base of support for a subperiosteal implant. On the other hand, although a dense cortical plate appears on the radiographs of (*B*) and (*C*), there is a definite lack of trabeculation, which of itself would negate the use of any implant procedure. Not only is the superficial topography of the residual ridge important, but as much as possible should be determined from radiographs as to the consistency of the inner aspect of this ridge.

preferable to place a subperiosteal implant on a site that reveals dense, compact mandibular bone. If alveolar bone remains, a subperiosteal implant should not be used, and a blade implant is thus indicated for the mandible (Fig. 2-12). If alveolar bone is present in an area that is to bear either the struts or the peripheral border of the subperiosteal implant, this bone must be removed before any bone impression can be made. In this situation, the standard waiting period of about 9 months is imperative before the healed osseous substructure can be used as an implant-bearing base.

It is the preference of the author to use the broad expanse of the subperiosteal implant in any cases that require a maxillary implant, so as to dissipate the forces over as great an area as possible because of the relative instability of the spongy bone (Fig. 2-13). Although the terminal and intermediary subperiosteal implants can be successful on the maxilla, the complete upper subperiosteal implant should be avoided unless it is absolutely considered to be "a last resort" (Fig. 2-14).

It is not only the nature of the supportive bone that must be considered with respect to implant determinations. For example, the maxilla may have an overbite relationship with the mandibular teeth, subjecting any complete upper implant to horizontal forces that are detrimental even in the most sound environment. Also, it is obvious that osteoporosis or the relative position of a sinus may preclude the use of any implant (Fig. 2-15). The relationship of a mandibular canal to the height of a ridge or to the depth of the body of a mandible may point the way for the clinician to either select the proper blade implant or to forego the blade implant in favor of the subperiosteal implant.

The Status of the Occlusion

The harmony of the occlusion must be such as to dissipate the forces of occlusion throughout as great an area as possible without any undue stresses on the implant that may, in whole or in part, support the occlusal tables. As previously mentioned, when the upper arch is in a severe overbite-overjet relation to the mandible, it is a poor candidate for a complete implant. In Class III skeletal crossbite cases, the mandible would be a poor candidate for a complete implant.

In an arch that has been edentulous for quite some time, the use of a temporary removable prosthesis over a complete implant is necessary and, at times, very revealing. The added proprioception through an occlusal surface that is in a stable position usually allows the patient to return to a true centric relation. This allows the permanent removable or fixed superstructure to be fabricated in a physiologically acceptable position. Any manipulation of the mandible by the dentist may not have attained this jaw-to-jaw relationship. *At no time should the clinician be so presumptuous as to fabricate a final prosthesis without the intermediary temporary (provisional) phase.*

Once the occlusion has been established at the proper vertical dimension in centric position, it appears to be preferable to have the superstructure in a group-function occlusion. The anterior segment should be in as much of an edge-to-edge relation as possible. The intermediary implant appears to be most successful in a group-function occlusion, whereas the free-end terminal implant appears to succeed best in a cuspid-rise for lateral jaw excursions. A minimum of two mesial abutment teeth is advised for all terminal implant abutments. These are clinical empiricisms.

Chair-side notes concerning the visual, palpatory, and occlusal aspects of examination should be made by a competent secretary as directed by the examiner. This examination outline may later be augmented with radiographic findings (Figs. 2-9, 2-16, 2-17).

The General Health Condition

Probably the best rule of thumb regarding the overriding issue of medical health status is the following: anyone who can

Morton L. Perel, B. Sc., D. D. S., M. Sc. D.

PRACTICE LIMITED TO PROSTHODONTICS

130 WATERMAN STREET
PROVIDENCE, RHODE ISLAND 02906
TEL. 401-861-1343

April, 19__

Mrs. X.Y.Z.--CONSULTATION
Dr. Morton L. Perel--April, 19__

The lower right edentulous area distal to the lower right second bicuspid shows moderate resorption with a broad external oblique ridge that slopes buccally to the same height as the ridge itself. In the lingual aspect toward the mylohyoid ridge there is a ledge of bone that extends inferiorly for about 5 to 6 mm prior to having any undercut. The soft tissue is pink, firm, and healthy with a nice band of attached tissue (3 to 4 mm); however the sublingual tissues at rest come to within 2 mm in the mucolingual fold area. Opposing this there is a first molar that has been held in place by mesial occlusal contact of the opposing second bicuspid. The second molar is in buccal version and has extruded with a marginal ridge discrepancy of about 3 mm.

Right lateral excursion is cuspid rise.

The second bicuspids anterior to this ridge are non-mobile.

MLP:lag

A

Fig. 2-16. A consultation examination report *(A)* is followed by a written report to the referring dentist *(B, opposite)*. The study and follow-through of even a single implant site is imperative. In this case, the considered implant site was in the lower right posterior quadrant in an arch that had multiple remaining natural teeth. It is important to note the sequence of procedures that has been delineated, aside from the determination of the implant site itself.

undergo the sophisticated procedures of modern periodontal treatment can also undergo the procedures for the subperiosteal and blade dental implants. In extensive implant procedures, it is advisable to have the patient undergo a series of blood tests and a physical examination. Thus, the hazards of improper clotting, improper healing, or a lowered resistance to the rigors of surgical implant procedures can be avoided. Also, the patient must be able to accept some form of sedation, because all implant procedures can be done under local anesthetic in the office operatory (unless the patient expresses a preference to undergo general anesthesia in a hospital). For the most part, local and oral conditions appear to have a more direct bearing on the potentiality for success; only the most obviously adverse systemic factors that would preclude any other type of surgery would preclude implant procedures.

Patients with certain classifications of systemic diseases are not amenable to im-

Morton L. Perel, B. S., D. D. S., M. Sc. D.

PRACTICE LIMITED TO PROSTHODONTICS

130 WATERMAN STREET
PROVIDENCE, RHODE ISLAND 02906
TEL.: 401-861-1343

April, 19__

Dear Doctor ____________:

On ______________, Mrs. X.Y.Z. was seen in this office for consultation regarding a possible placement of an implant in the lower right area quadrant. A copy of the examination is enclosed for your perusal.

Having also studied two radiographs of the area under consideration, I have concluded that Mrs. Z. can have a lower blade implant. The alveolar bone remaining in this area precludes the use of a subperiosteal implant. There are two additional favorable conditions relating to this area:

1. The cuspid rise lateral excursion should be left intact;

2. The two bicuspids mesial to the implant site are good candidates to serve as double abutments.

There are three facets that would have to be completed prior to insertion of the implant:

1. The orthodontic movement which has been initiated on the lower left posterior quadrant would have to have been completed;

2. Lower right 4 and 5 will have to have been temporized;

3. The upper right second molar should be reshaped occlusally so as to allow adequate room for the implant abutment and the eventual full-crown retainer which will serve as the distal abutment for the fixed bridge.

The usual risk factor was explained to the patient who was still most receptive to the idea that she is an implant candidate. As such, Mrs. Z. has made an appointment on September ______, in order to proceed with the implant insertion procedures.

B

Fig. 2-16B.

plant procedures. Diabetics and alcoholics are usually poor candidates, depending on the degree of disease progression and the degree of its control. Patients with heart problems must be questioned as to their present drug intake; if anticoagulants are to be decreased, permission must be obtained from the attending physician. The standard, yet important, questionnaire regarding allergic responses and sensitivities must be noted prior to the acceptance of a patient for an implant. Not only is the patient with a history of rheumatic fever treated with antibiotics prior to (and dur-

Morton L. Perel, B. Sc., D. D. S., M. Sc. D.

PRACTICE LIMITED TO PROSTHODONTICS

130 WATERMAN STREET
PROVIDENCE, RHODE ISLAND 02906
TEL.: 401-861-1343

December, 19____

Dear Doctor __________:

On November, 19____, Mrs. P. D. L., whom you so kindly referred for consultation, was seen in this office. Specific concern related to the lower posterior segments which were edentulous and might be amenable to distal implants. The upper arch supported a complete upper denture.

The examination revealed the following: The lower six anterior teeth are present, and included the presence of the first bicuspids. All of these teeth are stable. The bicuspids are rotated toward the distal with about a 60 degree angle of rotation. The labial aspects have gingival recession; and gingival free grafts have been placed just gingival to these areas. The lower left residual ridge has moderate to severe recession with a blunted, rounded ridge of about 3 to 4 mm in width. The mylohyoid ridge area is perpendicular, with no appreciable undercut. There is attached tissue of 2 to 3 mm in width along the height of this ridge. The lower right residual ridge has moderate to severe resorption with a blunted knife edge that is 2 to 3 mm in width. There is a prominent external oblique ridge; and there is a narrow band of attached tissue that is 2 mm in width at its narrowest point. The mylohyoid ridge is perpendicular for about 4 mm, under which there is a distinct concavity in the form of a prominent undercut.

In view of the results of such visual inspection, palpation, and radiographic interpretation, Mrs. L. appears to be a good candidate for mandibular bilateral blade implants. I should prefer having these done at two separate sessions. Firstly, it would be necessary to splint and temporize the mesial abutments, so that immediately upon insertion of any one implant, I can fabricate and attach a temporary fixed splint to such abutments. Therefore, as soon as you have completed temporization, please inform me and I will be happy to cooperate in appointing Mrs. L. for the individual sessions that require placement of such implants.

A

Fig. 2-17. Two examples of actual letters that were written after implant consultations. It is as important to note the rejection of an implant *(B, opposite),* as it is to determine the type of implant *(A)* that is to be selected for a suitable implant case.

ing) the initial surgical procedures; *all* patients are similarly premedicated. Penicillin is most often used; but erythromycin stearate may have to be resorted to in cases of possible allergic responses.

The debilitated patient should not necessarily be eliminated as a candidate for dental implants. If such debilitation was caused by the inability to masticate properly, then such a person may be a prime

Morton L. Perel, B. Sc., D. D. S., M. Sc. D.

PRACTICE LIMITED TO PROSTHODONTICS

130 WATERMAN STREET
PROVIDENCE, RHODE ISLAND 02906
TEL. 401-861-1343

August, 19______.

Dear Doctor ____________:

Only July, 19_____, I had seen Mrs. R. S. R. in this office for consultation regarding the possible use of dental implants.

I sincerely believe that this patient is not a candidate for oral implants. The upper right arch does not have enough supportive bone, and the residual ridge is in close approximation to the maxillary sinus. Also, the lower right posterior would have to await a period of nine months after extraction of the periodontally involved teeth prior to considering placement of any type of oral implant.

All in all, I explained to Mrs. R. that any dental implant involved a degree of unpredictability even under the best of circumstances. If there are more predictable avenues of dental treatment, I must in good faith advise same. Therefore, in this particular case, I would advise a combination of fixed and removable prostheses which would preclude the use of any dental implant.

B

Fig. 2-17B.

candidate to receive an oral implant. People who appear for implant consultations are often those who have not been able to chew properly and who thus have experienced weight loss and accompanying general debilitation. The use of implants for these people can create the stability of dentition that would make possible the proper mastication of a variety of foodstuffs. Thus, rehabilitation through implant prostheses could reestablish the patient's state of general well-being that may have existed prior to the loss of the natural dentition.

Therefore, weight loss and even mental depression—which are common in people who present to the office with edentulous mouths—do not in themselves preclude the use of implants. Neither is old age a factor; in fact, it is usually the geriatric patient who most often requires the use of a prosthesis, in general, and perhaps implants specifically. An acceptable level of general good health—aside from the inability to masticate and ingest food properly—however, *is* a prerequisite. In this regard, freedom from adverse occlusal habits and adverse tongue habits are factors for case selection in the context of the overall health picture.

Case Selection by Case Elimination

Following this survey, it becomes obvious that a process of elimination is necessary to establish a selection of cases that are best suited for dental implants. Those patients who are suited for dental implants represent a very select group.

The dentist may reject the patient as an

implant candidate on the basis of (a) the ability to restore the stomatognathic system to its optimum function by using only other forms of dental treatment; and (b) the unsuitability of an implant site due to local factors or due to a positive medical record.

The patient may decide against receiving an implant because of (a) the surgical procedures involved; and (b) the intertwined risks undertaken on his behalf (see Case Presentation). The patient's freedom of choice eliminates another segment of the population from possible implant restorative procedures.

Dentists and patients should be aware of the notice in the *A. D. A. Leadership Bulletin** that recommends that patients be informed of the limitations of endosseous implants.

Two scientific councils of the ADA will recommend in a joint report to the profession that patients be advised of the limitations of endosseous implants prior to their use whenever implantation is the chosen treatment procedure. For the protection of both the patient and the dentist using implants, the patient should be made aware "that the degree of success to be expected from an appliance designed specifically for the patient is at this time not known," according to the Council on Dental Materials and Devices (CDMD) and the Council on Dental Research (CDR).

CASE PRESENTATION: THE RISK OF COMPLICATIONS AND FAILURE

If the case selection is ideal for the type of implant intended, it is incumbent upon the dentist to outline the possibilities of implant failure to the patient. All things being equal, both the dentist and the patient must realize that there is always a risk of implant failure at any time after implant insertion.

The so-called "rejection syndrome" may take one of two avenues, months or years after the insertion of the implant. One of these avenues may be spontaneous infection, which at this time appears to be associated with the influx of bacteria through the soft-tissue collar surrounding the implant neck.

The more mysterious of these avenues of failure is spontaneous bone resorption, which may or may not be accompanied by pain. The clinical assessment of this situation tends toward the hypothesis that *a particular individual's functional forces, imparted to the supportive bone through the implant of choice, may not be tolerated by this same osseous structure.* Obviously, bruxers and clenchers are not candidates for any implant that is available at this time. Although clenching and bruxism cannot be determined in patients who have totally edentulous arches, the partially edentulous mouth may exhibit telltale signs of clenching and bruxism, such as extensive wear facets, that may preclude the inclusion of implants in the total treatment plan.

Imparting Information to the Patient

All of the facts must be presented to the potential dental implant patient. For example, there are some implant sites that have a greater predilection for success; the mandible generally is one such site. Any implant inserted in the maxilla has a greater chance of failure. Consequently, it is important to recall all implant patients periodically, to assess the stability of the implant and the condition of the supportive bone and surrounding soft tissues.

At this time in the development of oral implantology, it is foolhardy to compare its success rate to that of conservative endodontics. This would be as fallacious as comparing the success rate of open heart surgery to that of an appendectomy; that is to say, there is an inherently greater chance of encountering critical problems in one area of medical treatment when com-

*American Dental Association, vol. 4, no. 1, Jan. 7, 1974.

MORTON L. PEREL, D.D.S., M.Sc.D.

CONSENT TO OPERATION

PATIENT________________________________ AGE______________________

DATE________________________________

1) I hereby authorize Dr. Morton L. Perel and whomever he may designate as his assistants to perform surgery upon (name)__________________________, and if any unforeseen condition arises in the course of the operation calling on his judgment for procedures in addition to or different from those now contemplated, I further request and authorize him to do whatever he deems advisable.

2) The nature and purpose of the operation, the risks involved, and the possibility of complications have been fully explained to me. I acknowledge that no guarantee or assurance has been made as to the results that may be obtained.

3) I consent to the disposal by authorities of any tissues or parts which may be removed.

4) I consent to the taking and publication of any photographs or moving pictures before, after, or in the course of this operation for the purpose of advancing dental education.

5) For the purpose of advancing dental education, I also consent to the admittance of observers to the operating room.

I CERTIFY THAT I HAVE READ AND FULLY UNDERSTAND THE ABOVE CONSENT TO OPERATION AND THAT THE EXPLANATIONS THEREIN REFERRED TO WERE MADE.

Signature of patient__________________________

When patient is a minor or
incompetent to give consent:

Signature of person authorized
to consent for patient__________________________

Relationship to patient__________________________

Witness________________________________

Fig. 2-18. This consent form is not merely a legal document. It is a constant reminder to the dentist that implant procedures have been properly explained to the patient and to any other dentist that is involved in the treatment of this patient. (Courtesy of Dr. Mendell Robinson)

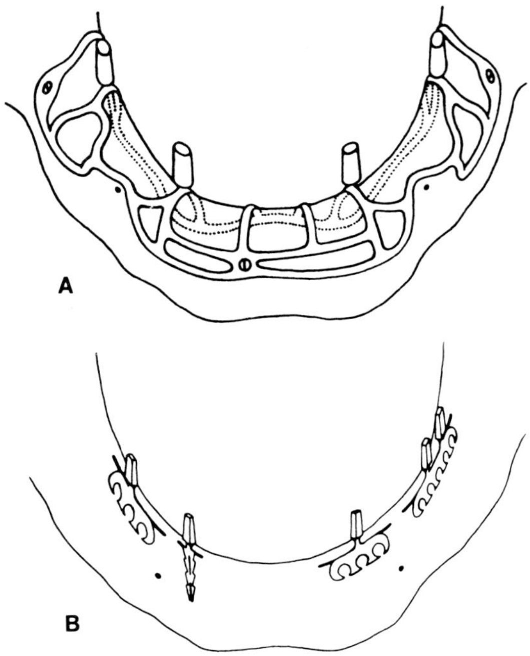

Fig. 2-19. The complete implant takes the form of a single subperiosteal implant (*A*) or multiple-blade implants (*B*), for a completely edentulous arch. These posts may support a fixed or a removable superstructure prosthesis. The same category of implants pertains to both the maxilla and the mandible.

pared with the other. As in any of the health sciences, not all treatments have the same predictability of short-term and/or long-term success.

The approach to the patient should not be negative, but rather *truthful.* The dentist must present all of the possibilities to the patient and then leave the choice as to whether the dentist should proceed with his selection of implant procedure to the patient. The idea is not to sell, but rather to present both the knowns and unknowns of oral implantology. The surgical procedures and postoperative sequelae of swelling and possible hematoma may in themselves be distasteful to the patient.

It is also important to warn the patient that if an implant has to be removed at any time in the future, there is an accompanying loss of bone that varies tremendously according to the type of implant (intra-osseous or supra-osseous) involved and according to the timing of such removal. Again, the point is not to scare the patient, but rather to inform him of the potential of the successful implant and of the possible accompanying problems of an implant failure. The dentist should also present the alternatives that may be available if success is not attained. After having explained all the general facts concerning implants—using visual aids—and noting those particular factors that are endemic to that particular patient, it is wise to have the patient sign a consent form. The form is not only a legal document, but also a reminder to the implantologist that he has properly informed the patient of procedures and of possibilities (Fig. 2-18).

The Modification of Patient Habits

In the course of such presentation at the initial office visit, the patient should be informed of his responsibilities regarding oral physiotherapy. The patient should also be informed that if he is in the habit of clamping a pipe between his teeth, continuance of this habit would endanger the retention of the dental implant. The consequence of all other such habits that become known to the dentist should be explained to the patient. Although the implant patient can, for the most part, eat normally, he may have to alter certain eating habits that might be injurious to the implant. A patient with a complete implant, for example, should be discouraged from eating whole fresh apples and corn on the cob. The transverse and horizontal forces imparted by these activities are not consistent with the vertical lines of force that should be transmitted through an implant in function.

Summation of the Case Presentation

At the initial appointment, the expectations and the fears of the patient should be completely and honestly dealt with by

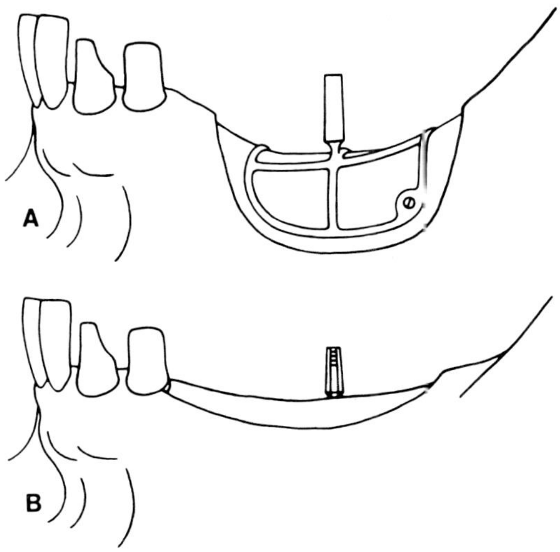

Fig. 2-20. A terminal implant abutment may take the form of either a supra-osseous (*A*) or an intra-osseous (*B*) design. The amount of bone loss and the type of remaining bone will determine which implant design should be used. In any case, a minimum of two mesial abutment teeth is needed. Therefore, the *smallest* fixed-bridge prosthesis would consist of four units (two natural abutment teeth; one pontic; and one implant abutment).

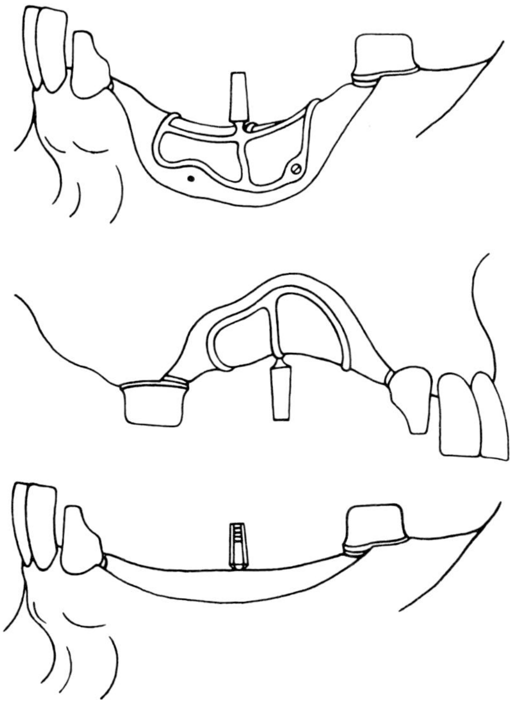

Fig. 2-21. An intermediary implant abutment is used in conjunction with a superimposed fixed prosthesis. In these cases, a long edentulous span between two or more natural abutment teeth may lead to the choice of either a removable partial denture, or an intermediary implant post that would allow for the fabrication of a fixed bridge.

the dentist. All the benefits *as well as* the potential shortcomings of an implant should be explained. Although case selection may allow the dentist to rule in favor of an implant procedure, certain fears and apprehensions of the patient may make him decide not to undergo implant procedures.

CATEGORIZATION OF IMPLANTS

All implants may be classified in three categories:

The Complete Implant

This may take the form of a single subperiosteal implant in a completely edentulous upper or lower arch. It may also take the form of the restoration of a completely edentulous arch by the use of multiple blade implants (Fig. 2-19).

The Terminal Implant

This may be either a subperiosteal or a blade implant that serves as a single distal abutment in a partially edentulous arch (Fig. 2-20). It may be either unilateral or bilateral. The latter takes the form of two separate implants. The classic use of terminal bilateral implants is to replace the mandibular bilateral free-end saddle removable partial denture.

The Intermediary Implant

This pier abutment is an implant that is affixed between two or more natural teeth to enable the superimposition of a fixed bridge over a long span of an edentulous ridge area (Fig. 2-21).

A modification of the subperiosteal implant may be designated as a fourth classification. This refers to the universal-type of subperiosteal implant which straddles both sides of an arch that is edentulous except for two to four remaining intervening natural teeth, usually in the anterior region. The design of such an implant covers a bilaterally edentulous arch with the continuity of the frame that circumvents the natural remaining teeth. The superstructure then consists of both the single-frame, multi-abutted implant and the remaining prepared natural teeth.

BIBLIOGRAPHY

Baylink, D. J., Wergedal, J. E., Yamamoto, K., and Manzke, E.: Systematic factors in alveolar bone loss. J. Pros. Dent., *31:*486-505, 1974.

Becket, L. S.: Partial dentures. The rebasing of tissue borne saddles. Theory and Practice. Australian D. J., *16:*340-346, 1971.

Becks, H., and Weber, M.: Influence of diet on bone system, with special references to alveolar process and labyrinthine capsule. J. A. D. A., *18:*197-264, 1931.

Cheraskin, E., and Ringsdorf, W. M.: Ecology of alveolar bone loss. Oral Surg., *30:*333-350, 1970.

Cheraskin, M. D.: Roentgenographic manifestations of osseous changes in the jaws. Oral Surg., Oral Med. and Oral Path., *12:*442-456, 1959.

Cranin, A. N., Cranin, S. L., and Dennison, T. A.: Physical evaluation of the patient presenting for implant surgery. Oral Implantol., *2:*183-189 (Part 1); 265-275 (Part 2); 1972.

Garn, S.: The Earlier Gain and the Later Loss of Cortical Bone in Nutritional Perspective. Springfield, Illinois, Charles C Thomas, 1970.

Goldman, H. M., and Cohen, D. W.: Periodontal Therapy. ed. 5. St. Louis, C. V. Mosby, 1973.

Jamieson, C. H.: Geriatrics and the denture patient. J. Pros. Dent., *8:*8-13, 1958.

Kabcenell, J. L.: More retentive complete dentures. J. A. D. A., *70:*116-120, 1970.

Kelly, E.: Changes caused by a mandibular removable partial denture opposing a maxillary complete denture. J. Pros. Dent. *27:*140-150, 1972.

Knight, N.: Reverse images and ghosts of Panorex radiography. J. Am. Soc. Preventive Dent., *3:*53-57, 1973.

Lammie, G. A.: Aging changes and the complete lower denture. J. Pros. Dent., *6:*450-464, 1956.

———Aging changes in the complete lower denture, J. Pros. Dent., *25:*152-161, 1971.

McKevitt, F. H.: Clinical and roentgenographic manifestations of atrophic changes in the jaws: endocrine and vitamin factors in the practice of prosthodontia. J.A.D.A., *19:* 1901-1917, 1932.

Massler, M.: Tissue changes during aging. Oral Surg., *9:*1185-1196, 1956.

Neufeld, J. O.: Changes in the trabecular pattern of the mandible following the loss of teeth. J. Pros. Dent., *8:*685-697, 1958.

Parfitt, G. J.: An investigation of the normal variations in alveolar bone trabeculation. Oral Surg., Oral Med. and Oral Path., *15:*1453-1463, 1962.

Prichard, J. F.: The roentgenographic depiction of periodontal disease. J. Am. Soc. Preventive Dent., *3:*44-50, 1973.

Schafer, S. A.: Alveolar bone loss associated with vascular disease, Northwest D. J., *51:*299-301, 1972.

Schei, O., Waerhaug, J., Lovdal, A., and Arno, A.: Alveolar bone loss as related to oral hygiene and age. J. Periodont., *30:*7-16, 1959.

Schweiger, J. W.: Prosthetic considerations for the aging, J. Pros. Dent., *9:*555-558, 1959.

Shafer, W. G., Hine, M. K., and Levy, B. M.: A Textbook of Oral Pathology. ed. 3. Philadelphia, W. B. Saunders, 1974.

Stahl, S. S. and Fox, L. M.: Histologic changes of the oral mucosa associated with certain chronic diseases. Oral Surg., *6:*339-344, 1953.

Stahl, S. S., Wisan, J. M., and Miller, S. C.: The influence of systemic deseases on alveolar bone. J. A. D. A., *45:*277-282, 1952.

Tallgren, A.: The reduction in face height of edentulous subjects during long term denture wearing. Acta odont. scandinav., *24:*195-239, 1966.

Thoma, K. H., and Goldman, H. M. Oral Pathology. ed 6. St. Louis, C. V. Mosby, 1970.

Thoma, K. H., and Robinson, H. B. G.: Oral and Dental Diagnosis. ed. 5. Philadelphia, W. B.. Saunders, 1964.

Updegrave, W. J.: The role of panoramic radiography in diagnosis. Oral Surg., *22:*49-57, 1966.

———: Right-angle dental radiography. D. Clin. North America, 571-579, November, 1968.

———: Right-angle dental radiography—common problems with solutions. J. Tennessee State D. A., *51:*205-210, 1971.

Weinmann, J.P., and Sicher, H.: Bone and Bones. ed. 2. London, Henry Kimpton, 1955.

Wical, K. E., and Swoope, C. C.: Studies of residual ridge resorption. Part II. The relationship of dietary calcium and phosphorus to residual ridge resorption. J. Pros. Dent., *32:*13-22, 1974.

Worth, H. M.; Principles and Practice of Oral Radiologic Interpretation. ed. 3. Chicago, Year Book Medical Publishers, 1972.

3 The Subperiosteal Implant—Nomenclature and Rationale of Design

THE SNOWSHOE EFFECT

The subperiosteal oral implant can best be compared to the snowshoe. Both are intended to dissipate, over as large an area as possible, the forces that are exerted on their frames. The design of any subperiosteal implant requires the encompassment of as much of a supportive bony area as is possible. This is referred to as a "snowshoe effect" (Fig. 3-1). According to the *Random House Dictionary of the English Language,* a snowshoe is "a contrivance that may be attached to the foot to enable the wearer to walk on deep snow without sinking, esp. a light, racket-shaped frame across which is stretched a network of rawhide." The analogy is appropriate. If the forces imparted through the implant abutments are spread over a large area, then the stress on the supportive bone is dissipated (Figs. 3-2 to 3-8). A 200-lb. (90-kg.) man may sink into fresh fallen snow; but wearing snowshoes, he may walk on top of the same texture of snow. Another analogy may be appropriate. On a hot summer day the asphalt of one's driveway may be softened. A 200-lb. male may walk on this asphalt without leaving indentations; however, a 100-lb. (45-kg.) female wearing spike-heeled shoes may walk on this same asphalt at the same time and would definitely leave imprints or indentations in the asphalt. The spike-heeled shoes created a concentration of forces in a small area; whereas, in the case of the male, there was a dissipation of larger forces over a larger area. The same principles of dissipation of forces appears to hold true in a broad outline of the peripheral border of a subperiosteal dental implant.

NOMENCLATURE OF PARTS OF THE SUBPERIOSTEAL IMPLANT

The subperiosteal dental implant consists of three distinct yet coalescent parts. These are the implant post (abutment), the implant neck, and the implant frame (body or crib) (Figs. 3-9 to 3-12).

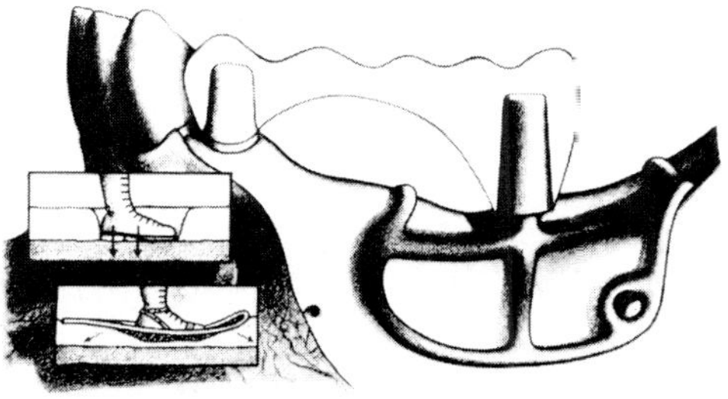

Fig. 3-1. Molar implant post abutment supported by an extensive frame outline. As much of the external oblique ridge is encompassed as is possible. The mesial aspect does not approach the mesial natural-tooth abutment, in order to avoid supportive impingement on alveolar bone. The "snowshoe effect" is comparable to a person walking on fresh-fallen snow *(insets).* The top inset exemplifies the concentration of forces by showing a person's foot sinking directly through snow. The lower inset demonstrates the efficacy of a snowshoe which, through its dissipation of forces, prevents the same person from sinking through the snow. The same principle is applicable to all subperiosteal implant designs.

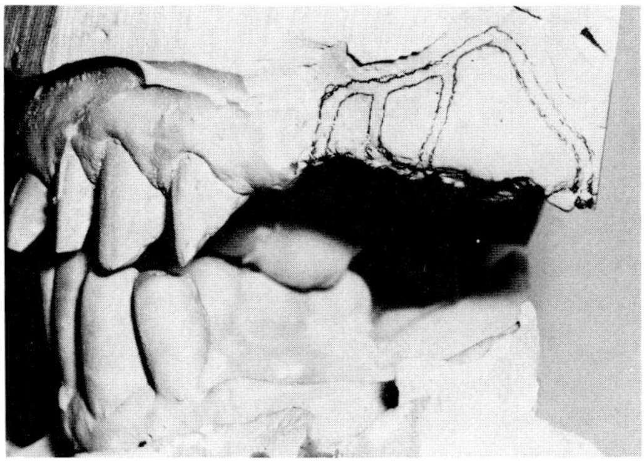

Fig. 3-2. Buccal view of the design of an upper left terminal subperiosteal implant. The broad outline form encompasses: the distal aspect which approaches the hamular notch; the apical extension to the concavity that begins to form the zygomatic arch; and a mesial extension that avoids the supportive structures of the natural cuspid-tooth abutment.

The Implant Post

The post (abutment) is totally within the environment of the oral cavity. Except for its base or gingival margin, it is covered by the crown retainer of the fixed superstructure or by the female portion of the removable superstructure. The form of the post is similar to a prepared natural abutment tooth that is to receive a full crown retainer. All posts are similar in size to a prepared natural premolar tooth, even if they are placed in molar areas. The narrow

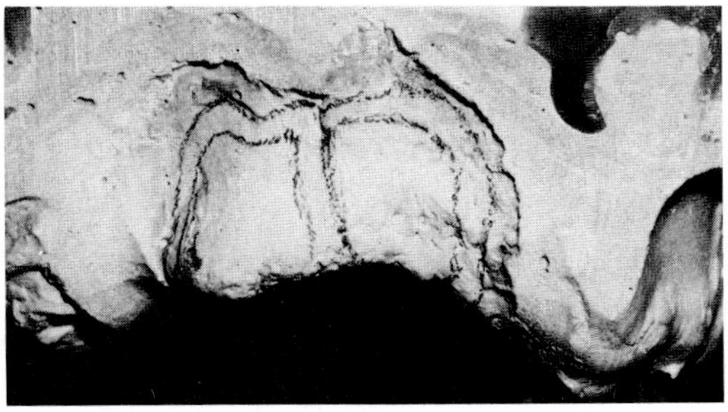

Fig. 3-3. Buccal view of an intermediary cuspid subperiosteal implant design. The distal extension avoids the supportive bone of the molar root that has been endodontically treated. The mesial extension of the peripheral border terminates distal to the mid-suture line of the premaxilla.

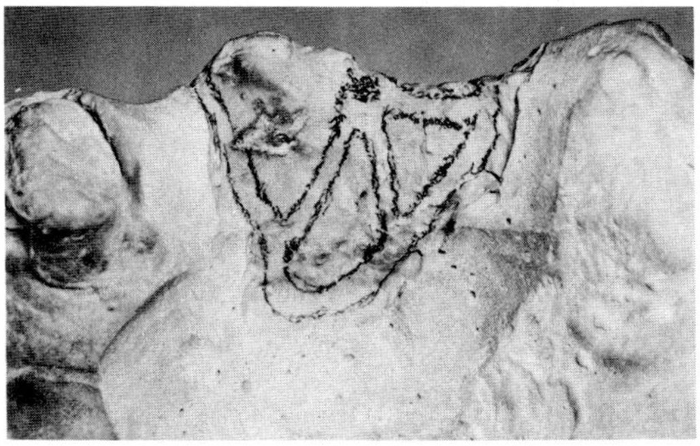

Fig. 3-4. Palatal view of the same implant outline shown in Figure 3-3 portrays: the crossing of the peripheral border extensions at the height of the residual ridge through valleys of bone; and the termination of the palatal extension at the concavity that delineates the hard palate from the residual ridge. A distinct effort is made to avoid the placement of struts or portions of the peripheral border on any osseous protuberance.

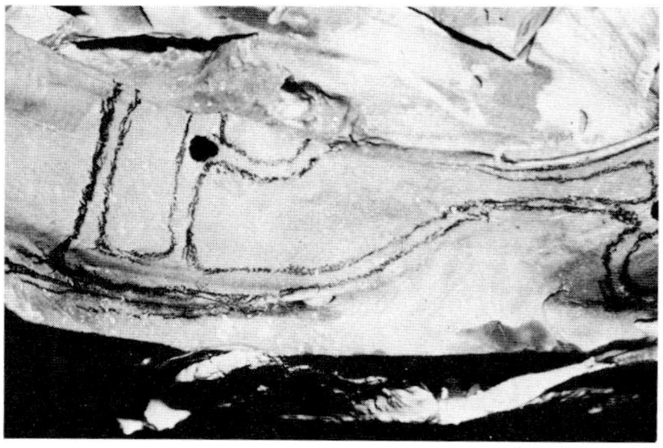

Fig. 3-5. Occlusobuccal view of the right distal extension of a complete lower subperiosteal implant design. The peripheral border actually embraces the outermost aspect of the external oblique ridge and lies under the retromolar soft-tissue pad. The broad expanse of the neurovascular bundle that emanates from the mental foramen is bypassed with a sweeping outline of the peripheral border. As much dense, compact bone is embodied as is possible, in order to fulfill the requirements of the snowshoe effect.

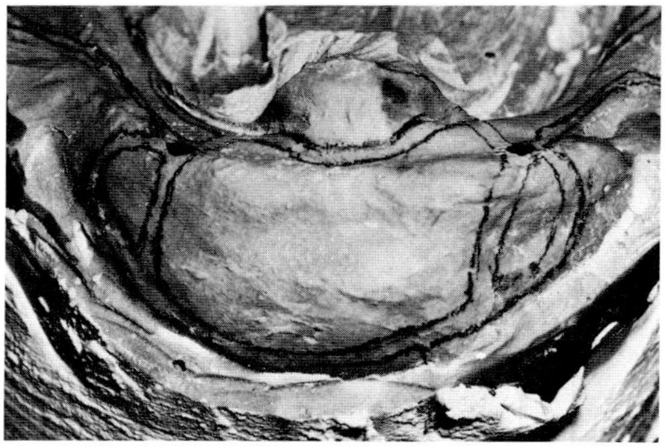

Fig. 3-6. Labio-incisal view of the anterior portion of a complete lower subperiosteal implant design. The lingual part lies at the junction of the genial tubercle and the remainder of the residual ridge. The broad expanse of the anterior symphyseal area is included inferiorly to the point where the operator can actually see the rounding of the bone under the chin. The distal aspects of the peripheral border are confined within the mesial borders of the two mental foramina.

cross section thus created by this size post allows for better oral-hygiene accessibility at the base of the post, than would posts of a larger horizontal dimension. Also, the narrow buccolingual aspect serves as a reminder to incorporate relatively narrow dimensions for the superimposed retainer food tables. There is no need to make an

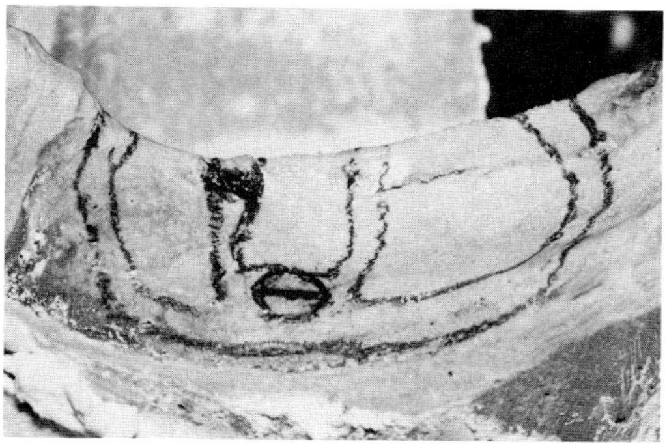

Fig. 3-7. Buccal view of a lower left terminal subperiosteal implant design. All accessible portions of the external oblique ridge have been incorporated. The distal portion terminates under the retromolar soft-tissue pad, and the mesial portion terminates just shy of the alveolar bone that surrounds the mesial abutment tooth. Minor undercuts such as that seen at the distobuccal border, are included in the design. Upon insertion of the implant, the metal is flexible enough to allow the frame to snap into place. The frame then rests passively on the supporting compact bone.

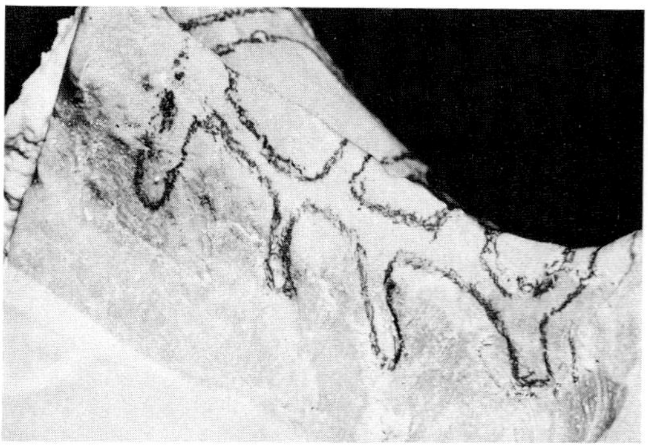

Fig. 3-8. Linguo-occlusal view of the lower left terminal subperiosteal implant design. The lingual fingers project between muscle bundles that are found in the mylohyoid ridge area. The secondary struts that link these fingers to the rest of the implant frame are lingual to, and below, the height of the residual ridge. This view portrays *(upper left)* the sweeping expanse of the peripheral border that extends over the convexity of the external oblique ridge.

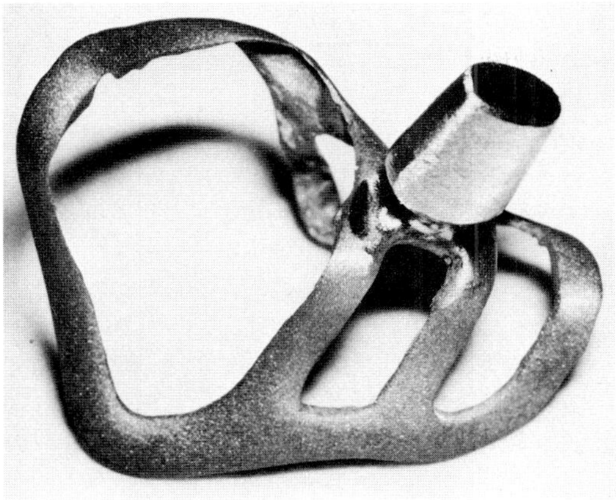

Fig. 3-9. Finished casting of an upper unilateral subperiosteal implant. The implant post is appropriately tapered to accommodate a superstructure fixed retainer. The post is joined to the implant frame by the highly polished neck that will extrude through the soft tissues. The implant frame—which will cover a broad area of bone—in this case consists of primary struts and a peripheral border.

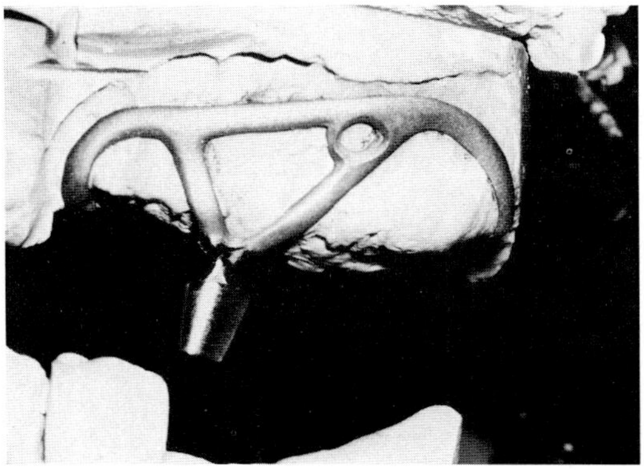

Fig. 3-10. Upper left terminal subperiosteal implant. The fabrication of the implant has taken place only on a hinge-mounted working model. Proper adaptation of all inner aspects of the casting to the supporting bone is exemplified by the stability of the implant in an inverted position. The screw hole may be left as is for connective-tissue ingrowth. A screw, however, should *never* be placed in any portion of any upper subperiosteal implant. If a screwhole has erroneously been incorporated into an upper implant casting, it should be left as is and used as is (*without* a screw).

implant molar abutment similar in appearance to a natural molar. If such were to be done, not only would broader occlusal surfaces negate the theory of vertical placement of forces, but plaque accumulation would abound at the gingival margins of the abutment base.

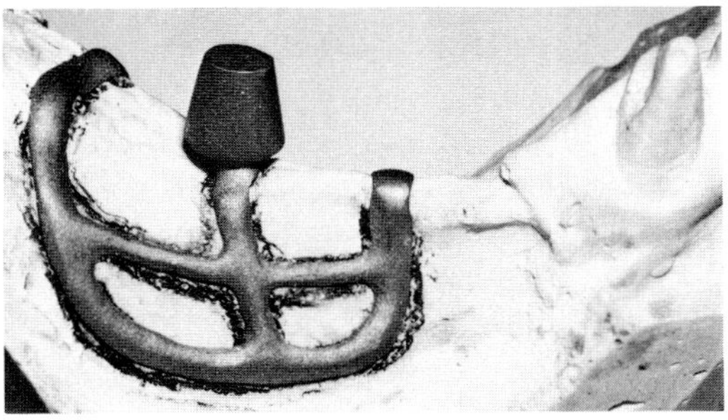

Fig. 3-11. Buccal view of a lower right terminal subperiosteal implant. A primary strut extends from the implant neck to the base of the peripheral border. Secondary struts extend both mesially and distally from the buccal primary strut to the peripheral border. In such cases, the secondary struts may add to the stability of the frame and allow for additional areas of connective tissue interweaving.

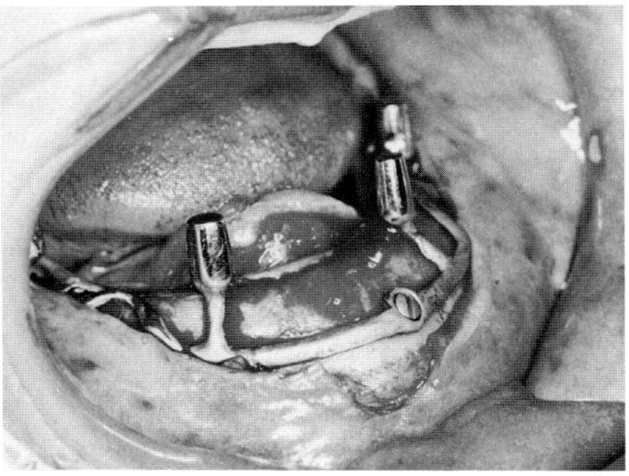

Fig. 3-12. Labial view of the anterior portion of a complete mandibular subperiosteal implant. The complete implant has just been inserted and the full-thickness flaps are to be approximated. The use of the screw within the peripheral border may be used for initial stabilization, in order to allow for uneventful healing. It is best to attempt to avoid the use of any screw by extending the peripheral border so as to "hug" the bone wherever possible. Primary struts extend from the peripheral border to the implant necks, which support highly polished posts that will bear a removable prosthesis.

The Implant Neck

The neck connects the post to the broad-based frame. By doing so, it passes through the soft tissues so as to form a link between the closed subperiosteal system and the open oral cavity environment. The neck has a smaller diameter than the post, so that—within the limits of nonflexibility and adequate supportive strength—it creates as small a channel as possible through the soft tissue. The tissue through which it passes should be of gingival consistency, and the neck's occlusogingival length should conform to the depth of this tissue. At no time should the neck be too short, so as to cause impingement of the post base on the gingival collar. Such impingement could be compared to the improper accommodation of the interproximal tissues between two adjacent natural abutment teeth by an inadequate major embrasure space.

The Implant Frame

The frame (body or crib) is the supportive structure that lies upon the bone and in itself contains the following elements:

The peripheral border delineates the outermost circumferential aspects of the frame. In much the same way as operative dentistry is concerned with outline form, there is a similar intrinsic necessity for the subperiosteal implant. The outline form here is the peripheral border, which determines the area of man-made attachment apparatus. This, in turn determines the extent of the "snowshoe effect." The outline circumvents bundles of nerves and blood vessels much as part of the outline form of tooth preparation would avoid the dental pulp.

Also, the expression "extension for prevention" applies to the implant situation. The extension of the peripheral border may either lock an implant mechanically in place or may be broad enough mesiodistally and buccolingually to sustain any adverse forces that are other than vertical in nature. The prevention thus achieved is a prevention from rocking the implant when the patient slides into any lateral excursion.

The outline of the peripheral border is determined by sound clinical judgment, bearing in mind the enhancement of the snowshoe effect. There are some areas that are preferable on which to lay the outermost extensions. These include such broad expanses as the external oblique ridge of the mandible, and the hard palate extension of the maxilla. Obviously, extension should be made to such areas as the genial tubercle of the mandible and the nasal spine of the maxilla, with the proper circumvention of these areas without overextension. Impingement should not occur on the contents of the major palatine foramen, the sublingual muscle attachment areas, and the mental foramen.

There is another modifying factor. The superimposed soft tissues must be taken into account when designing the peripheral border. If such extension on sound bone is made in areas where the soft tissues may be unduly taut and friable in consistency, the outline may have to be modified, as in the non-meeting of the peripheral border at the height of a ridge. It is for this reason that the *lingual fingers* have come into prominence (i.e., to avoid the possibility of peripheral border metal exposure, and to secure placement between muscle bundles) (Fig. 3-13).

The lingual fingers may be primary or secondary struts, or portions of the peripheral border that terminate as cul-de-sacs. There is no interconnecting peripheral border. There are variations of each of the above. For example, the peripheral border may be free-end with a double cul-de-sac at the height of a ridge, so that the buccal and lingual aspects may not necessarily join.

The primary struts are connectors that join the implant neck to the peripheral border. The primary struts usually number two to four. The goal is to have a stable, inflexible support of the implant abutment. This would prevent flexure from the frame through the supported prosthesis. Primary struts usually do not cross the height of a ridge in a mesiodistal direction. Such areas are susceptible to metal exposure, and all struts should be designed to avoid this critical area.

The secondary struts are reinforcements that join primary strut to primary strut, or primary strut to peripheral border. The implantologist may use many secondary struts or none at all; however, it is preferable to use secondary struts, for two reasons. First, they act as reinforcements to stabilize the frame against undue flexure. Second, they provide more areas for the weblike formation of connective-tissue attachments between the underlying bone and the overlying subperiosteum and soft tissues. The stability of the implant is not only predicated on a broad showshoe outline, but also on the interwoven effect of multiple struts and metallic borders amid a soft- and hard-tissue complex (see Chap. 6, on subperiosteal implant histology).

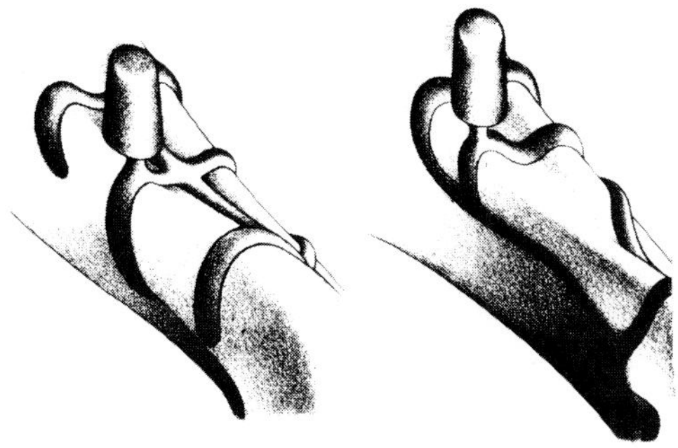

Fig. 3-13. (Left) Lingual fingers are modifications of the standard peripheral border. They extend between muscle origins and minimize the chances of metal exposure where the overlying soft tissues are thin and friable. *(Right)* The continuity of a peripheral border on the lingual aspect of a mandibular posterior area can be effected when there is no interference from muscle bundles and when the lingual tissues are loose but dense. In many cases, such a border extension can avoid the placement of metal crossings at the height of the ridge, which is usually necessary with lingual fingers.

The Implant Screw

The use of the screw (Fig. 3-12) depends, for the most part, on sound clinical judgment. The screw is intended to hold the implant in place throughout the healing process. It can be left with the implant indefinitely. The screw may eventually become a source of irritation, however, and subsequently may have to be removed. There are times when the unilateral implant would mechanically snap into place, especially on the lingual surface. This provides adequate mechanical retention even prior to suturing the flap over the implant frame. In such instances, it is unnecessary to insert a screw. A sound rule of thumb is to provide for a screw in each implant design. Thus, a decision as to its insertion may be made upon the insertion of the implant itself. The retention thereafter is provided by the healing and growth of tissue between the periosteum and the underlying bone.

THE RATIO CONCEPT

Mechanical decisions as to the design of the frame are graphically illustrated in this chapter. In its most simplistic manner, the spread of the crib should be related to the length of the implant abutment and its intended crown superstructure. This is not unlike the basic principle of fixed prosthodontics that stresses the need for a sound crown-root ratio.

The center of the implant neck is to be used as the radial center of a circle. The radius is determined by the occlusal height of the visualized crown retainer that is to be superimposed. A circle thus drawn to encompass the buccolingual plane will determine the buccal or lingual extensions of the peripheral border. The peripheral border should lie outside the circumference of such a circle, unless there is a positive mechanical lock that may be attained by

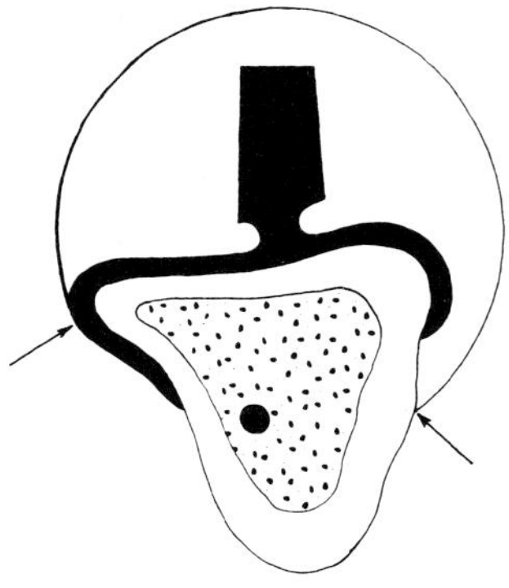

Fig. 3-14. The ratio concept can be exemplified best by visualizing a cross section through the mandible or the maxilla that supports a subperiosteal implant frame. A circle is drawn with a compass, with the neck of the implant as the center. The radius extends to the anticipated height of the occlusal surface of the superimposed prosthetic retainer. A circumference is then drawn. The buccal and the lingual borders should terminate at or beyond the points where the circumference of the circle meets the supporting bone. If an undercut exists on either side, then the border may terminate within the confines of this circle. For example, the buccal border *(right arrow)* would *not* be adequately extended if it were not for the existing undercut. It would, at least, have to extend to that arrow. The lingual border *(left arrow)* would suffice in extension even if no undercut were present, because it extends adequately beyond the confines of the circumference of the circle.

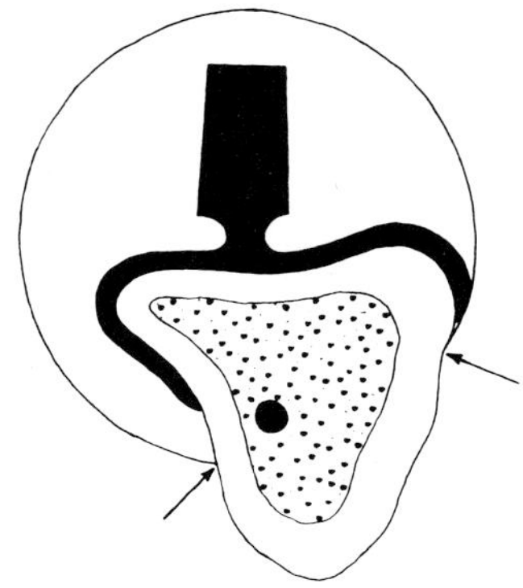

Fig. 3-15. The center of the circle is shifted lingually by the lingual placement of the implant neck. The buccal extension *(right arrow)* would suffice even if no undercut existed. However, the lingual border *(left arrow)* is adequate only because an undercut exists in the mylohyoid ridge area. If such were not the case, the lingual border would have to extend to the border of the circumference *(left arrow).*

an osseous undercut (Figs. 3-14 to 3-17). If the border would lie within the circumference of the circle, lateral forces would tend to rock the frame in a buccal or lingual direction. It is obvious that a proper initial surgical incision would preclude such concern regarding the mesial and distal portions of the peripheral border. This concept applies as much to the complete edentulous

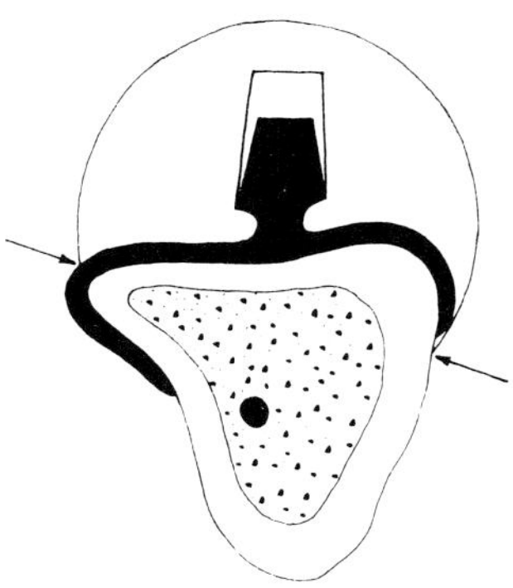

Fig. 3-16. The radius of the circle must extend from the center of the implant neck to the height of the occlusal table even if a cast coping intervenes. In this case all buccal *(right arrow)* and lingual *(left arrow)* extensions would be adequate with or without existing osseous undercuts. It is important to note that although an implant frame may have to snap into place to accommodate such undercuts, once seated, the implant lies passively over the bone.

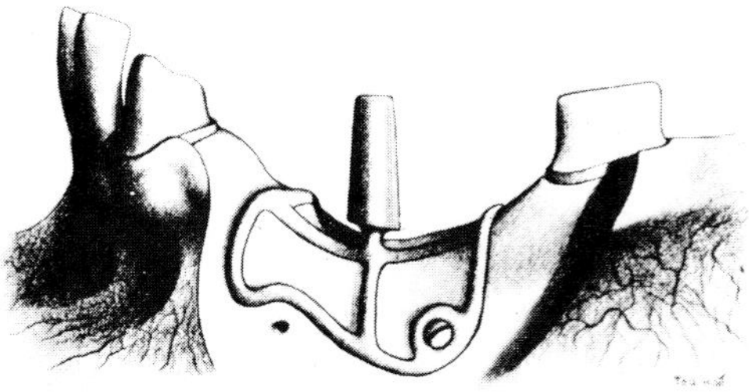

Fig. 3-17. This intermediary subperiosteal implant would not fulfill the ratio concept of design. It is obvious that if an imaginary circumference of a circle were to be drawn, the buccal peripheral border would lie well within the confines of the circle. Therefore, the peripheral border would have to be extended inferiorly towards the buccal aspect. Otherwise, the implant would be top-heavy. Usually, by following the basic tenet of the snowshoe effect, the fulfillment of the ratio concept is generally achieved.

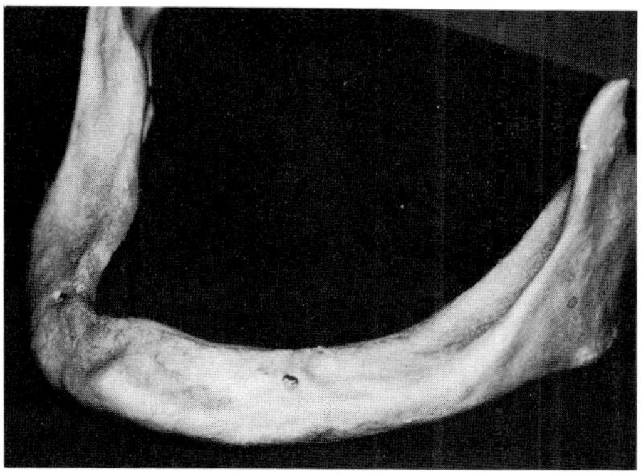

Fig. 3-18. A dry specimen of a highly resorbed mandible. It is just such dense, compact bone that is appropriate for the support of a subperiosteal implant. It is through all the facets of examination that the examiner attempts to visualize such supportive structures prior to surgical entry (See Chap. 2, on case selection). It is not until actual surgical exposure, however, that such a true three-dimensional image can be revealed. Radiographs alone would not suffice.

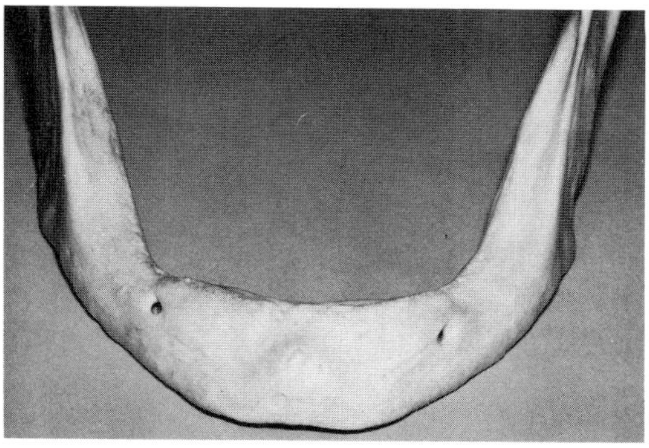

Fig. 3-19. A dried specimen of an edentulous mandible. This mandible may support a complete subperiosteal implant. Although there is moderate to severe resorption of the residual ridges in the external oblique areas, the broad anterior portion also exhibits a loss of the alveolar ridge. Such a situation may lead us to consider the use of a standard well-fabricated complete lower denture rather than any implant.

arch as it does to a unilateral implant site. The exceptions to this rule are those cases wherein a definite mechanical lock is achieved on the lingual aspect of a unilateral subperiosteal implant. Such retention may even be achieved in the complete mandibular implant, but not in a complete maxillary implant.

CONVENIENCE FORM PRINCIPLES

G. V. Black's convenience form for tooth preparation is also appropriate for implants. The surgical procedures that expose the bone for the impression are, in essence, convenience form, because once entry has been made subperiosteally, it is important to expose an adequate amount of bone. In the same manner that convenience form in the preparation of a tooth allows proper access for acceptable cavity preparation and restoration insertion, the surgery for implant impressions should expose broad expanses of bone so that the subsequent impression can capture areas beyond which the peripheral border would extend. A comparison of the technique employed for crown and bridge procedures is in order (i.e., to have an impression that extends beyond the margins of the inlay, onlay, or crown preparation).

Adequate surgical exposure of bone is equal to adequate reduction of any tooth surface during preparation for a retainer. Once one has committed oneself to cut a tooth surface, it is important that this be done to a depth that would prevent the eventual restoration from having to be overly contoured. Similarly, once we have committed ourselves to cut the soft tissues, such incisions and the subsequent blunt dissections should allow us to see those areas of bone over which we intend to extend our implant. This does not imply radical surgery, but rather adequate surgery.

BONE SUPPORT

Mandible

The bone that underlies the subperiosteal implant should be of a hard cortical consistency. It is for this reason that the highly resorbed mandibular ridge exhibits the greatest potential for the success of this type of implant (Figs. 3-18 to 3-21). Alveo-

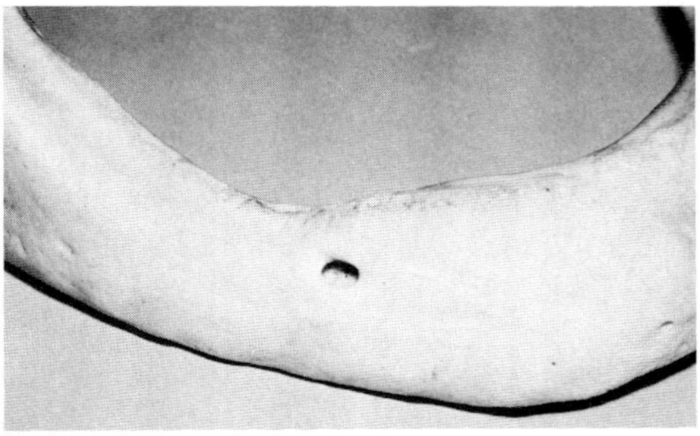

Fig. 3-20. Buccal close-up view of the lower right mental foramen area. The proximity of the neurovascular bundle to the height of the residual ridge may preclude the fabrication of a comfortable, well-fitting, tissue-bearing, complete lower denture. As long as dense, compact bone is available for the support of the subperiosteal implant frame, an implant denture—which would be supported by this frame—may be indicated.

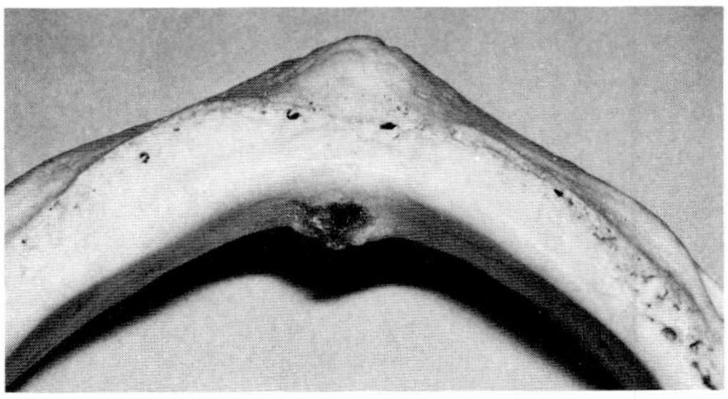

Fig. 3-21. Incisal view of the anterior portion of dried edentulous mandible. Although the ridge is moderately resorbed to the extent that alveolar bone is not present, the remaining compact bone is not dense and has many perforations, tunnels, and dehiscences. Most often, these anomalies are not seen radiographically. Therefore, upon surgical exposure for the bone impression, it may be necessary to halt the procedure, suture the flaps, and revert to a complete lower denture. Such initial surgical entries may terminate as exploratory operations.

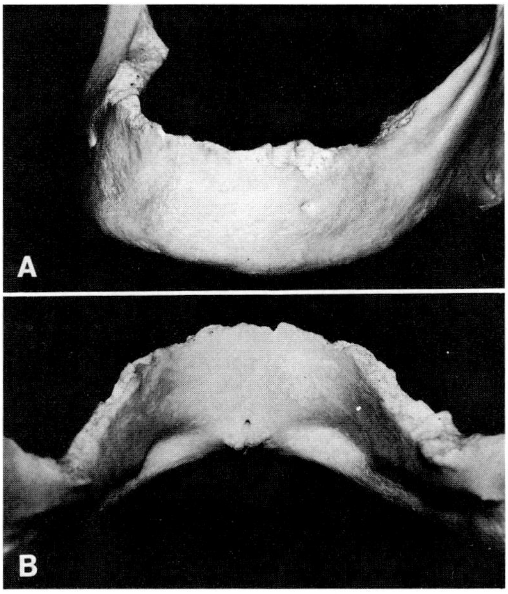

Fig. 3-22. The buccal *(A)* and lingual *(B)* views of a dried edentulous mandible. There is a continuous ridge of alveolar bone that is very narrow and even knife-like in the anterior region. Any alveolar bone would be nonsupportive for a subperiosteal implant. The narrowness of the ridges in *(A)* and *(B)* would also preclude the use of intra-osseous implants. Only a standard complete lower denture would be indicated in this instance, and only after ridge modification in the form of osseous plasty is performed.

lar bone offers inadequate long-term support for all or any of the struts of a subperiosteal implant (Fig. 3-22). Therefore, it would stand to reason that the most successful subperiosteal implants are found in the highly resorbed mandibular ridge areas, which offer little support and no resistance to lateral movement for any conventional complete denture. It is not coincidental that the subperiosteal implant was originated on a rather grand scale. That is to say, the use of the complete mandibular subperiosteal implant historically preceded the use of any terminal or intermediary single implant.

It is reasonable to conclude that in many cases of highly resorbed mandibular ridges, the mandible may be very thin; this would definitely preclude the intra-osseous placement of blade-type implants. Often, such highly resorbed ridges may exhibit mandibular canal dehiscences and/or a virtual "relocation" of the mental foramina at the height of such ridges. In these situations, only the subperiosteal implant would be of value. Its struts and borders may be so designed as to circumvent and avoid all impingements on the vascular and neurologic contents of such areas. It would naturally follow that as complete a resolution of the bone pattern as possible should be anticipated prior to any bone impression. As such, timing is of the essence. At no time should any osseous recontouring be instituted at the time of any bone impression.

Also, if extractions are necessary, an immediate denture should be worn during a reliable, essential waiting period. To wit, if extractions are to be instituted, a proper alveolectomy may be necessary at the time of extraction. This may aid in creating a more favorable osseous architecture at the site of the intended implant. (No doubt, if the struts of a subperiosteal implant are not to cross such an area, then a waiting period would not be necessary.) Extractions and/or necessary alveolectomies should be followed by a transitional 9-month waiting phase (Fig. 3-23). After that time, all structures should be reevaluated and reassessed, to determine the eligibility of the patient for an implant.

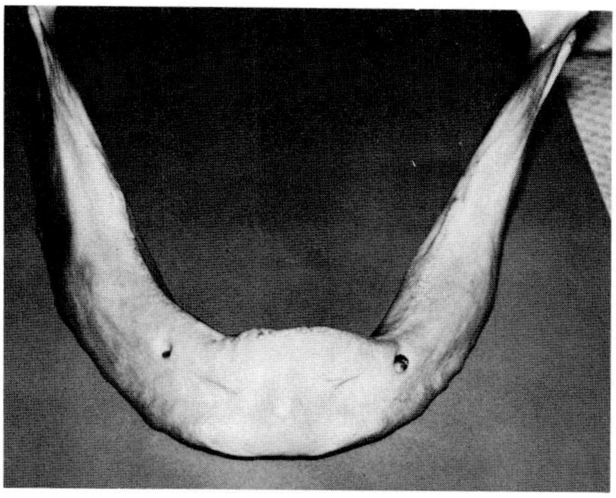

Fig. 3-23. Dried specimen of an edentulous mandible. Except for a small portion of the anterior region, the residual ridge is highly resorbed to the extent that the left mental foramen is almost at the height of the ridge. In such a case, it is best to perform a minor alveolectomy in the anterior region. After a transitional 9-month phase, procedures for a subperiosteal implant may be undertaken.

Maxilla

The very nature of the spongy bone of the maxilla makes it a poor candidate to receive a complete subperiosteal implant (Figs. 3-24 to 3-26). The success rate of the complete subperiosteal maxillary implant is poor. It should only be attempted if the patient so insists, and only *after every other prosthetic treatment has been attempted* and rejected physically or psychologically by the patient. Even then, the patient must be aware that the failure rate of the complete subperiosteal maxillary implant is high. The terminal and even the intermediary upper subperiosteal maxillary implants, however, have been successful. The use of periodontally acceptable natural-teeth abutments leads to a more favorable prognosis.

The complete lower subperiosteal implant tends to fall into a more favorable mechanical pattern with respect to the stresses of occlusion. The very nature of the opposition of maxilla and mandible appears to have a positive vertical seating direction on the frame of the mandibular subperiosteal implant. Contrary to this, the maxilla, with its usual inherent direction of forces that accompany various degrees of overjet and of overbite, is subject to adverse effects on the supporting bone. To date, those patients with successful complete subperiosteal maxillary implants come closest to an edge-to-edge occlusion together with fairly short replacement teeth required in that same arch. It should be noted that these observations are strictly clinical empiricisms and are not as yet substantiated by research.

SOFT–TISSUE CONSIDERATIONS

Regardless of the soundness and density of the underlying bone, many patients have a friable and delicate soft-tissue covering in the potential implant site. This may exist throughout the implant site and may dictate that an implant not be inserted. In other cases, such tissue may be

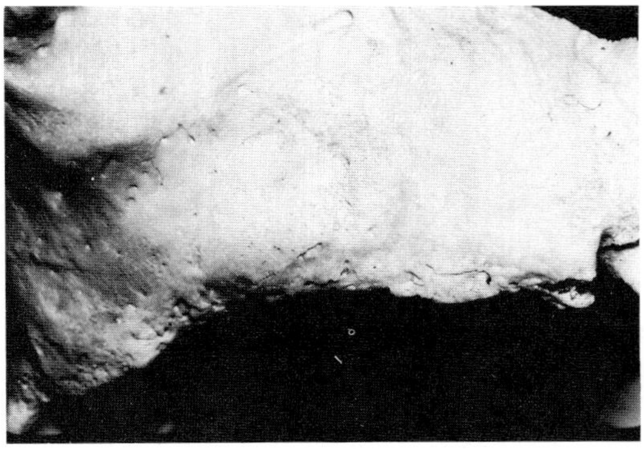

Fig. 3-24. Buccal view of the left posterior portion of a dried maxilla specimen. The view encompasses the zygomatic arch *(upper left)* and the hamular notch *(lower right).* The unpredictable supportive capacity of the spongy bone requires specific extensions of maxillary implant designs through the hamular notch and below the zygomatic arch. Such extension applies as much to the unilateral implant as to the complete implant.

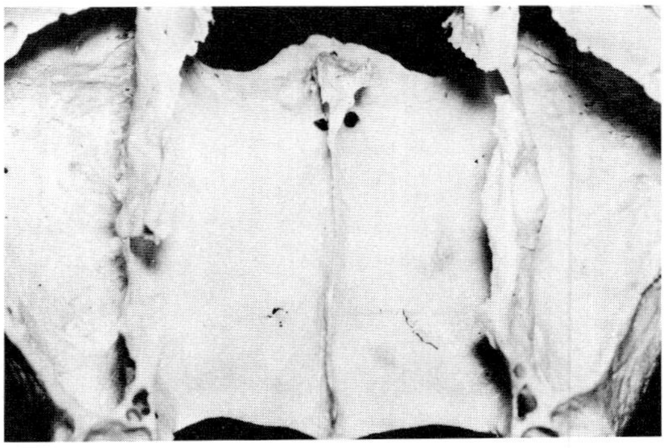

Fig. 3-25. Coronal view of a horizontal section through the maxillary sinuses. This dried specimen includes the hard palate and the nasal area *(top center).* The thinness of the hard palate, and the proximity and thinness of the sinuses are two hazards that add to the unpredictability of maxillary implants. Such dimensions cannot be determined radiographically. Therefore, *intra-osseous* maxillary posterior implants are rarely indicated, and subperiosteal implants in these areas should be approached with caution.

prevalent in only a certain area of the intended implant site. Most often, the tissue is thinnest on the lingual aspect of the mandibular ridge and may often result in the exposure of part or all of any one strut. Such potential exposures have often led to

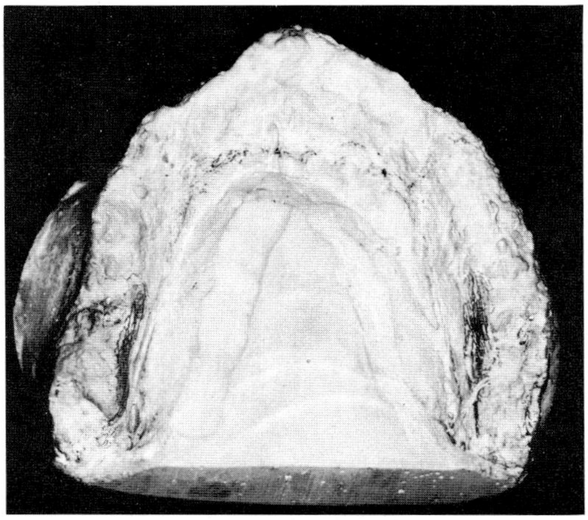

Fig. 3-26. Model of a maxillary bone impression for a complete subperiosteal implant. The buccal and lingual borders extend to the concavities that border the residual ridges with the zygomatic turn and the palatal turn. The hamular notch areas are crossed, as they would be in any unilateral case.

modifications of designs. In designing the outline of the subperiosteal implant, therefore, soft-tissue areas should be considered separately, aside from the normal osseous anatomic landmarks. It should be noted that the mere exposure of a strut without any concomitant information and/or symptoms should not be considered as a failure of the implant. The exposure of a strut may be left as is. Exposure with symptoms or with inflammation, or both, may be conservatively treated by the removal of the involved strut.

Most importantly, pain, mobility, uncontrollable infection, gross radiographic bone resorption, or any combination of these, would necessitate the removal of the entire implant. Thus, implants have a better chance for success if the necks of implant abutments extrude through sound, attached-type, gingival tissue (Figs. 3-27, 3-28). Therefore, in designing the outline of the subperiosteal implant frame, it is imperative to delineate for the technician not only where the screw is to be inserted, but from where the implant abutment is to originate.

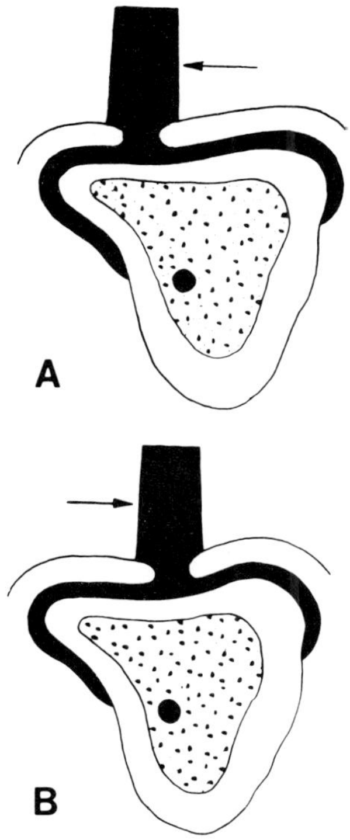

Fig. 3-27. In order to accommodate an opposing occlusion, the subperiosteal implant provides flexibilility in the placement of the implant post. The post may be placed toward the lingual *(A)* or toward the buccal *(B)* aspects. It may not even be at the height of the residual ridge, as long as the implant neck extrudes through sound attached-type of gingival tissue. Naturally, such alternate placements of the neck would alter the extensions of the peripheral border, according to the ratio concept.

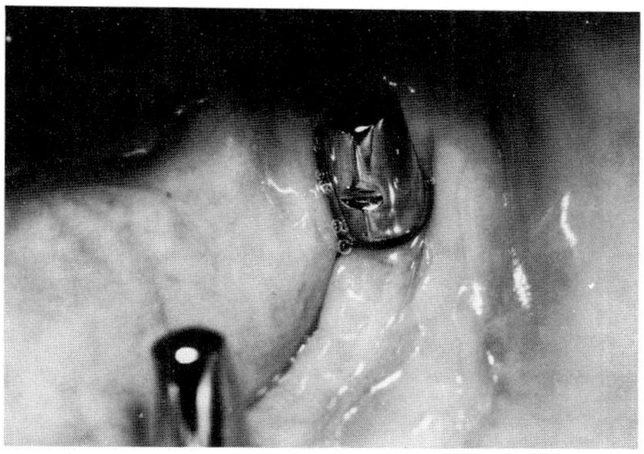

Fig. 3-28. Posterior post of a complete subperiosteal implant extrudes through sound gingival tissue rather than through pliable mucosa. The following should be noted: (1) The sublingual tissues and the mucobuccal fold tissues are higher than the residual ridge. (2) Such a patient would find it difficult to retain a complete lower denture, and so an implant may be indicated. (3) Even if the supportive bone is of a dense and compact nature, it is necessary for the implant neck to extrude through attached-type of tissue. (4) If such tissue is not present, it is possible, at times, for the periodontist to transfer a free gingival graft. Otherwise, an implant would be contraindicated.

In all aspects of prosthodontic treatment, one is always reminded of the need for complete and adequate prescriptions from the dentist to the technician with whom he works. At no time should this consideration be overlooked with respect to the design of the subperiosteal implant. It is incumbent upon the dentist to designate all outlines and all measurements for the technician to appropriately follow through.

BIBLIOGRAPHY

Ackerman, F.: Equilibrium with subperiosteal complete denture implants. J. Pros. Dent., *9:*1049-1055, 1959.

Atwood, D. A.: Some clinical factors related to rate of resorption of residual ridges. J. Pros. Dent., *12:*441-450, 1962.

——: Reduction of residual ridges: a major oral disease entitity. J. Pros. Dent., *26:*266-279, 1971.

Barandes, J., *et al.*: Technical details of a new approach to the full maxillary subperiosteal implant. Oral Implantol., *4:*420-430, 1974.

Carlsson, G. E., Bergman, B., and Hedegard, B.: Changes in contour of the maxillary alveolar process under immediate dentures. A longitudinal clinical and x-ray cephalometric study covering 5 years. Acta odont. scandinav., *25:*1-31, 1967.

DeAngelis, V.: Observations on the response of alveolar bone to orthodontic force. Am. J. Orthodontics, *58:*284-294, 1970.

Edwards, L. F.; The edentulous mandible. J. Pros. Dent., *4:*222-231, 1954.

Foldvari, I.: Functional correlation of abutments of subperiosteal implant dentures. J. Pros. Dent., *12:*796-799, 1962.

Gabriel, A. C.: Some anatomical features of the mandible. J. Anat., *92:*580-586, 1958.

Gershkoff, A., and Goldberg, N. I.: Implant Dentures. Philadelphia, J. B. Lippincott, 1957.

Goldberg, N. I., and Gershkoff, A.: The lower implant denture. D. Digest, *55:*490-494, 1949.

———: A six year progress report on full denture implants. J. Implant Dent., *1:*13-16, 1954.

Hobkirk, J. A.: The management of gross alveolar resorption. J. Pros. Dent., *29:*397-404, 1973.

Jermyn, A. C.: Technique and problems of placing implant screws. J. Implant Dent., *2:*36-40, 1956.

Kapur, K., and Shklar, G.: The effect of complete dentures on alveolar mucosa. J. Pros. Dent., *13:*1030-1037, 1963.

Kelsey, C. K.: Alveolar bone resorption under complete dentures. J. Pros. Dent., *25:*152-161, 1971.

Knowlton, J. P.: Masticatory pressures exerted with implant dentures as compared with soft-tissue-borne dentures. J. Pros. Dent., *3:*721-726, 1953.

Kratochvil, F. J., and Boyne, P. J.: Combined use of subperiosteal implant and bone-marrow graft in deficient edentulous mandibles: a preliminary report. J. Pros. Dent., *27:*645-653, 1972.

Lammie, G. A.: The reduction of the edentulous ridge. J. Pros. Dent., *10:*605-611, 1966.

Landsberg, I.: Subperiosteal implants. Clinical observations during an 18 year period. Israel J. D. Med., *22:*16-26, 1973.

Laskin, D. M.: A sclerosing procedure for hypermobile edentulous ridges. J. Pros. Dent., *23:*274-278, 1970.

Linkow, L. I.: Some variant designs of the subperiosteal implant. Oral Implantol., *2:*190-205, 1972.

Lytle, R. B.: Soft tissue displacement beneath removable partial and complete dentures. J. Pros. Dent., *12:*34-43, 1962.

Mack, A.: Reactions of the oral tissue to subperiosteal appliances. Internat. D. J., *18:*779-789, 1968.

Manson, J. P., and Lucas, R. B.: A microradiographic study of age changes in the human mandible. Arch. Oral Biol., *7:*761-769, 1962.

Mentag, P. J.: Subperiosteal prosthesis after skin graft into the oral cavity. D. Clin. North America, *14:*169-172, 1970.

Nakamoto, R. Y.: Bony defects on the crest of the residual alveolar ridge. J. Pros. Dent., *19:*111-118, 1968.

Nedelman, C., Gamer, S., and Bernick, S.: The alveolar ridge mucosa in denture and non-denture wearers. J Pros. Dent., *23:*265-273, 1970.

Ortman, H. R.: Factors of bone resorption of the residual ridge. J. Pros. Dent., *12:*429-440, 1962.

Pernell, W. E.: History of implant work and a report on mandibular implants by the direct impression method. J. Pros. Dent., *2:*51-54, 1952.

Sicher, H.: Oral Anatomy. St. Louis, C. V. Mosby, 1960.

Sissons, H.: Bone as a Tissue. New York, McGraw-Hill, 1960.

Stein, I., Stein, R. O., and Beller, M. L.: Living Bone in Health and Disease. Philadelphia, J. B. Lippincott, 1955.

Steinhauser, E. W.: Free transplantation of oral mucosa for improvement of denture retention. J. Oral Surg., *27:*955-961, 1969.

Tallgren, A.: Alveolar bone loss in denture wearers as related to facial morphology. Acta odont. scandinav., *28:*251-270, 1970.

Turck, D.: A histologic comparison of the edentulous denture and non-denture bearing tissues. J. Pros. Dent., *15:*419-434, 1965.

Weiss, C.M., and Judy, K. W. M.: Severe mandibular atrophy—biological considerations of routine treatment with the complete subperiosteal implant. Oral Implantol., *4:*431-469, 1974.

Wical, K. E., and Swoope, C. C.: Studies of residual ridge resorption. Part 1. Use of panoramic radiographs for evaluation and classification of mandibular resorption. J. Pros. Dent., *32:*7-12, 1974.

4 The Subperiosteal Implant—The Bone Impression and the Laboratory Prescription

The subperiosteal implant is most commonly used in the restoration of the completely edentulous, highly resorbed mandible (Fig. 4-1). Herein, dense cortical bone is the only discernable supportive osseous base for an implant frame. In such cases, the implant posts may support a complete, fully removable, lower denture or a complete, fixed, lower-arch cast splint.

More recently, the smaller terminal and intermediary subperiosteal implants have been used on similar osseous structures to aid in the support of fixed prostheses (Figs. 4-2 to 4-5). These terminal and intermediary subperiosteal implants have been equally successful in sharing the support of prostheses in the upper arch. The complete upper subperiosteal implant, however, has a more guarded prognosis and a more limited selectivity in its prescription. This appears to be caused by the following factors:

1. The thrusts exerted in the labial direction by the tongue and the predominant Class II occlusions may both be detrimental to the stability of the complete upper subperiosteal implant. (Class II occlusions, however, may be favorably altered in some cases by placing the prosthetic superstructure dentition in an edge-to-edge occlusion.)

2. The upper arch has a relatively weaker osseous infrastructure of spongy bone. This bone, therefore, may not be capable of supporting a complete-arch implant because of the resultant forces placed on it and on the thin bony plates in the palatal and sinus areas. This is why, in the upper arch, the smaller terminal and intermediary subperiosteal implants, which combine with natural teeth to support a prosthesis, have a higher success rate than the complete subperiosteal implant.

In any case, implants alone or the combination of implants and natural teeth can support a removable or a fixed prosthesis,

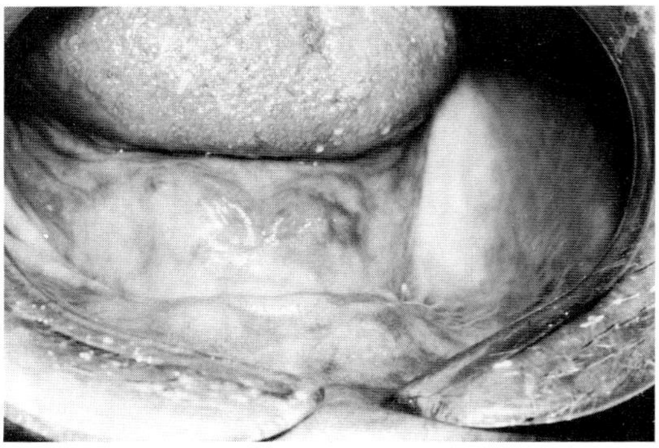

Fig. 4-1. Highly resorbed edentulous ridge of a mandible. Specific notation is made of (a) the posterior ridges, which coalesce with the depth of the mucobuccal folds; (b) the depressions in the vicinity of the mental foramina, which are below the lingual and buccal soft tissues; and (c) the lingual tissues surrounding the genial tubercle, which are higher than the anterior residual ridge. This degree of ridge resorption is most amenable to a subperiosteal implant.

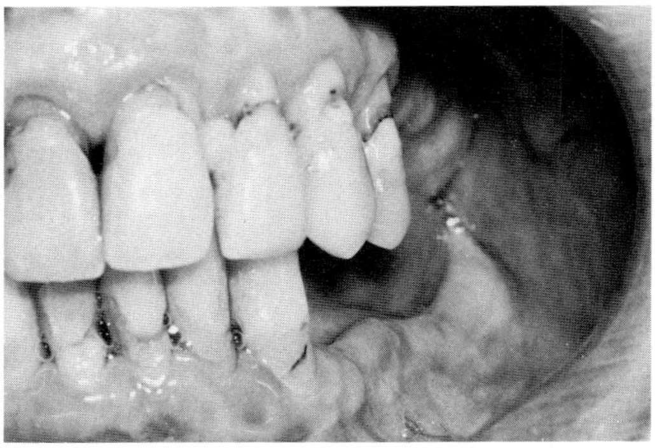

Fig. 4-2. The left segment of an oral cavity that is to receive combined treatment. Sequential therapy should consist of initial periodontal preparation, provisional temporization, finite periodontal surgery, and implant procedures for the edentulous areas. (See Figs. 4-3 and 4-4.) In this case, the upper arch is to receive a terminal subperiosteal implant, and the lower arch is to receive a terminal endosseous blade-vent implant. (See Plate 4-1.)

but *never* a combined fixed-removable prosthesis. Torque, especially in excess, adversely affects the positive vertical long-axis seating forces that should predominate. Any twisting, rotational, or lateral force placed on an implant would tend to dislodge the implant from its anchorage within bone or within a connective-tissue network. A combined fixed-removable prosthesis, regardless of its design, would tend to apply such adverse forces on the implant. Naturally, some lateral forces are always to be expected; however, intense, continuous lateral, rotational, or twisting forces placed on an implant eventually

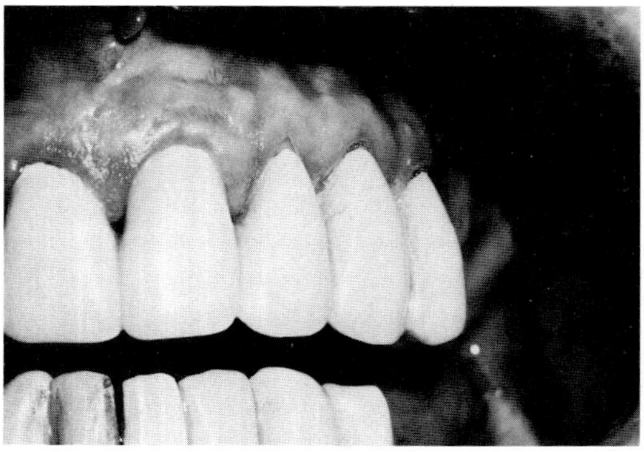

Fig. 4-3. Prior to periodontal surgery, the dentition has received customized acrylic-resin temporary full coverage. Initial periodontal preparation, followed by temporary splints carved chair-side, have already created a better environment for the soft tissues. An optimum environmnet now exists for periodontal surgery. (See Plate 4-2.)

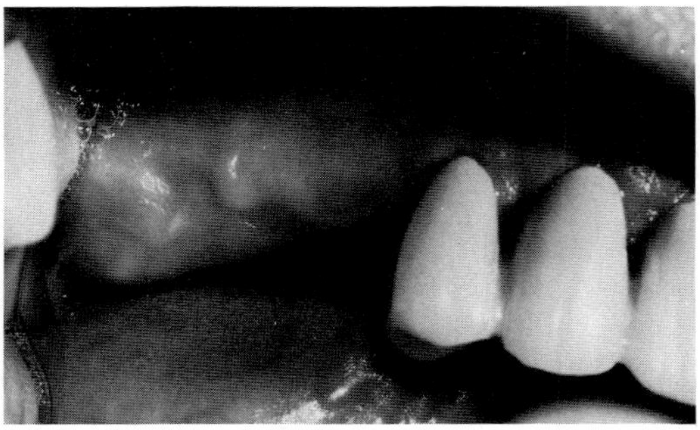

Fig. 4-4. Mirror view of the upper left posterior edentulous area that is to receive a subperiosteal implant. All preparatory procedures have been performed, and the soft tissues are deemed to be firm and sound. The broad edentulous residual ridge has an adequate amount of attached-tissue coverage in every dimension. (See Plate 4-3.)

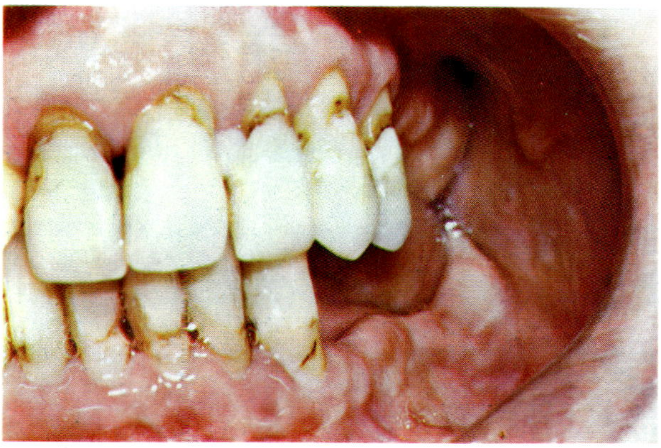

Plate 4–1. See Figure 4–2.

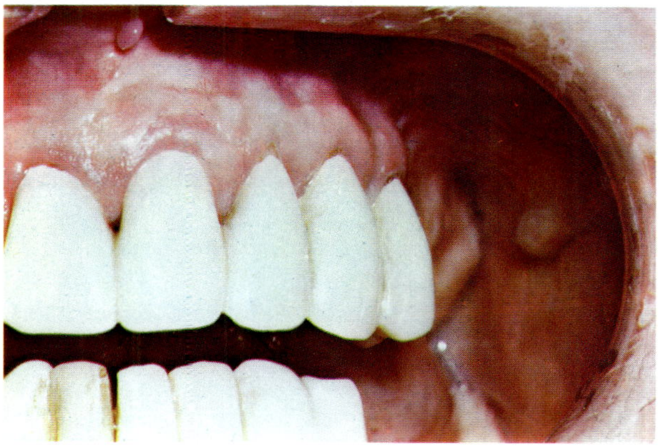

Plate 4–2. See Figure 4–3.

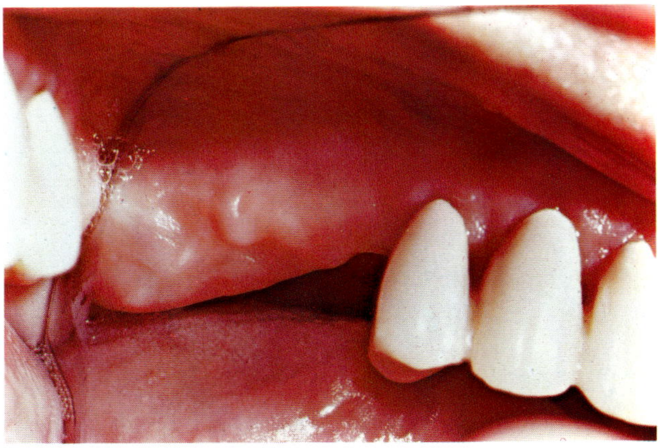

Plate 4–3. See Figure 4–4.

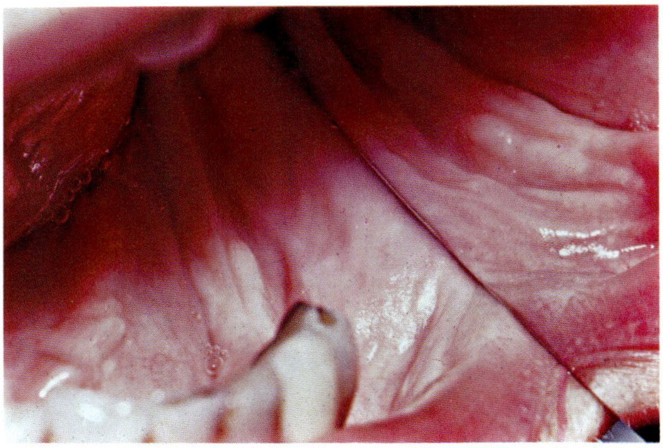

Plate 4–4. See Figure 4–5.

cause a deterioration of the hard and soft structures that support the implant.

Regardless of the type of prosthesis that will be superimposed on the complete subperiosteal implant, there is no difference in the initial procedures of implant fabrication. Similar surgical and impression procedures—with minor modifications—are used in the fabrication of the terminal and pier implants.

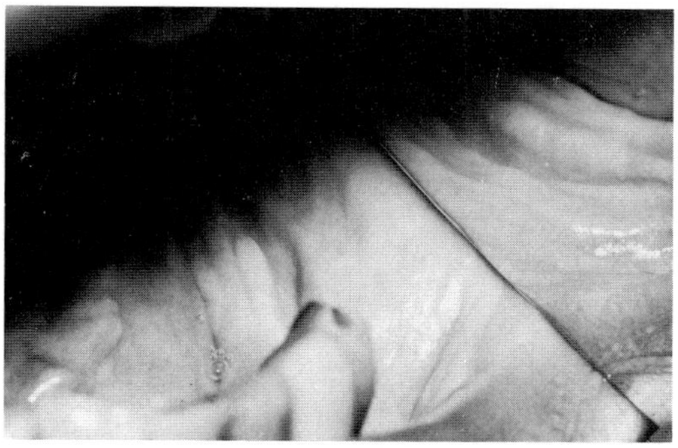

Fig. 4-5. Mirror image of a different case, showing the lower left residual ridge. The amount of ridge resorption has left no remaining alveolar bone, so that a subperiosteal implant is indicated. Periodontal preparation of this ridge consisted of free gingival grafts in order to create a wider buccolingual band of attached gingival tissue. Such grafts may be equally important in a longitudinal direction, where a delicate and thin mucosal coverage can eventually rupture over an implant frame. (See Plate 4-4.)

THE BONE IMPRESSION

The choice of the technique for the bone impression is based on the ability to encompass and to accurately duplicate all of the exposed osseous areas. The vehicle for the impression material is a custom acrylic-resin tray that is fabricated directly in the mouth for unilateral impressions and on a stone study model for a complete implant impression. The preferred impression materials are the light- and heavy-bodied rubber bases. Prefabricated trays should not be used for the initial direct bone impression.

Surgical Bone Exposure of the Supportive Residual Ridge

Many of the principles of sound crown and bridge technique are also applicable in procedures for the subperiosteal implant impression. For example, for fixed prostheses, it is a cardinal rule to retract tissues in order to see the margins of tooth preparations that are to be captured by the impression technique of choice. Likewise, in subperiosteal implantology, it is imperative to adequately retract the soft tissues above all bony structures that are to be encompassed in the bone impression. The operator must be able to see all the bony structures of which a stone model will be made later. Obviously, the surgical technique of combined sharp and blunt dissections serves as an "access form."

The initial incision is made in a vertical plane in order to create full-thickness flaps (Fig. 4-6). The vertical incision is extended through the buccolingual center of the gingiva-type tissue in order to create flaps that have mucogingival margins and are mucoperiosteal in depth. In performing the initial incision, the operator must bear in mind the necessity to retain and to preserve the gingival tissue at the height of the residual ridge, because the implant posts will eventually extrude through this thick and firm tissue. The initial incision varies as follows:

1. For the complete subperiosteal implant, either mandibular or maxillary, the incision is extended from retromolar area to retromolar area through the height of the tissues on the residual ridge. This constitutes a single U-shaped incision.

2. The intermediary subperiosteal implant requires an incision, through the gingiva-type tissue, that approximates the adjacent natural teeth within about 5 mm. In this manner, no surgical disturbance is inflicted on the prepared periodontal supportive tissues of the remaining natural teeth. Also, in this manner, the struts of the subperiosteal implant frame would not lie upon the supportive alveolar bone of these remaining natural teeth.

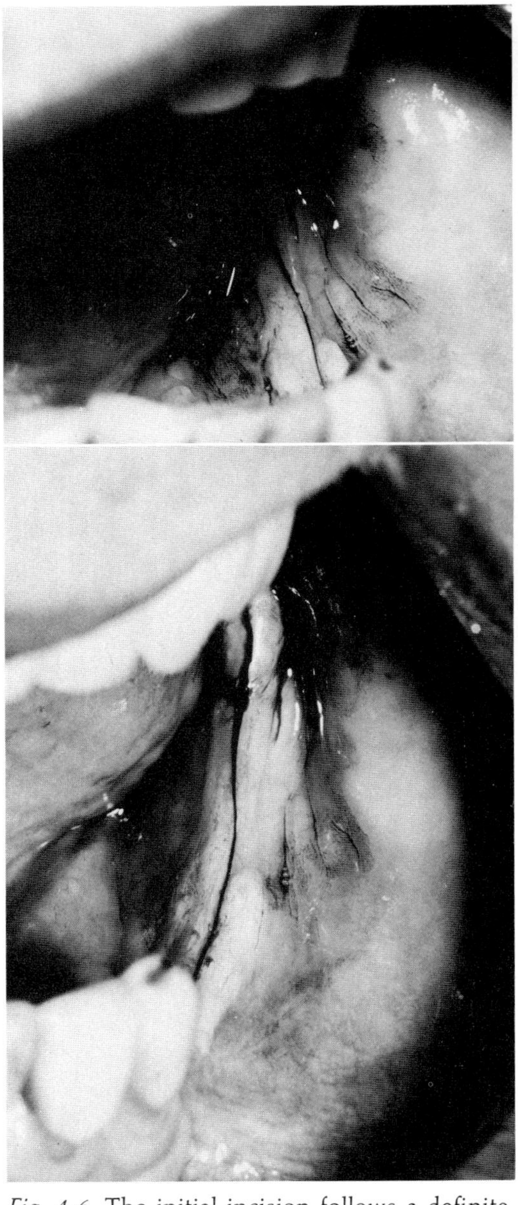

Fig. 4-6. The initial incision follows a definite, clean path through the attached gingival tissue on a lower left posterior edentulous ridge. This is created with a No. 15 scalpel blade in order to form full-thickness mucoperiosteal buccal and lingual flaps. Except for the minor horizontal incisions that are required to lay back such flaps for bone exposure, all further instrumentation is by blunt dissection.

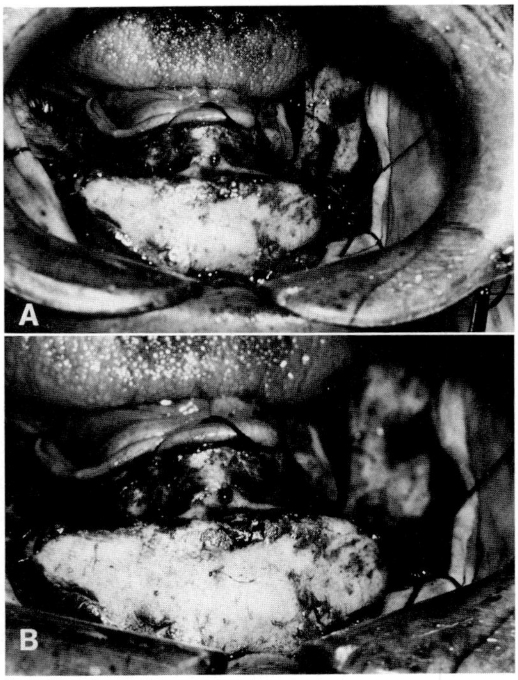

Fig. 4-7. Full view (*A*) and a close-up view (*B*) of a freshly dissected mandible. Adequate osseous exposure reveals all the landmarks that are necessary for a bone impression for the fabrication of a complete subperiosteal implant. Adequate exposure has been followed by necessary retraction by means of suspensory temporary sutures, so that a bone impression can be taken.

3. The terminal implant incision should extend from the distal aspect of the retromolar area to within 5 mm. of the distal aspect of the mesially retained natural tooth.

The horizontal incisions that follow the initial vertical incision are necessary in order to provide full exposure of the osseous structures that are to support the extremities of the implant frame. For the complete subperiosteal implant, in both the maxilla and the mandible, five horizontal relaxing incisions are usually made. Three of these are buccal horizontal incisions that are extended into the mucobuccal fold areas: one each at the distal-most parts of the initial incision, and one at the anterior symphyseal region. The other two are lingual horizontal incisions that are extended through about 4 to 5 mm., lengthwise, of soft tissue. For the terminal and intermediary subperiosteal implants, only

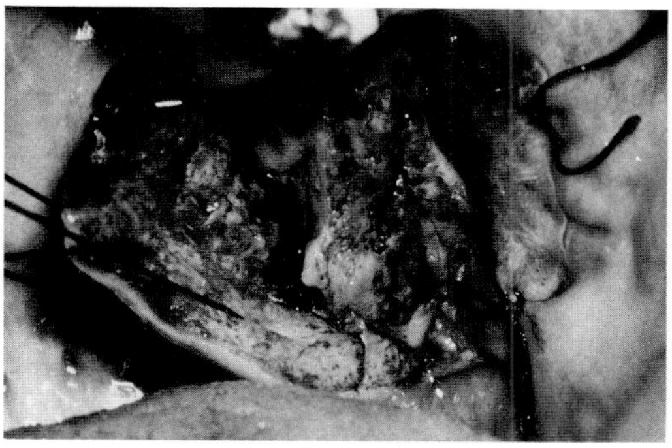

Fig. 4-8. Occlusal view of the exposed left posterior residual ridge of an upper arch. Retraction for exposure has been accomplished by (a) the temporary suturing of the buccal flap to the inner aspect of the mucosa of the cheek; and (b) the cross-arch temporary suturing of the lingual full-thickness flap to the temporary splint on the right side of the same arch. It is interesting to note that such bony configuration can never be fully revealed by radiographs.

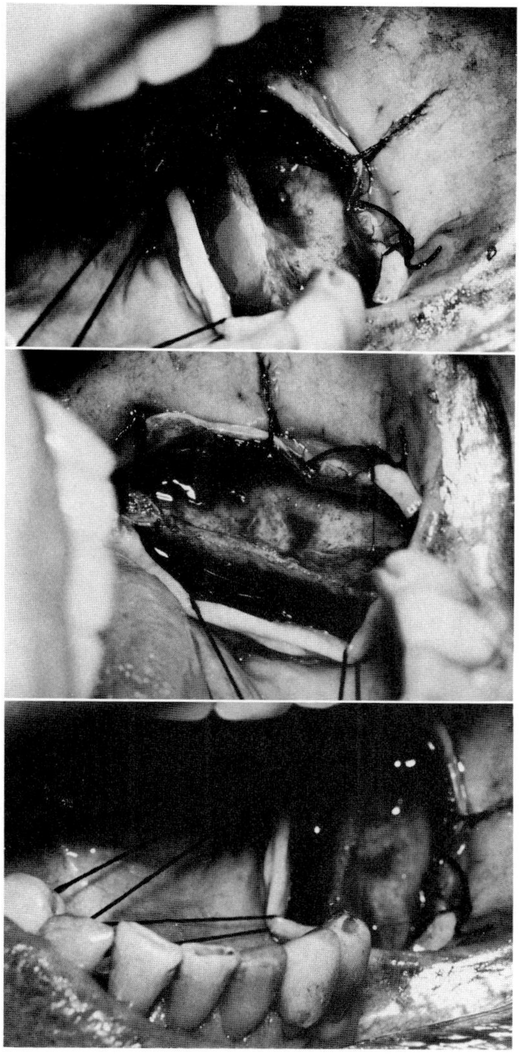

Fig. 4-9. Different views of an exposed edentulous area of the lower left posterior segment of a mandible. In this case prior provisional splinting was not necessary. Tooth preparation and temporization, however, should be completed prior to implant insertion in order to have a base for the immediate attachment of the acrylic-resin splint upon implant insertion.

two horizontal relaxing incisions are required for each of the lingual and buccal flaps.

Both the vertical and the horizontal incisions are performed with the No. 15 scalpel blade. Each of the flaps thus outlined is raised with mucoperiosteal elevators. After the initial outline incisions, all further dissection should be blunt, using mucoperiosteal elevators that are convenient and comfortable to the operator.

The "access form" thus achieved must be supplemented by a "convenience form." The retraction of the soft-tissue flaps serves as this "convenience form" and is accomplished by suturing the borders of the flaps to the mucous tissue of the inner aspect of the cheek, and to each other in the sublingual area (Fig. 4-7). If natural teeth remain, the retraction sutures are placed through the embrasures of temporary acrylic-resin splints that are placed diagonally opposite to the surgical site within the same arch (Figs. 4-8 to 4-10). Thus, just as in fixed prosthodontics, retraction thread or a contoured copper band is used to retract tissues in order to see crown margins; in implantology, the surgical-suture retraction techniques serve a similar pre-impression role.

The Custom Acrylic-Resin Impression Tray

In fixed prosthodontic procedures, the most preferred vehicles for impression ma-

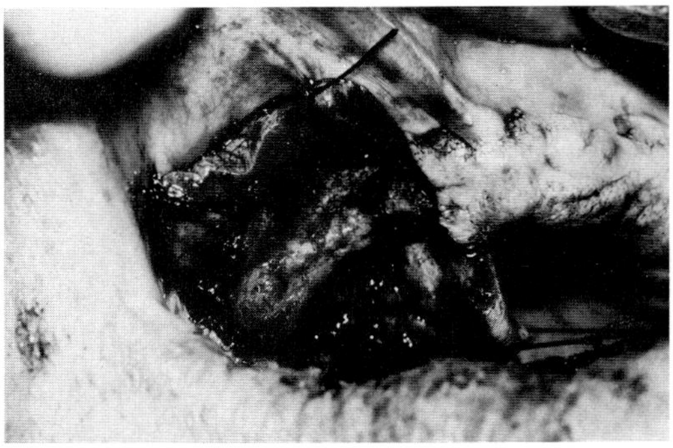

Fig. 4-10. Buccal view of the exposed ridge of an upper right intermediary implant site. The exposed area is temporarily retracted and will be bathed in normal saline solution prior to taking the rubber-base impression.

terials are customized acrylic-resin trays or individually contoured and adapted copper bands. Likewise, in subperiosteal implantology, a custom acrylic-resin tray is the best vehicle to use for the materials for the bone impression. In cases where a singular terminal or intermediary subperiosteal implant impression is to be taken, this tray is fabricated directly on the bone at the time of tissue retraction. Obviously, the extensive nature of the complete-arch subperiosteal impression does not lend itself to the direct fabrication of such a tray at the time of bone exposure. Therefore, in the full-arch procedure, it is necessary to fabricate the custom acrylic-resin tray on a stone model that has been obtained previously from an overextended alginate impression of the intact residual ridge.

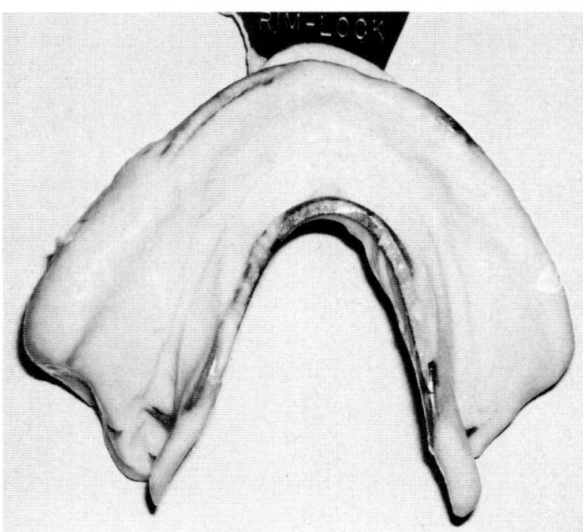

Fig. 4-11. An overextended alginate impression of an edentulous mandibular arch. Although such an impression distorts the overlying soft tissues, it is necessary, in order to encompass all the osseous landmarks on which the subperiosteal implant frame is to rest.

The Custom Tray for the Complete Subperiosteal Implant

If the use of a complete subperiosteal implant is indicated, an alginate impression is taken of the edentulous arch. This impression is useful both as a study model and as a preliminary model for the fabrication of a custom acrylic-resin tray. In order to create an accurate and useful final impression, the preliminary alginate impression must encompass at least four key landmarks on the lower arch and should extend beyond the retromolar pad areas. The landmarks include the external oblique ridges, the mylohyoid ridges, the anterior symphyseal protrusion, and the genial tubercle. An overextended tray is necessary to order to encompass all of these areas and to mechanically retract the pliable soft tissues simultaneously (Fig. 4-11). (This overextended tray impression would be considered too large for the mouth under the normal objective of fabricating routine study models.) At this same session, an opposing-arch alginate impression is taken; the stone model obtained from this impression serves as a study model and as the working countermodel that is to be mounted for the fabrication and the placement of the implant posts.

Subsequent to the examination and the preliminary impressions, the patient should be told when to return for the initial surgical procedure for the bone impression. The patient should also be told that he will be premedicated and therefore should arrive at the office about $^{1}/_{2}$ hour prior to the arranged appointment. Premedication is advocated for all implant surgical procedures, in order to calm the patient and to raise his threshold of discomfort. Conscious sedation can be administered orally, in pill or capsule form. It is not necessary to place a patient under general anesthesia unless he has a palsied condition or his emotional status requires such action. Sedation and local anesthetics usually suffice for all surgical procedures for implants. The patient should also be told to have a companion accompany him home after the initial surgical appointment. This is done (a) because of the patient's possible discomfort, which may make him unable to function freely and safely; (b) because of the possible drowsiness that may accompany the sedation, and (c) so that the patient can be free to apply external ice packs immediately after insertion of the sutures. The patient is also given a prescription for antibiotics, which he must begin taking 2 days prior to the surgical session.

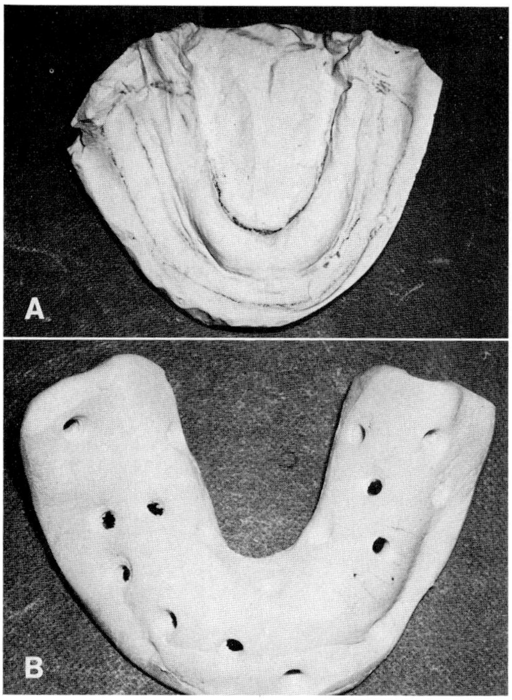

Fig. 4-12. A stone model (*A*) is obtained from the overextended complete-arch impression. A custom acrylic-resin tray (*B*) is fabricated on this model so that it encompasses as much as possible of the external oblique ridges, the anterior symphyseal area, the genial tubercle, and the mylohyoid ridge segments. Perforations are made randomly throughout the tray in order to acquire a mechanical lock (in addition to the rubber-base adhesive) for the heavy-bodied, rubber-base impression material.

Laboratory Procedures for the Complete Subperiosteal Implant Prior to Surgery

The model that is poured from the overextended alginate impression is used for two laboratory procedures. First, the custom acrylic-resin tray is fabricated, encompassing the extremities of the captured tissues (Fig. 4-12). Although this tray will serve as a vehicle for the rubber-base impression materials, there is no need to establish artificial relief. It is customary to relieve custom acrylic-resin trays for rubber-base impressions with layers of asbestos or base-plate wax. This purposefully provides a space to accommodate an adequate amount of the rubber-base material. The tray that is fabricated for the bone impression of a complete implant, however, has a natural relief, from the soft tissues. These soft tissues are retracted during the final impression. Thus, the mucoperiosteum, which is present at the preliminary alginate impression but is not present at the final rubber-base bone impression, serves as a buffer and holds the rubber-base impression material.

It is preferable to perforate this customized tray in order to provide added mechanical retention for the heavy-bodied rubber base. It is not necessary to have a handle; this is a matter of personal preference. The tray may be set aside, because it is not cold-sterilized until just prior to the surgical session. After sterilization, the tray is coated with rubber-base adhesive on its inner surface and slightly beyond its peripheral border, to maximize the retention of the impression material.

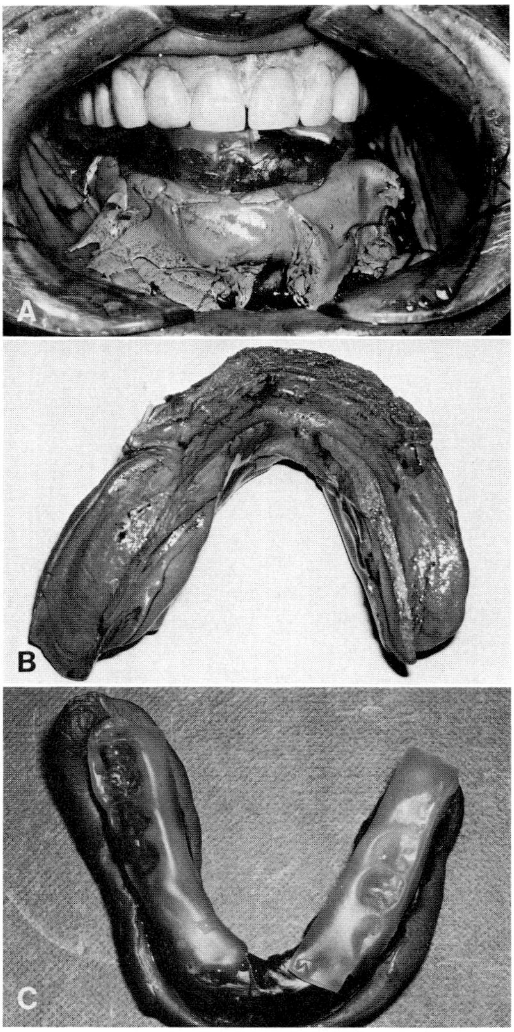

Fig. 4-13. At the time of surgical retraction, prior to the impression, the surgical bite is registered by relining the initial bite-block registration, which is obtained prior to any surgical procedures. This is merely relined on the basal portion of the base plate in order to get proper seating on the exposed bone (*A*). After removal from the oral cavity, the flash of the reline material is trimmed, and a neat, compact bite-block remains (*B, C*). It is important to note that this registration is strictly for the placement, alignment, and height of the implant posts; it is *not* to be used for the fabrication of the final superstructure prosthetic appliance.

The second laboratory procedure is the fabrication of a baseplate on which a wax bite-block is superimposed. The baseplate is fabricated and shaped on the same study model that is obtained from the original alginate impression. The bite-block serves as the surgical bite registration. Such registration captures both centric relation and the occlusal vertical dimension upon exposure of the osseous structure of the complete arch (Fig. 4-13). The bite registration helps to establish the proper relationship of the implant posts to the opposing arch as well as the relative length of these posts.

Meanwhile, the opposing study model may be mounted on any hinge articulator, without the aid of a face-bow. The reason for the relative simplicity of this opposing mounting is that no occlusion is established at this time from this mounting. The bite registration and the mounting for articulation are used only to ascertain the relevant positions and lengths of the implant posts, which are to bear the superimposed prosthesis.

The Impression Technique for the Complete Subperiosteal Implant

The heavy- and light-bodied rubber-base materials are used simultaneously (Fig. 4-14). The heavy-bodied rubber-base material should be of a putty-like consistency so that it can be readily molded with the fingers when it is inserted in the tray. Also, this consistency facilitates the placement of additional portions of this material into the mouth, directly over the light-bodied material, in areas in which it is difficult to gain access. The purpose of the heavy-bodied rubber-base material is to compress the light-bodied material, so that every fine detail of bone topography can be duplicated. While the heavy-bodied material is being mixed, the light-bodied material is spatulated and inserted in a syringe. Next, while the tray is being filled with the heavy-bodied material, the syringe is used to express the light-bodied material onto all areas of exposed bone. It should be noted that the light-bodied material will not displace mucus, saliva, or blood; therefore, the exposed bone should be gently washed with saline solution just prior to the injection of this material (Fig. 4-15). While the

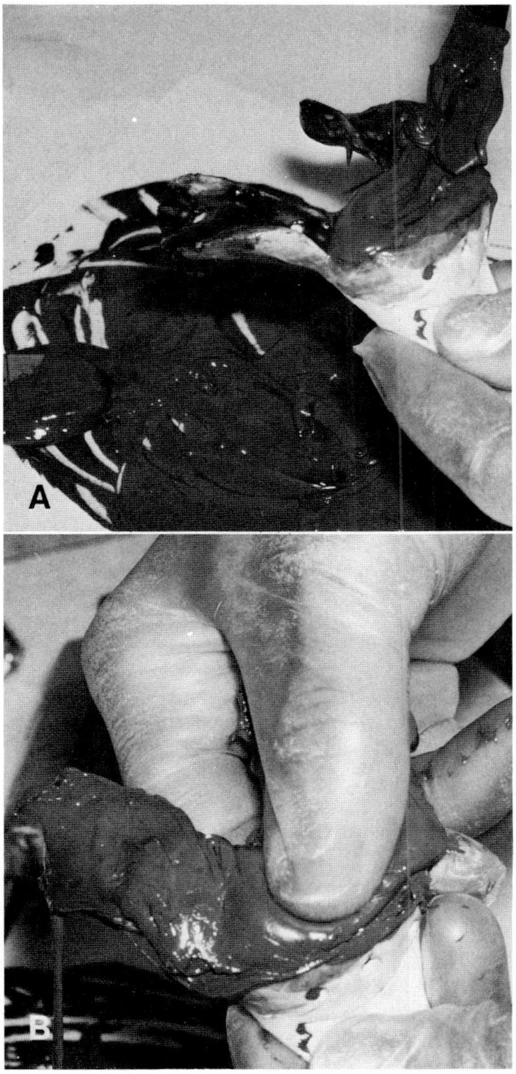

Fig. 4-14. (A) Heavy-bodied rubber-base impression material being inserted into a custom acrylic-resin tray with a second spatula. *(B)* Once the heavy-bodied material has passed the tacky stage, this specific heavy-bodied rubber base (Neo-Plex*) can be molded with the fingers, to achieve the desired shape prior to the insertion of the tray in the mouth. While the assistant is performing this procedure, the dentist places the light-bodied rubber-base material on the exposed bone surfaces by means of syringes.

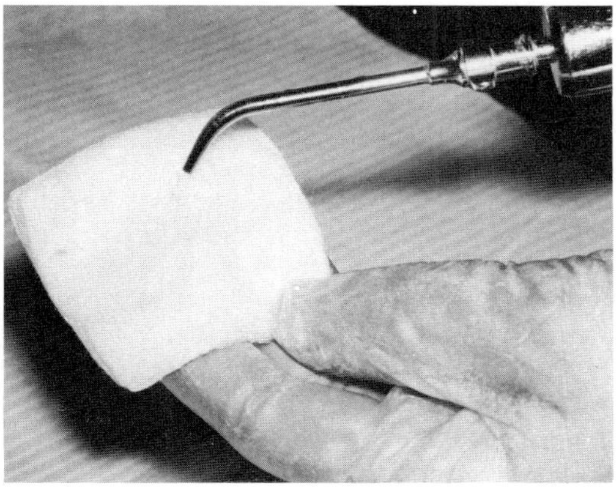

Fig. 4-15. Sterile surgical sponges are kept freshly and constantly replenished with normal sodium chloride solution. These sponges are used to prevent the desiccation of bone and tissues while any laboratory procedures are being performed to modify the custom tray. The syringe may be used intra-orally to wash the surgical areas as well.

filled tray is being seated in the mouth, it should provide some compression, and a flow of light-bodied material should be seen along the periphery of the tray. This procedure, using both heavy- and light-bodied rubber-base materials, is the same for both complete and partial subperiosteal implant impressions.

In the partially edentulous arch, the custom tray has a positive stop on the prepared natural tooth. In the completely edentulous arch, however, there is no such similar guide, so the operator must carefully judge the positioning of the tray. In either situation, the tray should be held in place for at least 7 minutes (Figs. 4-16, 4-17).

The Custom Tray for the Terminal or the Intermediary Subperiosteal Implants

A cold-cured, acrylic-resin tray material may be used intra-orally as long as it has

*Lactona Corp., Philadelphia, Pennsylvania.

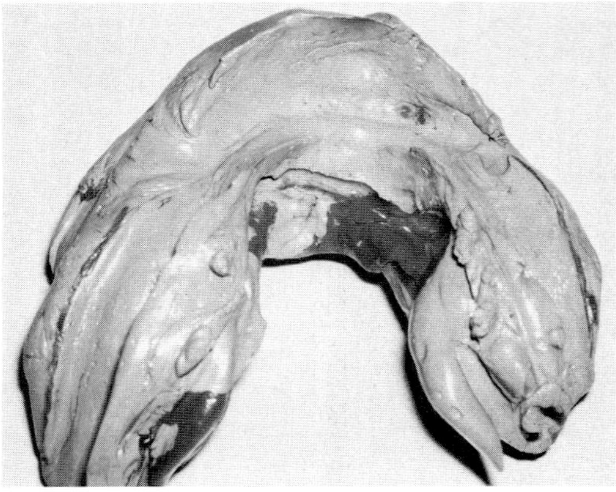

Fig. 4-16. A complete lower-arch bone impression for a subperiosteal implant. The light-bodied rubber-base material covers all the necessary osseous components and has been properly compressed into place by the heavy-bodied material that was carried into the mouth by means of a custom acrylic-resin tray. The layers from top to bottom are: the light-bodied rubber base, the heavy-bodied rubber base, and the acrylic-resin tray that has been coated with adhesive.

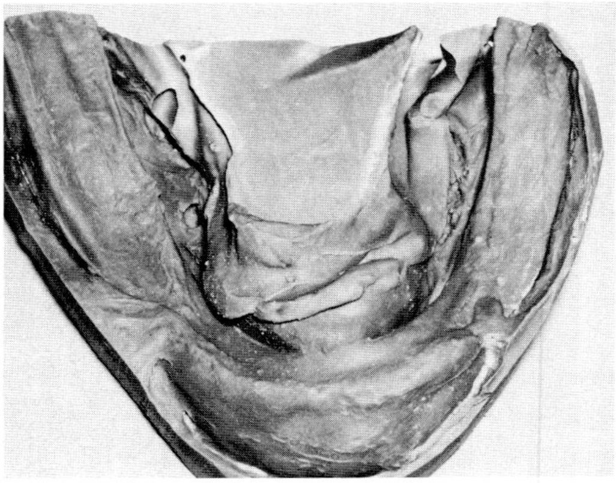

Fig. 4-17. The trimmed die-stone model for a complete subperiosteal mandibular implant. This model reflects the accuracy and clarity of the impression. It is best to pour such a model by means of a vacuum mixing machine, in order to avoid porosities.

a doughy, but not tacky, consistency. This material should be easy to handle, so that it may be compressed with gentle finger pressure and molded over all the exposed bone (Fig. 4-18). *Undivided attention is essential at this point.* As soon as heat is generated through the material, the amorphous mass of acrylic resin should be removed from the mouth and chilled under tap water. This prevents any bone from being burned, and prevents the material from being caught in any undercut areas. It is best to overextend the tray material either mesially or distally in order to include any adjacent prepared natural teeth, because these teeth serve as an index and

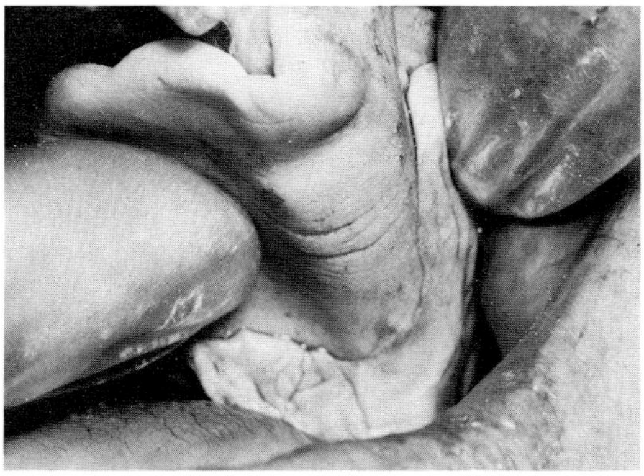

Fig. 4-18. A terminal subperiosteal impression tray being customized directly on the bone at the time of flap reflection. The bulk of acrylic resin has been molded while it had a doughy consistency, over the exposed bone. The tray encompasses a portion of the prepared teeth anterior to the edentulous ridge.

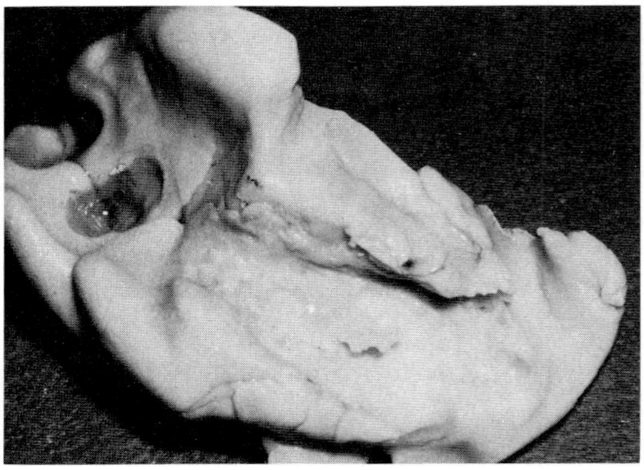

Fig. 4-19. The custom acrylic-resin tray that has been fabricated intra-orally is almost a good impression in itself. This upper terminal tray extends from the hamular notch (*lower right*) through to the prepared natural tooth that is to serve as one of the mesial abutment teeth.

as a positive stop when the tray is finally filled with the chosen impression material (Fig. 4-19). Before the untrimmed tray is reinserted in the mouth to check for any possible distortion, it should be rinsed in normal saline solution. Then it may be safely reinserted for try-in.

The mass of acrylic resin is then brought to the lathe for trimming in order to accomplish the following (Fig. 4-20):

1. The flash is removed.
2. The tray is thinned on its outer aspect to allow for the later superimposition of a full-arch tray. The tray should not be made so thin, however, that it becomes flexible.
3. The inner aspect of the tray is relieved in order to accommodate both light- and heavy-bodied rubber-base materials. This relief is not extended to the prepared-tooth area that serves as the positive stop and index.
4. The tray is randomly perforated with a large, round, No. 6 steel bur in order to create mechanical locks for the heavy-bodied rubber-base impression material.

It should be noted that during the trimming procedures, the retracted soft tissues should be constantly bathed with sterile gauze pads saturated with saline solution. After the trimming is completed, the tray should be wiped with alcohol solution and washed with normal saline solution, prior to another try-in in the mouth (Fig. 4-21). Upon try-in, any overextension of the tray may be removed. If there is an underextension of the tray, it is very simple to add cold-cured acrylic resin in the same manner as in the initial fabrication of the original tray.

The custom acrylic-resin tray will not adversely affect the exposed structures, providing that:

1. The material is allowed to adequately set prior to insertion in the oral cavity, so as to minimize the amount of time that the tray material is in contact with the bone.
2. An excess of the monomer liquid is not created.
3. The acrylic resin is constantly and copiously chilled and washed by the dental assistant while it is in the oral cavity.

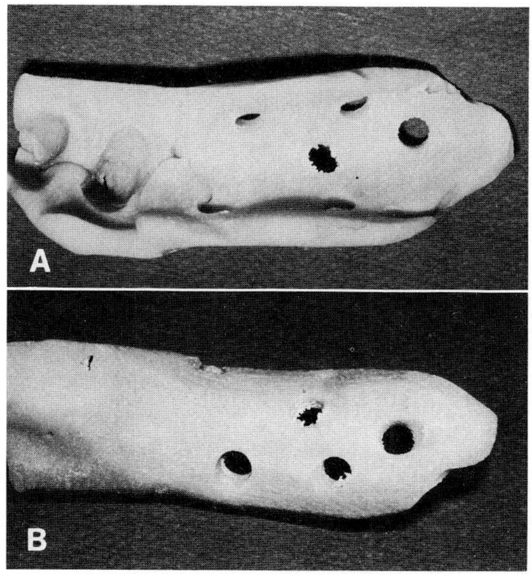

Fig. 4-20. Inner (*A*) and outer (*B*) aspects of the custom acrylic-resin tray after trimming procedures. The flash (excess material) has been removed. The inner portion has been relieved in order to accommodate both light-bodied and heavy-bodied rubber-base materials. Perforations have been placed at random for mechanical retention of the rubber-base impression materials. The outer aspect has been trimmed in order to accommodate a second overall impression tray.

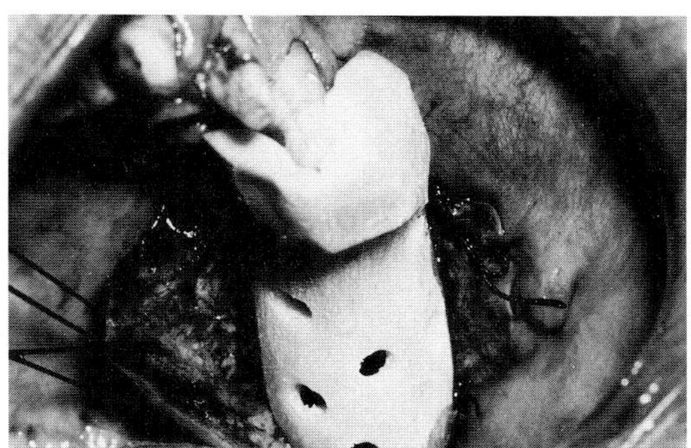

Fig. 4-21. A try-in of the trimmed custom acrylic-resin tray, prior to the taking of the impression. A guideline for seating is the positive stop on the prepared natural abutment tooth.

4. The material is removed immediately when it begins to warm in the mouth.
5. The tissues are subsequently bathed in a normal saline solution.

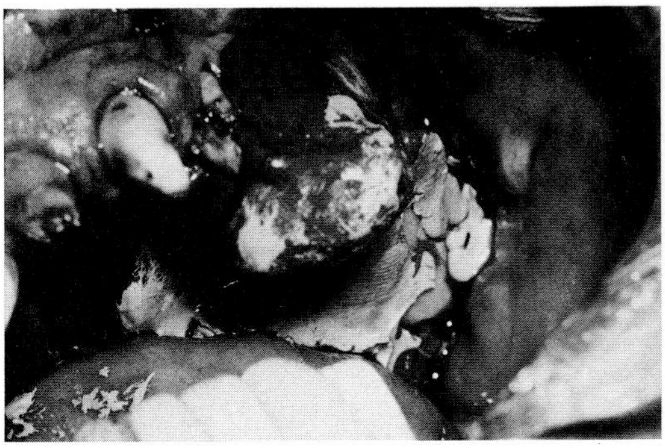

Fig. 4-22. The impression materials for this terminal subperiosteal implant are setting intraorally. This tray is *not* removed for visual inspection. The sutures are severed prior to the second complete-arch superimposed impression.

The tray is then sterilized and coated with the adhesive bonding agent, as is done for the customized impression of the complete-arch implant.

The Impression Technique for the Terminal or the Intermediary Subperiosteal Implants

The light-bodied rubber-base impression material is introduced into the exposed area with a syringe, and the customized tray is filled with the moldable heavy-bodied material. The heavy-bodied material then compresses the light-bodied material so that the latter flows over and around all of the bony structures and around the periphery of the custom tray (Fig. 4-22).

In order to achieve a good impression of the bone, it is necessary to adequately retract all soft tissues. Such retraction is accomplished by the temporary suturing of the surgically created soft-tissue flaps, to reflect and invert their positions. Such suturing is done to the inside of the cheek (as would pertain to the buccal flaps) or to each other (as would apply to the lingual flaps). Constant, adequate, osseous exposure is the key to a good impression. Bathing the bone with normal saline solution and expediting all intermediary steps are key factors in preventing traumatization of the bone.

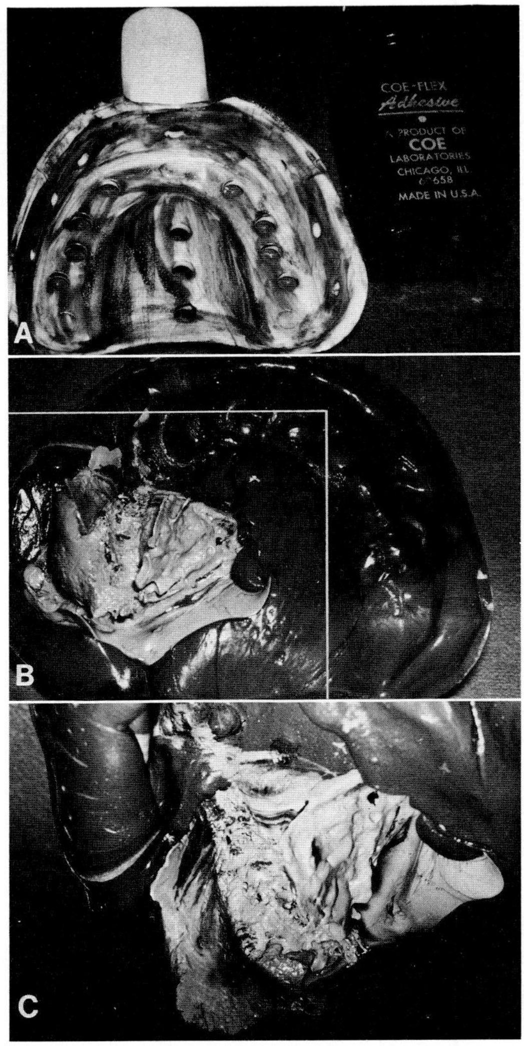

Fig. 4-23. A prefabricated acrylic-resin tray coated with adhesive material. This tray is filled with heavy-bodied rubber-base material only. It is inserted over the existing terminal custom impression. (B, C) After setting, the complete-arch impression (*B*) will carry the terminal impression (*C*) with it upon removal. (*C* is a close-up view of the blocked-in area of *B*.)

In cases involving a terminal or intermediary bone impression, the impression is left to set in the mouth and is not removed after it has completely set. A full-arch, heavy-bodied, rubber-base impression material is then superimposed to accommodate the bone impression and the remaining teeth in the same arch (Fig. 4-23). Thus, only after the second impression has set should the whole impression be removed from the mouth. The smaller initial impression should firmly adhere to, and be seated in, this second impression. Only in this manner can the implant post(s) and the prepared teeth be aligned (Fig. 4-24). It is not necessary to use a custom acrylic-resin tray for the secondary impression, nor is it necessary to include a light-bodied material in the secondary impression. A rigid, preformed, full-arch tray is used in combination with an adhesive bonding agent and heavy-bodied rubber-base material only.

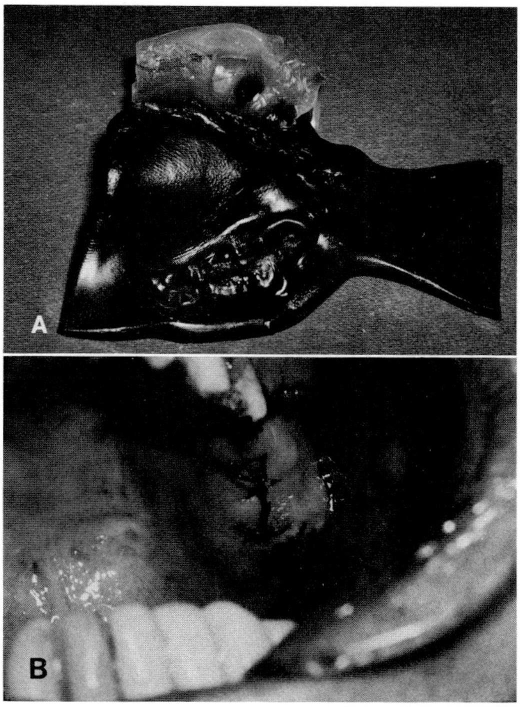

Fig. 4-24. Prior to closure of the surgical wound, a complete-arch wax bite (*A*) is taken. This bite registration includes the exposed bone and is used only for the fabrication of the subperiosteal implant. Primary healing is obtained by the close approximation of the mucoperiosteal flaps with individual sutures(*B*).

THE LABORATORY PRESCRIPTION

The accurate, mounted model of the bone impression must be accompanied by an explicitly detailed laboratory prescription (Fig. 4-25).

The Bone Model

The bone model is obtained by pouring an accurate die stone material, such as Vel Mix,* into the bone impression. The resultant model should be trimmed, and all areas that prevent accessibility to the exposed bone should be removed (Fig. 4-26). Specifically, those parts of the model that form the reflected soft-tissue flaps should be removed with trimming stones in a laboratory handpiece, and with the appropriate laboratory knives. The resultant model should have a clearly visible and accessible bony area, in order to facilitate the outline drawing of the implant frame by the dentist and the subsequent wax-up by the technician. It is preferable to include the complete arch in this model, in order to obtain the proper relationship with the prepared teeth in the same arch and to obtain an occluding relationship with a model of the opposing arch. The dentist then mounts the case and draws the outline of the subperiosteal implant frame.

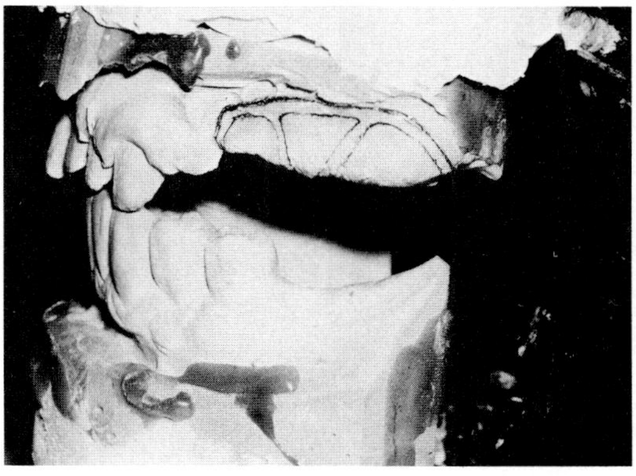

Fig. 4-25. Buccal view of the drawing of an upper left terminal subperiosteal implant frame. The drawing was done after the opposing models had been mounted on a simple hinge articulator. The mounting is necessary for the determination of post placement, alignment, and length.

*Kerr Sybron Corp., Romulus, Michigan.

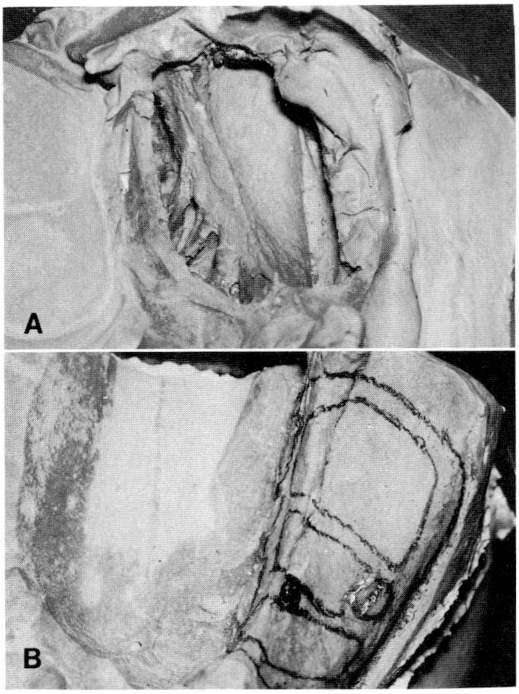

Fig. 4-26. A bone model of the lower left portion of the arch in die stone (*A*) is part of a complete-arch working model. Careful trimming of the superfluous stone reveals the full extent of the bone impression. The trimming procedure provides accessibility for the frame drawing (*B*) and the subsequent laboratory wax-up. These photographs are of the *same* model.

The Subperiosteal Implant Frame Drawing

There is a definite sequence of procedures for the subperiosteal implant frame drawing (Fig. 4-27). In order to indicate the placement of the post(s) and neck(s), the model of the bone impression should first be mounted with the opposing arch. Only after this has been done are the pencil markings to be undertaken. At this stage, the dentist should have: (a) a clean, full-arch model of the bone; (b) a full-arch model of the opposing arch; and (c) a surgical wax bite.

No face-bow or adjustable articulator is needed. A simple hinge mounting serves the stated purposes. Mounting the bone impression model with its opposing arch enables the implant post to conform to its buccolingual and mesiodistal positions relative to the opposing arch. Naturally, for the particular case at hand, the operator should have noted the buccolingual width of the attached tissues at the time of the initial surgical procedure, in order to ascertain the latitude of implant neck positioning. Also, it is preferable to place the post in a slight depression of the bony architecture rather than on a prominence. All parts of the implant that rest on bone should be placed in valleys, rather than on peaks, of bone in order to establish a smooth coalescence of the cast frame with its supporting and surrounding bone. This in turn allows for a more intimate adaptation of the superimposed soft tissues, thereby preventing these tissues from being stretched tautly over prominent parts of the subperiosteal implant frame and, consequently, minimizing the potential exposure of struts.

After the bone impression model and its opposing arch have been mounted, the peripheral border is outlined. The peripheral border must encompass as much as possible of the exposed bony area. While drawing the outline of the peripheral border, the operator must bear in mind the dissipation of forces and must avoid neurovascular bundles such as those in the areas of the mental foramina.

After the peripheral border is outlined, the primary and secondary struts are drawn. The primary struts join the implant neck to the peripheral border. There should be two to four primary struts for each implant neck, to prevent any flexure at this critical area. The secondary struts reinforce the flexible frame and, more importantly, serve as areas for the interweaving of connective tissue for the mechanical retention of the implant frame.

The Written Laboratory Prescription

It does not suffice to send this drawing and mounted model to the laboratory with a request for a subperiosteal implant. Written supplementary instructions must ac-

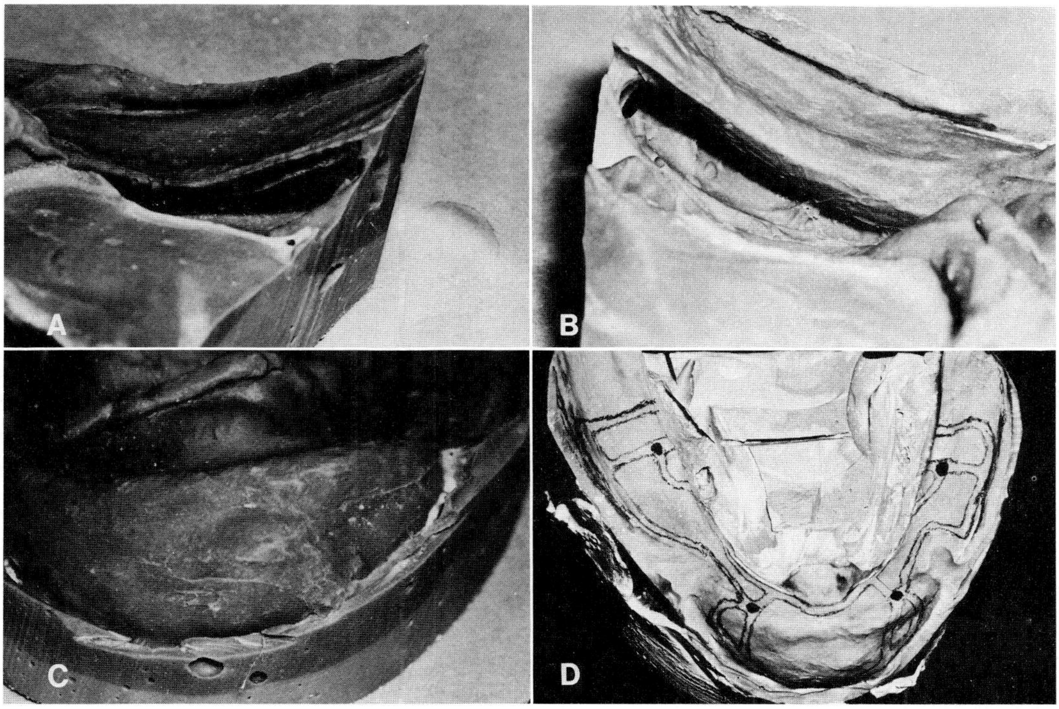

Fig. 4-27. The accuracy and completeness of all bone casts are of paramount importance. For example, the delineation of the mylohyoid ridge areas (*A*) and the fluidity of contour that encompasses the outermost portions of the external oblique ridges (*B*) are obtained. A close-up view of the anterior portion of a complete subperiosteal bone model (*C*) reveals the lingual extension to the genial tubercle and the buccal extension through the inferior portion of the curvature of the chin. These combined details form the complete model (*D*), which is mounted and designed by the operator for the laboratory technician.

company this graphic prescription. The occlusogingival height of the implant neck should be specified; as previously described, this would depend on the thickness of the tissue in the area of extrusion of the implant post. It should be noted that the neck is to be polished. References to the post should include:

1. The desired occlusogingival length
2. The alignment with appropriately prepared existing natural teeth
3. A sand-blasted finish to accommodate a fixed prosthesis
4. A highly polished surface to accommodate a removable prosthesis.

The frame should be about 0.3 to 0.4 mm. thick, which would provide a limited flexibility of the frame. If any screw hole is necessary, it should be outlined on the model, because the laboratory technician is not familiar with the anatomic topography of the bone and the underlying structures.

When requesting a return date for the implant, allow for a few days prior to the date of insertion. It is imperative to examine the implant closely after it is returned, to evaluate the execution of the prescription instructions and the quality of the implant casting.

BIBLIOGRAPHY

Archer, W. H.: Implant dentures: surgical—unfavorable—qualified. J. Pros. Dent., *10:*1127-1131, 1960.

Barandes, J.: A new approach to the full maxillary subperiosteal implant. Oral Implantol., *1:*175-193, 1973.

Bodine, R. L.: Implant dentures—follow-up after seven to ten years. J.A.D.A., *67:*352-363, 1963.

Bodine, R. L., and Kotch, R. L.: Mandibular subperiosteal implant denture technique. J. Pros. Dent., *4:*396-412, 1954.

———: Perfect mandibular subperiosteal implant denture technique. New York D. J., *20:*193-207, 1954.

Doner, A. G.: Implant dentures: surgical—favorable. J. Pros. Dent., *10:*1118-1126, 1960.

Killebrew, R. H.: The mandibular implant denture. J. Pros. Dent., *2:*618-624, 1952.

Kratochvil, F. J., and Boyne, P. J.: Combined use of subperiosteal implant and bone-marrow graft in deficient edentulous mandibles: a preliminary report. J. Pros. Dent., *27:*645-653, 1972.

Lee, T. C.: Subperiosteal implants—20 years' experience. J. California D. A., *47:*36-37, 1971.

Lew, I.: Progress report on full implant dentures. J. Pros. Dent., *3:*571-575, 1953.

Mack, A. O.: Histological investigations of effects of subperiosteal dental implants in monkeys. Brit. D. J., *108:*217-224, 1960.

Reisbick, M. H., and Benson, D.: Ceramic-coated subperiosteal implants. Part I. A pilot study. J. Pros. Dent., *31:*204-210, 1974.

Weinberg, B. D.: Subperiosteal implantation of a Vitallium artificial abutment. J.A.D.A., *40:*549-554, 1950.

5 The Subperiosteal Implant—Evaluation of the Castings; the Insertion and Temporization

EVALUATION OF THE LABORATORY CASTING

Six Key Aspects of Analysis by the Dentist

Any implant casting should be analyzed and evaluated as carefully as one would evaluate a partial- or full-coverage cast retainer for an abutment tooth. The quality of an implant casting is as important as the quality of a cast retainer (Fig. 5-1). An

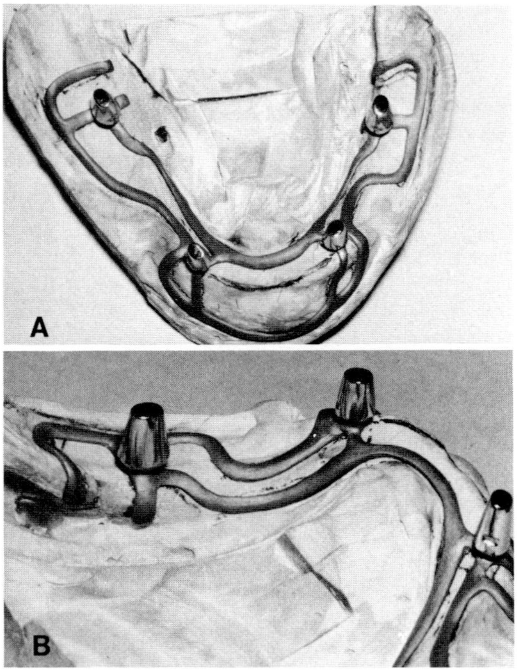

Fig. 5-1. An occlusal view *(A)* of a complete mandibular subperiosteal implant casting, and a lingual view *(B)* of a portion of the same casting. A clean, measured casting is well-adapted to the die-stone model. If the bone impression was properly taken, and the stone model poured shortly thereafter, then this casting should seat accurately upon surgical reentry and insertion. Note in the lingual view *(B),* that the mylohyoid muscle insertions and the genial tubercle have been removed on the diestone only; this affords better access for wax-up procedures.

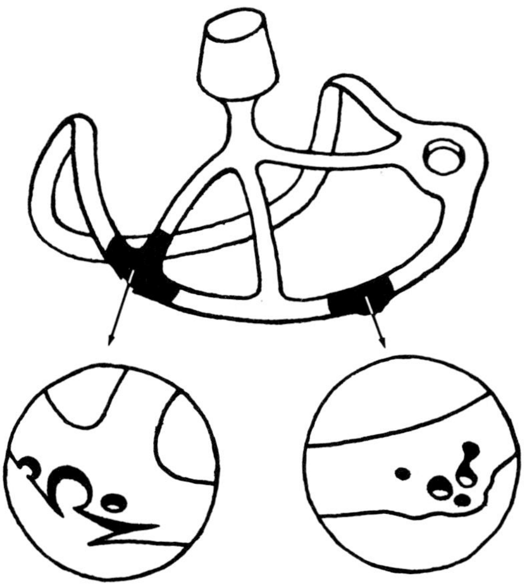

Fig. 5-2. A subperiosteal implant with flaws in the casting. Such discrepancies require the fabrication of a new casting. The flash and voids *(left inset)* can be removed by narrowing the peripheral border, but this may render a weakness in the width of the casting. The removal of porosities *(right inset)* would require excessive thinning of a portion of the casting; this would render a weakness in the thickness of the casting.

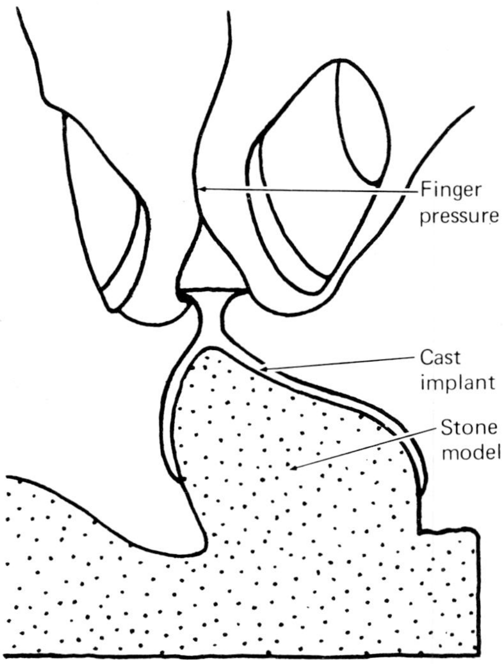

Fig. 5-3 The implant post is held between the thumb and index finger upon the stone model. Then, direct pressure is exerted downward, and an attempt is made to rock the implant while it is being positively seated. Should any movement of the frame occur, the casting should be examined for warpage. If there is any warpage, the implant cannot be used.

improperly adapted implant frame is as useless as an ill-fitting crown. The following checklist should be used for every subperiosteal implant, no matter how intricate or how simple its design may be:

1. Is the casting clean? Any spurs or any flash can be removed without harm to the implant. If the casting has any pits or similar voids, however, it should be discarded (Fig. 5-2).

2. Is the implant frame positively seated and immobile upon the stone model? There should be absolutely no play or rocking motion when finger pressure is placed on the post or on any part of the subperiosteal frame. If the casting is at all warped, it cannot be used (Figs. 5-3, 5-4).

3. Are there any voids between the im-

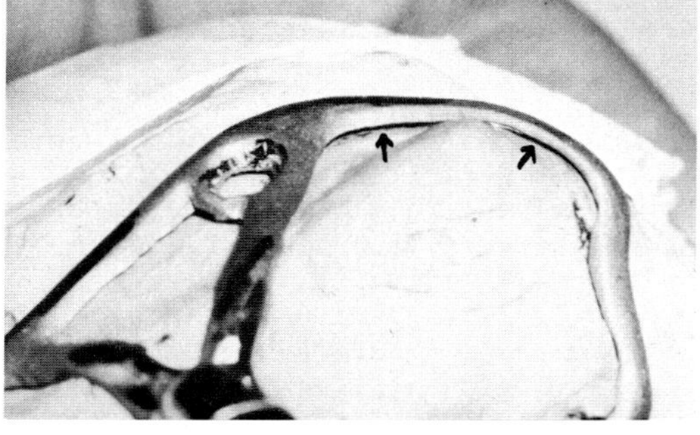

Fig. 5-4 Occlusal view of a maxillary unilateral terminal subperiosteal implant upon a stone model. The peripheral border appears to have a close adaptation to the stone at the buccal *(left)* and distopalatal *(right)* aspects. However, the entire segment *(arrows)* of the peripheral border distal to these areas *(top)* is $^{1}/_{2}$ mm. to 1 mm. away from the stone. This casting had to be remade.

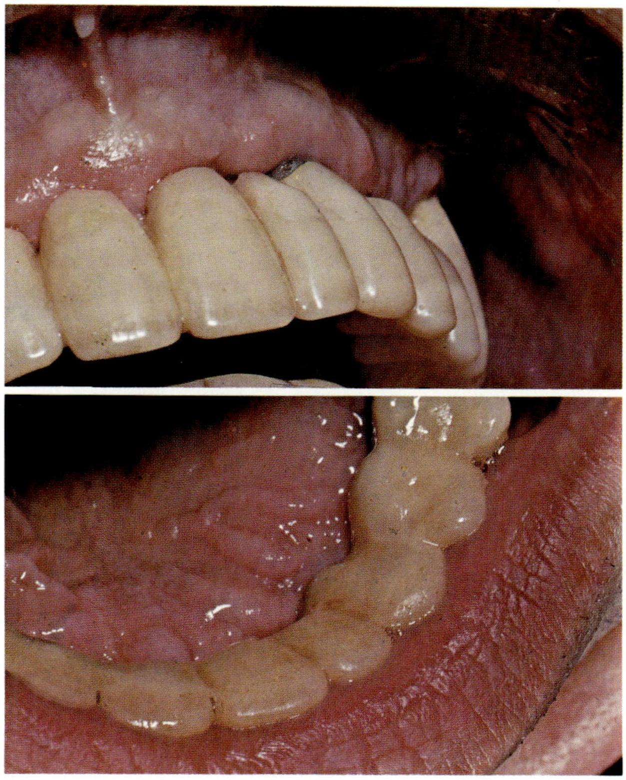

Plate 5–1. See Figure 5–12.

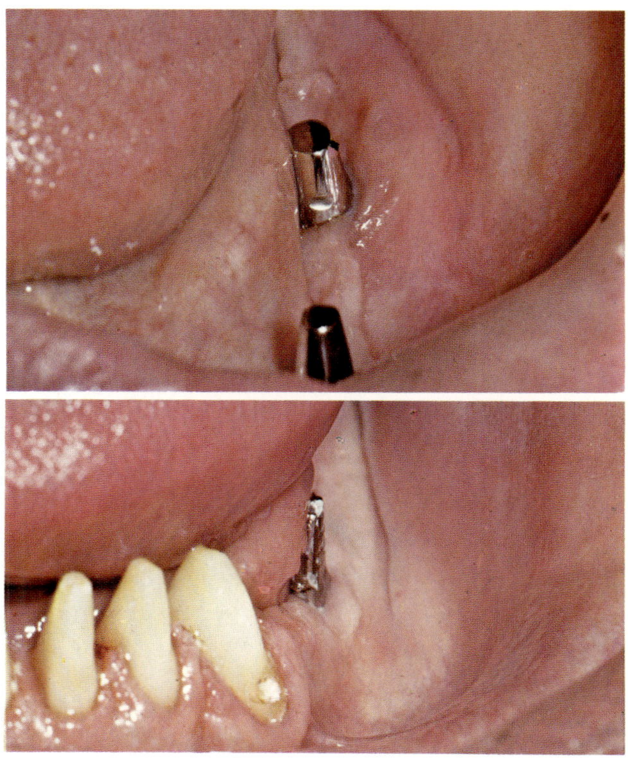

Plate 5–2. See Figure 5–13.

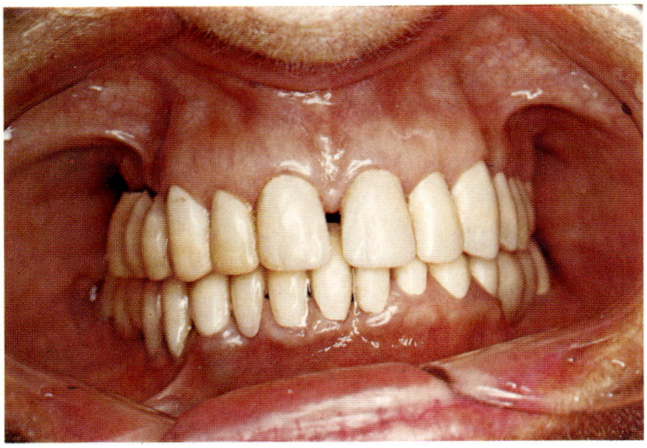

Plate 5–3. See Figure 5–15.

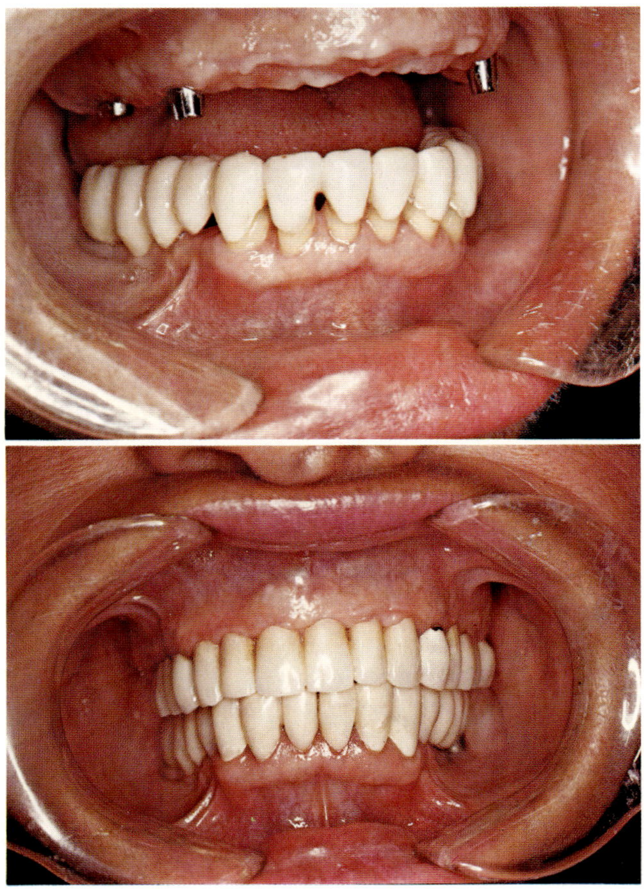

Plate 5–4. See Figure 5–16.

plant frame and the underlying bone? Often, although there may be no noticeable movement of the implant frame (see No. 2 above), there may be one or more voids, which represent an ill-fitting casting. The implant frame should be so closely adapted to the underlying bone that a sharp explorer could not be inserted between the implant frame and the supportive bone. (This is similar to the evaluation of the marginal integrity of a cast crown.) Even if the implant casting is stable, any void may lend itself to the formation of granulation tissue, or the eventual exposure of the metallic area in question (Fig. 5-5).

4. Is the frame casting of uniform thickness? The struts or peripheral border areas should never be thicker than 0.5 mm. It is preferred that the casting be 0.3 mm. thick and have a smooth outer surface, with no sharp protuberances. Thus, the casting should be strong and of limited

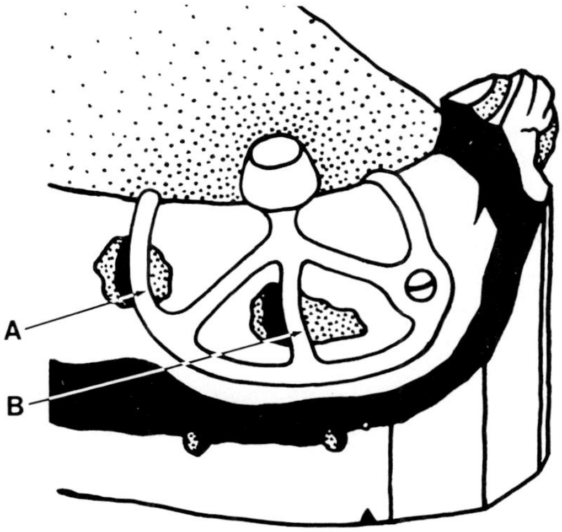

Fig. 5-5. A lower left unilateral terminal subperiosteal implant seated on a stone model. Although such a casting may be stable and proportionate on the model, its undersurface should be checked for adaptation to depressions in the osseous architecture. For example, the peripheral border *(A)* and the primary strut *(B)* should be concave in order to properly adapt to surface depressions of the osseous support.

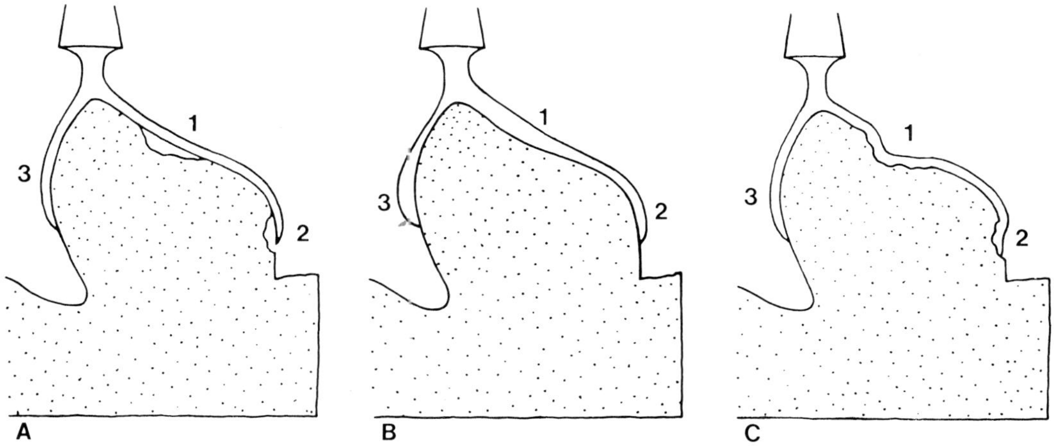

Fig. 5-6. (A) shows a subperiosteal implant frame of uniform thickness; however, even though this frame may be within the preferred 0.3-mm. to 0.5-mm. range in thickness, the only area of proper adaptation is at point *(3)*. At point *(1)* the casting is not adapted to the contours of the bone. At point *(2)* there is an overextension and a lack of adaptation of the casting. *(B)* shows a well-adapted casting; however, there is a lack of acceptable uniformity of thickness of the casting. At point *(3)* the unnecessary thickness may be a causative factor in the perforation of overlying tissue. Although the thickness at point *(2)* is proper and acceptable, point *(1)* is unnecessarily thick. There is no apparent need to approach the 1.0-mm. to 1.5-mm. range of thickness. *(C)* shows a well-adapted frame casting of uniform thickness, within an acceptable range; however, the overlying soft tissues have been considered only at point *(3)*. Points *(1)* and *(2)* both require thicker metal in order for a smooth and undisturbed superimposition of the overlying soft tissues.

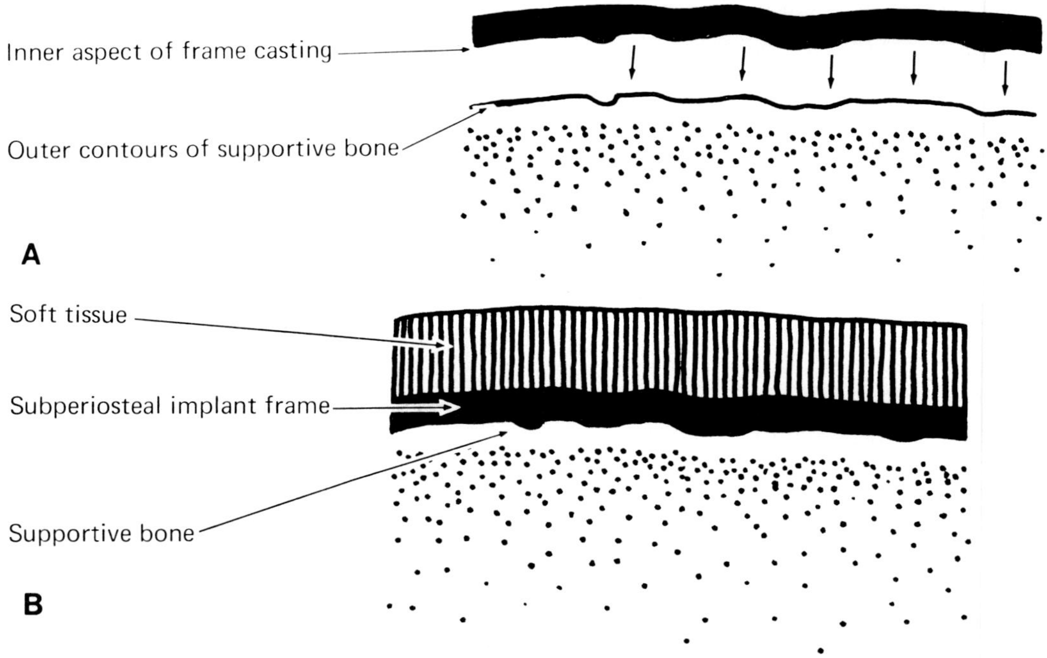

Fig. 5-7. (A) A portion of a subperiosteal frame casting being placed on its supportive bone. The outline of every contour, the depressions, and the protuberances of the bony architecture are duplicated within the inner portion of a well-adapted casting. Such configurations are especially noted in the maxillary arch. *(B)* A subperiosteal implant frame has been "sandwiched" between the osseous support and the soft-tissue covering. The following criteria have been met: the thickness of the casting is within acceptable limits; the base portion of the casting is adapted to the configuration of the osseous support; and the outer aspect of the casting is smooth enough to provide a passive adaptation of the mucoperiosteum.

flexibility. The thickness can be measured; the flexibility, at this time, however, is strictly a matter of subjective clinical judgment.

There is an exception to the rule of uniform frame thickness. If there is a concavity in the bone, the base of the frame should be adapted to the concavity, and the gingival aspect of the frame should lend itself to a harmonious adaptation of the overlying soft tissue. In such a case, the frame is made thicker basally to fill an osseous void; therefore, there would be no protuberance on the gingival aspect of the frame. Such a protuberance could cause an indentation into the full-thickness gingival or mucosal tissues. The idea is to place a prosthetic frame between hard and soft tissues with as little disturbance to the architectural configurations of these tissues as possible (Figs. 5-6 to 5-8).

5. Is the neck of the implant of the prescribed length (Fig. 5-9)? The neck of the implant is considered to be the critical link between the supportive structures and the oral cavity. In spite of this, there is a slight amount of leeway for the length of the neck. If the neck is longer than the thickness of the tissue that surrounds it, the implant is still acceptable because this area would still be accessible to oral-hygiene procedures. On the other hand, if the neck of the implant were shorter than the thickness of the tissue that surrounds it, the implant post may have detrimental effects on the soft tissues because the base

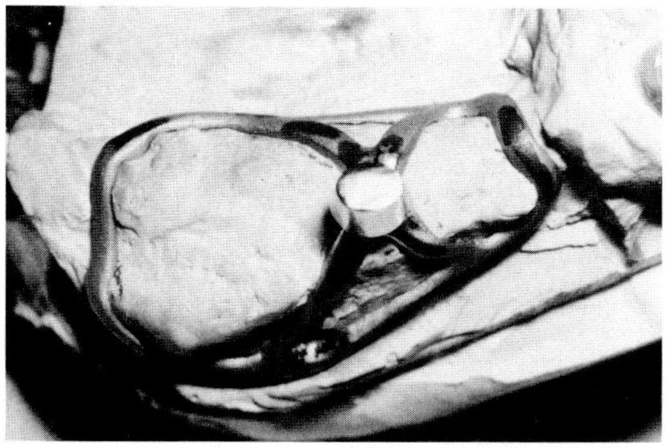

Fig. 5-8. Although this implant frame was properly adapted to the stone model, its thickness was unacceptable because: (a) the mesial aspect of the peripheral border *(right)* was 1 mm., and (b) the four primary struts were excessively thick (1.5 mm.) as they approached the neck of the implant. These areas would have to be thinned and refinished before the implant could be inserted in the mouth.

of the post would encroach upon them. This can best be compared to the importance of the architecture of a major embrasure, which should passively accommodate the interproximal soft tissues. A closed embrasure makes oral-hygiene procedures unmanageable and impinges upon the interproximal soft tissues, resulting in a deterioration, with cyanotic manifestations, of the tissues due to mechanical compression.

6. Is the implant post properly aligned with the prepared abutment teeth, and is the post of the prescribed length? If the implant post is poorly aligned to a minor degree, the dentist may correct this in his laboratory by milling and tapering the post on its nonaligned side. If the post is poorly aligned to a major degree or if correction of such nonalignment would cause too great a taper of the post, the dentist may then fabricate either: (a) a cast coping to create a new alignment, or (b) a complete new casting. The dentist may correct the length of any implant post by following these same procedures.

The Laboratory Responsibilities of the Implantologist

At the laboratory level, prosthodontics and implantology are similar and equally important. The prosthodontist must take accurate impressions and should pour his own models. This provides maximum control over all procedures—including ditching dies and defining margins—prior to sending the dies to the laboratory. The prosthodontist should also mount his models. He should not send ill-defined dies along with models and bite registrations to the laboratory with the expectation that "a textbook casting" will be returned. Likewise, the implantologist must take an accurate and detailed impression and must pour his own model. He must also trim the model and draw the implant design on this clean master cast. The implantologist should also mount the model so that the technician can concentrate on using the skills for which he has been trained. The implantologist must assume the responsibility of the

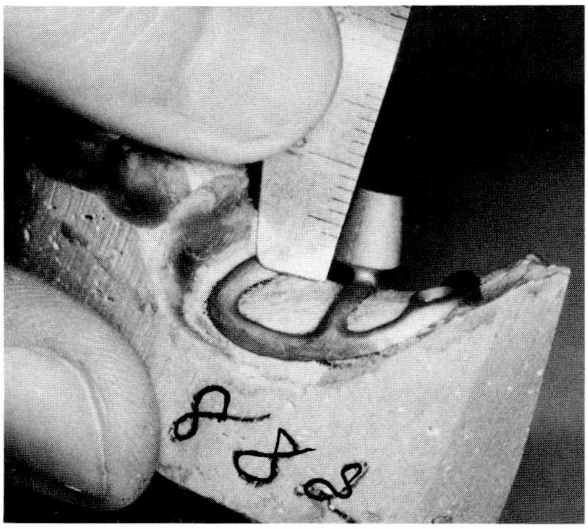

Fig. 5-9. A millimeter ruler is used to measure the length of the implant neck. This dimension should be noted in the written prescription that is sent to the laboratory technician. Here, the length of the neck is being verified after the implant has been delivered to the dentist. In any case, it is important to avoid impingement of the soft tissues by the base of the implant post. The length of the implant neck should be equal to the thickness of the tissue through which the neck protrudes.

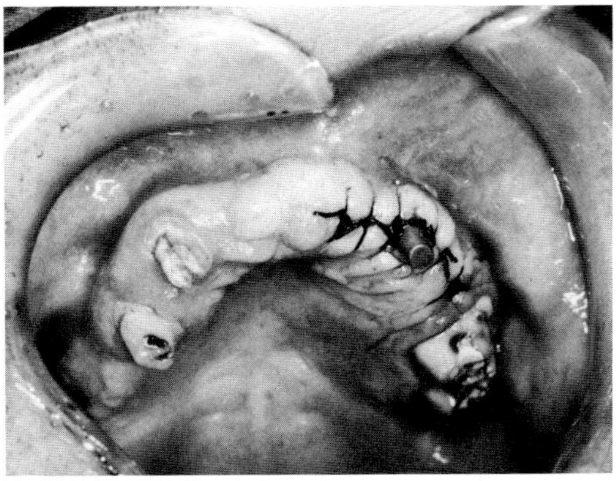

Fig. 5-10. A maxillary unilateral intermediary subperiosteal implant has been inserted. A single incision at the height of the ridge was made, followed by blunt dissection, in order to accommodate the implant frame. This surgical procedure is modest and conservative, compared with that which is needed for the bone impression. The individual sutures approximate the full-thickness flaps, to enable rapid healing. The close adaptation of the gingival cuff around the implant neck is mandatory.

preparatory laboratory stages. Pouring models is not demeaning; to the contrary, it is the duty of the dentist to control as many of the stages involved in dental implantology as is practicable.

INSERTION OF A SUBPERIOSTEAL IMPLANT

Presurgical Preparation

Surgical procedures for the insertion of the implant are usually done 6 to 8 weeks after the bone impression. Prior to the insertion appointment: (a) the sutures from the initial surgery should have been removed about 1 week after taking the bone impression; (b) the patient should have begun the oral intake of appropriate antibiotics; and (c) the dentist should have checked the implant casting. The casting should then be autoclaved and set aside as part of the instrument set-up for insertion. For terminal or intermediary subperiosteal implant abutments, it is advisable to have an acrylic-resin index (or jig) fabricated prior to the insertion. This index can be used during insertion to ensure the proper positioning of the implant on the bone by relating to the prepared natural teeth in the immediate vicinity. The index is readily fabricated with cold-cured acrylic resin. The index may take the form of a simple block or of a carved section of teeth including the pontics. After the insertion of the implant, the index in the form of a carved section including pontics may be luted to the acrylic-resin temporary crowns to form a fixed bridge.

Surgical Reentry and Implant Seating

The incisions for the insertion of the implant should be as long mesiodistally as the initial incision for the bone impression. For implant insertion, however, it is not necessary to make as many horizontal relaxing incisions that were made for the initial bone exposure (Fig. 5-10). Often, with just a single vertical incision and a single small (4- or 5-mm.) mesial-horizontal relaxing incision, adequate blunt dissection can be achieved in order to slide the implant into position.

In cases involving single-abutment implants, the flexible frame may actually snap into place as it is pressed over minor undercut areas. A similar situation may occur in the seating of a complete mandibular subperiosteal implant, because the opposing distolingual aspects of the implant in the mylohyoid ridge areas most often have opposing undercuts. Because of the slight flexibility of the metal frame, mechanical retention may be achieved by snapping the implant into position. This should not be mistaken to be a form of constant pressure on the supporting bone; once seated, the implant should rest passively, with no pressure on the underlying bone. This seating is accomplished with finger pressure. Then, much as one would use a bite stick for appropriate initial pressure in seating a crown casting, a similar procedure is used for seating the subperiosteal implant. A bite stick is placed on the implant post and is tapped gently with a mallet, as are the primary struts at the points at which they radiate from the implant neck. The peripheral border of the implant is then checked with an explorer, much as one would check the marginal seating of a crown on a prepared tooth structure. Sometimes, a primary or secondary strut may not come in close contact with the underlying bone. This most often occurs at the height of a ridge. At this time, such a situation should not be of concern, but it should be noted in order to appropriately evaluate later radiographic checkups.

It is reasonable to assume that the mere exposure of an osseous structure during the impression, with the attendant mechanical manipulations, may cause minor bone resorption, such as occurs during the manipulation of bone in certain periodontal procedures. If the initial implant procedures were executed properly and the subsequent healing was uneventful, then no bone resorption, or only minor resorption at the height of the ridge, should have occurred. Any gross resorption may cause a rocking movement of the implant or a negative seating in the peripheral border areas, rendering the implant useless.

Prior to using the bite stick and mallet, the aforementioned acrylic-resin index may be used. In the case of the complete implant, however, no relationship with adjacent prepared natural teeth can be established. Nevertheless, in view of the many anatomic landmarks and various nuances of bony architecture, there should be no problem in the positive positioning of the frame of a complete implant. Usually, the superstructure removable frame accompanies the complete subperiosteal implant casting. The superstructure removable frame may be placed in the mouth and used for placing pressure along the entire implant frame, from abutment post through abutment post, in order to assist in the seating of the implant casting. Seating is accomplished by facing the patient, placing the forefinger and middle finger of each hand on the superstructure frame, placing the thumb under the chin, and manipulating the frame from the end of either ramus to the symphyseal midline.

The Insertion of Implant Screws

It is not uncommon to have screw holes prepared in the frame to serve as a measure of security, even if they are not used. It is preferable not to use screws, because they may be a source of irritation. In most cases, whether it be in terminal, intermediary, or complete subperiosteal implants, it is not necessary to use screws. As long as a positive mechanical lock is achieved so that there is no lateral or occlusogingival movement of the implant, there is no need to use a screw for retention. The screw should *never* be used on an upper-arch subperiosteal implant because of the hazard of unwittingly placing a screw in a sinus. Screws may be used, primarily for initial stabilization, in two possible areas in the mandible: the external oblique ridges and the anterior symphyseal area.

Once healing is complete, it is a moot point whether the screws serve any long-lasting retentive function. It is not uncommon to find subsequent minor soft-tissue swelling or even minor bone resorption around the screws. In such instances, the screws should be removed, and the healing thereafter should be uneventful. That is not to say that every screw that is placed in the arch should be removed. Many screws can be left in place as if they were an integral part of the implant frame, with no adverse clinical or radiographic reactions.

The screw holes are prepared in the bone by initial entry with a No. 2 round carbide bur. At all stages of the hole preparation, copious amounts of water and intermittent pressure are applied. A No. 701 tapered

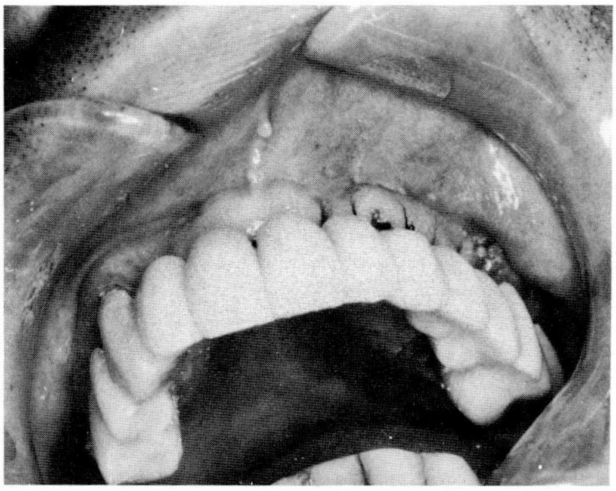

Fig. 5-11. At the same appointment of implant insertion, stabilization has been achieved by means of a customized acrylic-resin complete-arch splint. Certain precautions have been taken: (a) The sutures have been lubricated prior to retainer reline. (b) The base of the implant post has been blocked out with soft wax in order to avoid undercut retention of the retainer reline. (c) The pontics adjacent to the implant retainer have been relieved, to allow for any postoperative swelling of the soft tissues. (d) Cementation by means of a temporary cementing agent has been done on all natural abutment teeth, but not on the implant abutment at this time.

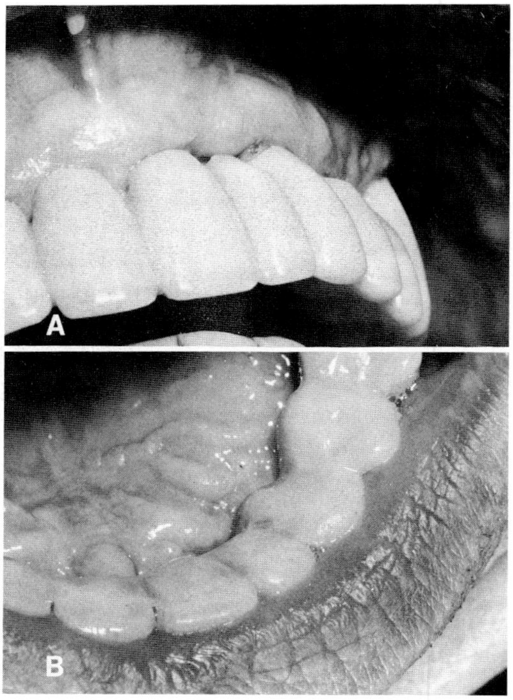

Fig. 5-12. Buccal *(A)* and palatal *(B)* views of an upper-arch provisional acrylic-resin splint in the area of an intermediary subperiosteal implant. The gingival margins of the crown retainer have been purposely kept short of the surrounding soft tissues. The adjacent pontics have been kept shy of gingival adaptation. Major embrasures have accommodated the contours of the healthy soft tissues. (See Plate 5-1.)

carbide bur completes the preparation, and the screw is inserted with a similarly metal-tipped screw driver. The head of the screw should be flush with the soft-tissue aspects of the screw hole in the implant frame.

Closure of the Surgical Incision

The suturing of the soft tissue over the implant frame should be done with utmost care. Either a continuous suture technique or an interrupted individual suture technique can be used. The aim of either technique should be to approximate the opposing flaps in such a manner as to enable healing by primary intention. The most important goal is to establish a snug cuff of tissue around the implant neck (Fig. 5-10). To this end, irrespective of the technique used, individual sutures are usually placed both mesially and distally to the implant neck to establish a proper housing of the soft tissue just below the base of the implant post. The tissues in this immediate area can be properly manipulated and tucked into place with a blunt instrument during suturing. The operator must always remember the critical nature of this area; that is, the soft-tissue cuff should be so tightly adapted around the implant neck that the passage of fluids or debris below the soft-tissue covering is minimized.

THE ROLES OF TEMPORIZATION

Stabilization

An important procedure during the insertion appointment is the temporization of the area being treated (Figs. 5-11, 5-12). For the intermediary or terminal implant,

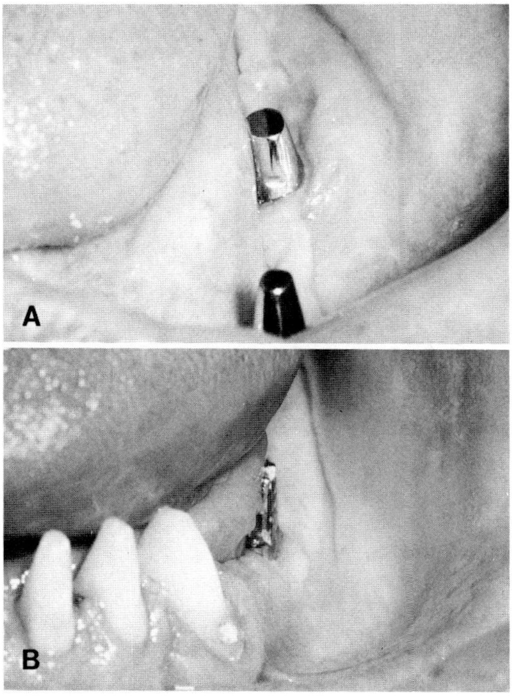

Fig. 5-13. A lower left subperiosteal implant *(A)* and a lower left blade-vent implant *(B)* serve as unilateral abutments in two different cases. Although the tongue was at rest in both individuals at the time these photographs were taken, it is easy to see how pressures can be exerted on these implants toward the buccal aspect. Not only do the sublingual tissues lie against these implants upon removal of the provisional splints, but the musculature of the tongue can play a dynamic role in exerting adverse forces upon nonsplinted implant posts. (See Plate 5-2.)

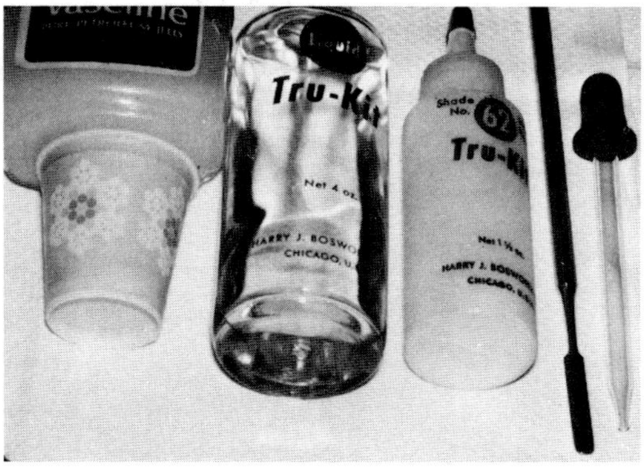

Fig. 5-14. The armamentarium for the chair-side fabrication of an acrylic-resin fixed splint. The liquid and powder are mixed and are allowed to set to a doughy consistency. The fingers should be lightly lubricated with petroleum jelly before handling the acrylic resin to form a workable block.

temporization is a form of stabilization or splinting (see Chap. 10). In the same manner as a fractured limb is immobilized with a cast, the implant is stabilized, not only by its mechanical retention on bone, but also by the placement of a temporary acrylic-resin superstructure, which is joined to a splint that has already been placed on the natural abutment teeth. Thus, the sequence of therapy plays a major role. For example, if a unilateral terminal implant abutment is to be inserted as part of a complete-arch periodontal-prosthetic fixed splint, the natural abutment teeth should have been prepared and temporized prior to the first implant procedure. This sequence not only helps to establish the alignment of the implant post with the path of insertion of the prepared natural teeth, but provides an acrylic-resin splint to which the distal section can be luted in order to stabilize the implant post. The use of this splint is most important in the mandible, where an enlarged area of the tongue, or the sublingual tissues, or a hyperactive tongue can play a major role in transmitting adverse horizontal forces during the initial healing of tissues around the frame of an implant (Fig. 5-13).

The Periodontal Environment and Occlusion

Acrylic-resin temporary fixed bridges are not only for the stabilization of the implants. Temporization should never be relegated to a minor role in implant prostheses. The author prefers to customize acrylic-resin temporary fixed bridges with chair-side carvings made from cold-cured acrylic resin (Fig. 5-14). This maximizes the operator's control of contours, adaptation, occlusion, margins, and periodontal subtleties, thereby providing optimum predictability in carrying any prosthetic treatment from preparation to appliance insertion. If laboratory-processed acrylic-

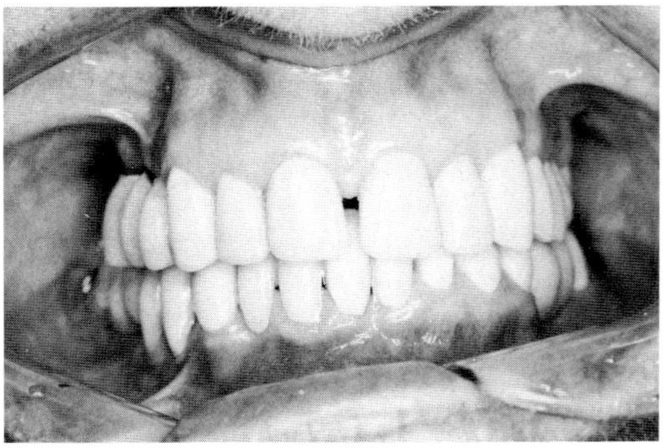

Fig. 5-15. Customized acrylic-resin provisional splints in place throughout the mouth. This case of periodontal prosthesis, with a subperiosteal implant in the area of the upper right first molar, is now ready for the taking of impressions in order to fabricate the castings. The contours and embrasures that have allowed for the maintenance of periodontal health will be simulated as closely as possible in the final prosthesis. (See Plate 5-3.)

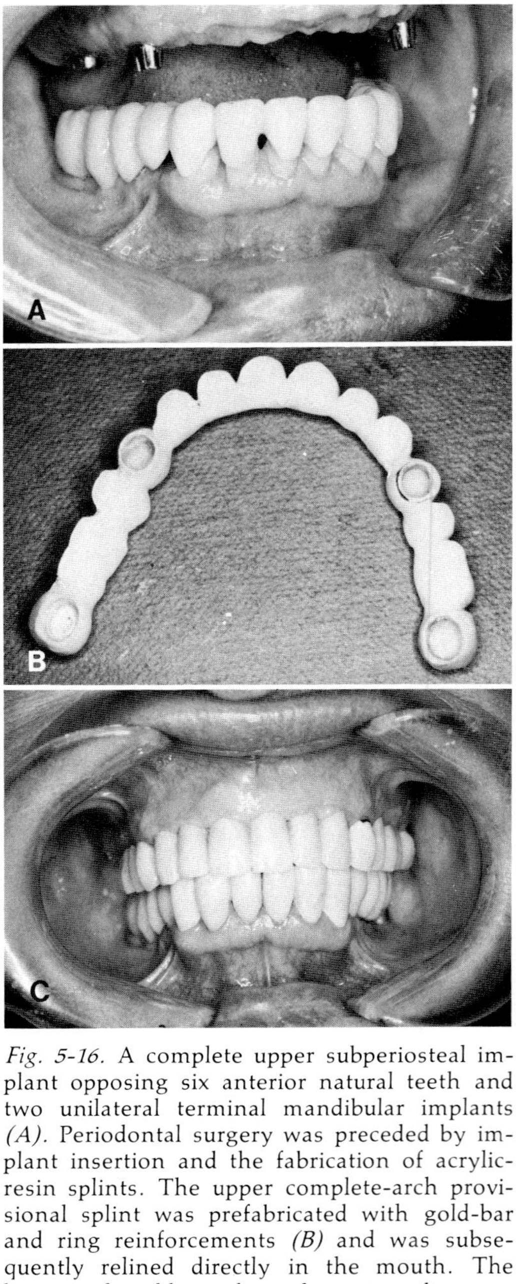

Fig. 5-16. A complete upper subperiosteal implant opposing six anterior natural teeth and two unilateral terminal mandibular implants *(A)*. Periodontal surgery was preceded by implant insertion and the fabrication of acrylic-resin splints. The upper complete-arch provisional splint was prefabricated with gold-bar and ring reinforcements *(B)* and was subsequently relined directly in the mouth. The lower-arch cold-cured acrylic-resin splint was fabricated as a chair-side procedure, followed by treatment by a periodontist *(A)*. After an appropriate healing period, the lower anterior teeth were reprepared, and the splint was relined and recarved *(C)*. (See Plate 5-4.)

resin splints are used, it is important that the dentist reline and recarve the embrasures and curvatures at the chair side.

The acrylic-resin splint should allow the patient to function comfortably and serves as a guide to the design of the final prosthesis. The embrasures and contours of the splint should closely resemble those structures that are encompassed in the final acrylic-veneered or porcelain-fused-to-metal prosthesis (Figs. 5-15, 5-16). The retainers and pontics of the splint should be designed to provide accessibility to soft-tissue areas and to enable proper home care by the patient. It is necessary to establish proper centric relation at the appropriate occlusal vertical dimension at this stage, so that these functional entities can be transferred during the fabrication of the final product. When carved and finished, the temporary fixed splint can be used on a provisional basis. This provisional use of a temporary splint provides an interval during which the operator can constantly evaluate the course of healing. The provisional temporary splint becomes a diagnostic tool. After a discretionary length of time, once the dentist is assured that healing of the tissues around the implant has been successful, the temporization phase will have fulfilled its purpose. *This temporization phase applies as much to the blade im-*

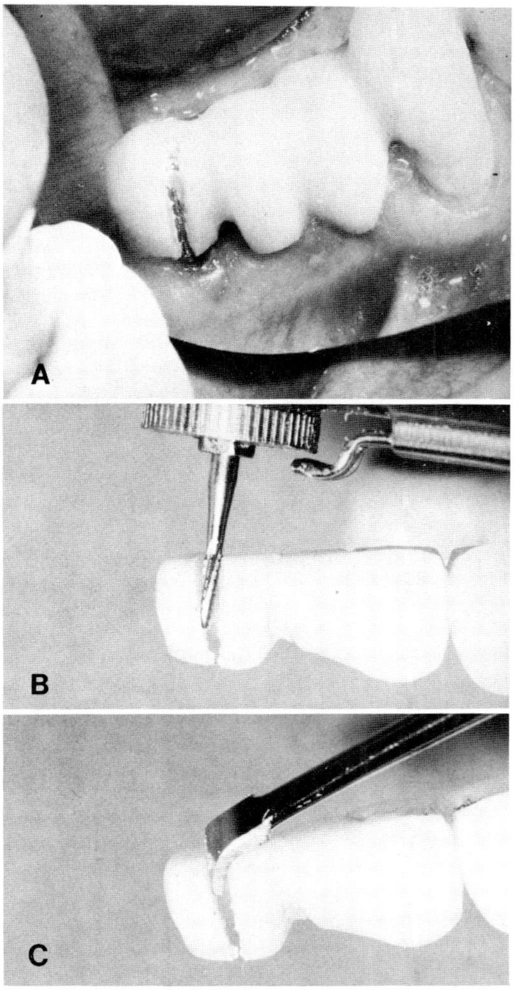

Fig. 5-17. Mirror view of the mandibular left area *(A)*. The temporary acrylic-resin splint has been worn with temporary cementation throughout the course of treatment. At each impression and try-in phase, the buccal and occlusal cuts have been created for the removal of the temporary prosthesis. This is done only on the implant retainer. The use of a carbide bur *(B)*, followed by the separation of the parts and the breakage of the cement seal *(C)* avoid undue forces from being placed on the implant abutment when the temporary splint is removed. The procedures shown in *(B)* and *(C)* are done while the splint is in the mouth, in order to facilitate its removal.

plant as it does to the subperiosteal implant. The temporary acrylic-resin splint is usually left in place a few weeks or a few months before the impressions are registered for the final prosthesis. This splint serves as a valuable diagnostic tool in the form of a provisional prosthesis. Throughout this transitional period, the splint can also aid in the establishment of esthetic patterns, which can be duplicated by the laboratory technician from mounted study models of the temporary acrylic-resin fixed bridges.

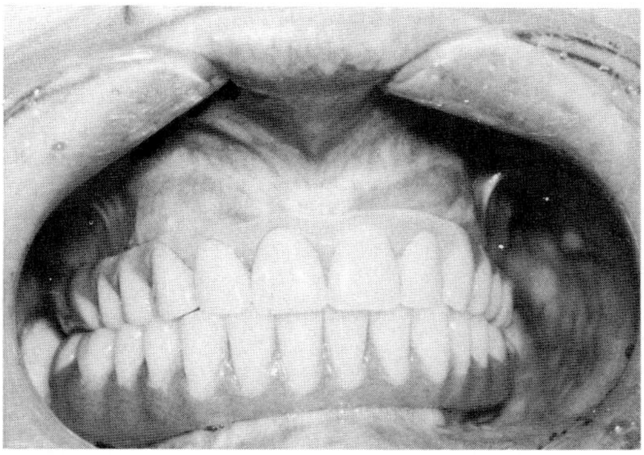

Fig. 5-18. Complete upper-arch and complete lower-arch temporary removable prostheses borne by complete upper- and lower-arch subperiosteal implants. The temporary removable prosthesis is in harmony with the soft tissues in that no impingement by the denture bases occurs upon these tissues. The appliances are maintained in place by the supportive implant posts and do not rely on flange extension for denture retention.

Manipulation of Acrylic Resin

The manipulation of the acrylic resin during insertion should be minimal, in order to prevent the implant from being dislodged. There are appropriate steps that should be taken to minimize trauma to the bone and soft tissues. First, the sutures should be well-lubricated with Mucolube* or Masque.† Second, the area around the neck of the implant should be blocked off with soft wax, so that acrylic resin does not get caught in the undercut area at the base of the implant post. This will also keep the cement from flowing into extraneous areas and interfering with healing.

*Cosmos Dental Products, Inc., New York, New York.

†Harry J. Bosworth Co., Chicago, Illinois.

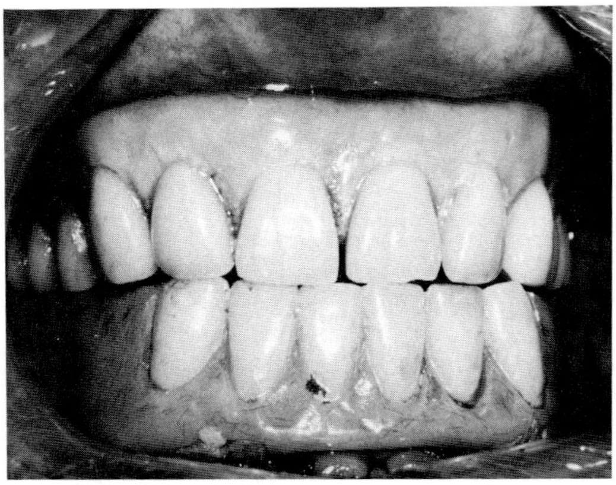

Fig. 5-19. A mandibular temporary removable complete-denture is tried in at the time of implant insertion. In this case, a standard complete upper denture opposes the implant prosthesis. (Note the presence of sutures below the lower denture base.) Prior to the dismissal of the patient at this appointment, the denture will be adapted to the implant posts, and posterior teeth will be carved to the opposing occlusion.

It is wise to keep the gingival margin of the acrylic-resin retainer at least 1 or 2 mm. away from the base of the post. Then, the occlusal aspect of the temporary splint should be placed in proper centric position in relation to the remaining teeth in occlusion. There should be no high spots or any interferences in lateral excursions. It is inappropriate to take the splint out of occlusion in this area, because doing so would create a torque that would tend to lift the retainer on the implant post in an occlusal direction.

Cementation and Removal Procedures for the Temporary Fixed Splint

The temporary prosthesis should be cemented with a smooth-flowing temporary cement such as Temp-Bond* or Opotow.† The removal of the splints at any time throughout treatment should not be done with the reverse-action bridge remover, because this method can harm the implant, is traumatic to the patient, and may break the splint.The most appropriate method of removal is a two-fold procedure (Fig. 5-17). First, a No. 700 carbide straight-fissure bur is used to penetrate the buccal and occlusal aspect of the retainer on each implant abutment. This exposes the cement line. Then, a separating instrument is used to break the cement seal in these areas. Second, hemostat is used to grip the acrylic-resin retainers on the natural abutment teeth; and, in a combined buccolingual and occlusal movement, the cement seal is broken on these teeth. This is readily achieved because of the flexibility of the acrylic resin, combined with the properties of the temporary cementing medium. Before the cement is cleaned out of the retainers, each retainer should be visually examined. There should be no washout. If washouts or plaque accumulations are prevalent in certain areas, the temporary splint may have to be redesigned. The operator can then transfer this design of knowledge to adjust the design of the final prosthesis. It is easy to place cold-cured acrylic resin in the seams created at the implant retainers, using the brush technique, in order to repair the opened areas. These areas are then relieved of any flash and are polished, prior to recementation at the end of the appointment.

The Temporary Removable Prosthesis

In cases that require placement of a complete removable superstructure denture on a complete implant, the principles of temporization are similar to those for fixed splinting (Fig. 5-18). At the time of insertion of the complete implant, a temporary complete-arch denture is inserted. If this were not done, the exposed implant posts could be traumatized by the opposing occlusion.

The temporary denture should be made of acrylic resin and should occlude harmoniously with the opposing arch. This transitional denture can be made just subse-

*Kerr Sybron Corp., Romulus, Michigan.
†Opotow Dental Manufacturing Corp., Brooklyn, New York.

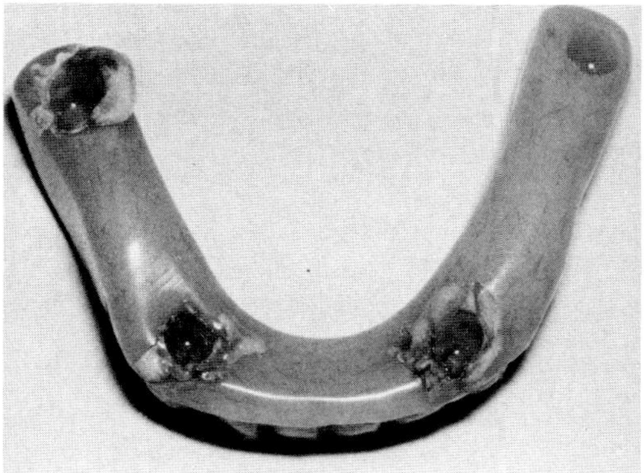

Fig. 5-20. The base of a temporary removable prosthesis for a complete lower implant. Three of the four post areas have been relined with cold-cured acrylic resin. The flash material will be removed after the fourth post space has been relined. It is safe to concentrate on the reline of one post area at a time, to prevent the acrylic resin from setting in an undercut.

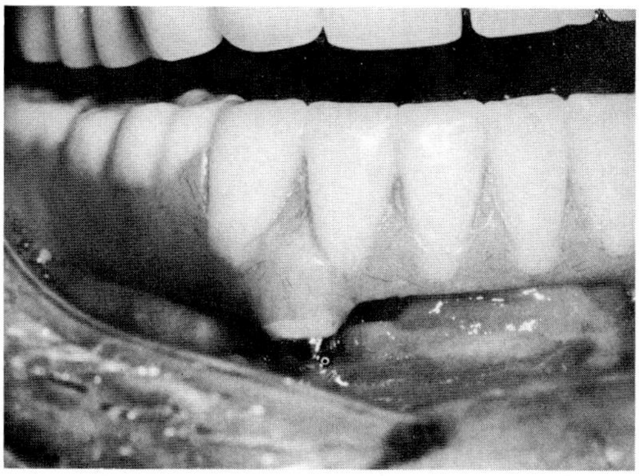

Fig. 5-21. The temporary removable complete implant denture 1 month after insertion. The relined post areas have been kept away from the base of the implant posts. The denture base has been grossly relieved to allow for postsurgical swelling. The permanent removable denture will conform more closely to the contours of the residual ridge.

quent to the fabrication of the implant frame, using the same mounted articulation model obtained from the surgical wax bite. It is best to have only the six anterior teeth in place, with full acrylic-resin posterior segments (Fig. 5-19). In this manner, a customized occlusion can be established in the posterior areas with cold-cured acrylic resin at the time of insertion of the implant.

There are three points of concern in the use of the transitional complete denture.

1. The denture must sit passively over the four abutment posts. In order to accomplish this, it is necessary to relieve the undersurface of the post areas of the denture and to reline these areas with cold-cured acrylic resin (Figs. 5-20, 5-21). The operator must be careful to withdraw the denture before the acrylic resin sets completely, so that there is no binding to the implant posts. It is important to realize that the implant posts primarily stabilize the implant denture against lateral movement. It is not as critical to stabilize against vertical displacement.

2. The posterior acrylic-resin areas are relieved on their occlusal surfaces (Fig. 5-22). Wafers of cold-cured white acrylic resin are placed on these surfaces. The patient is then instructed to and aided in closing his mouth in centric relation with the appropriate occlusal vertical dimension noted in the anterior section. The posterior areas are carved to correspond to the occlusal anatomy of the opposing arch during this transitional phase of treatment.

3. It is imperative that the denture be borne only by the posts, and *not* by any soft tissues (Figs. 5-23, 5-24). There is no need for any flanges or for any adaptation to the residual ridges. Any pressure on the residual ridges would only compress the soft tissues between the framework of the subperiosteal implant and the base of the removable superstructure. All stability is achieved by the implant posts. At this stage of temporization, the areas that are closest to the ridges should be overrelieved, to allow for postoperative swelling of tissues without impingement of the denture base on these tissues. Also, as in the case of the temporary fixed retainers, the margins around the implant posts of the removable denture should be shy of the bases of the implant posts.

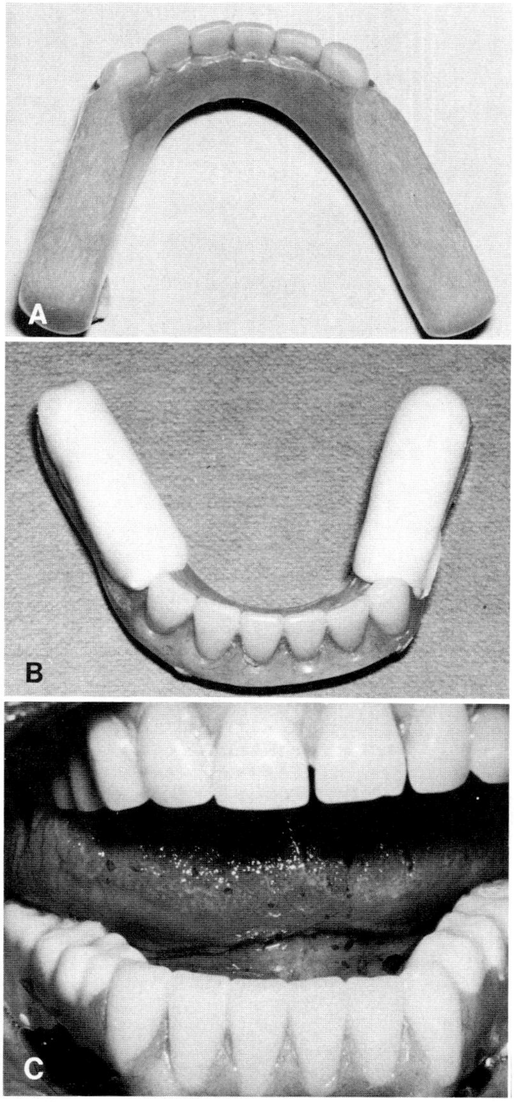

Fig. 5-22. After the reline of the implant posts at the base of the denture, the posterior occlusal surfaces are stripped of the pink processed base *(A)*. Wafers of cold-cured acrylic resin are placed in the posterior areas *(B)*, and the appliance is inserted in the mouth to determine occlusal patterns for chair-side carving. The posterior occlusion has been carved and polished for the temporary removable complete denture *(C)*.

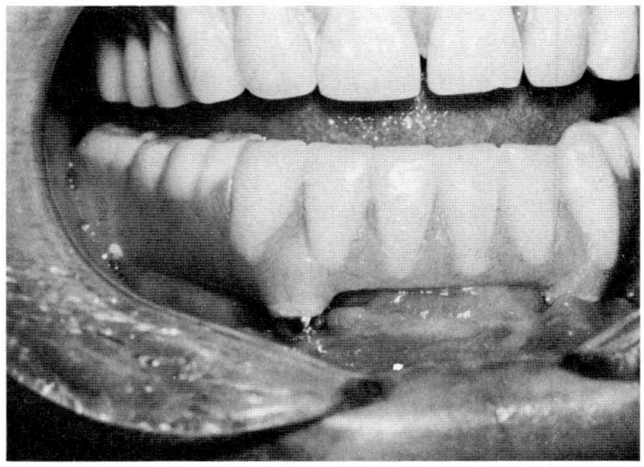

Fig. 5-23. Anterior view of the temporary removable complete implant prosthesis. Although the base has been relieved to allow for postoperative swelling, it may be relined after initial healing, during this transitional phase.

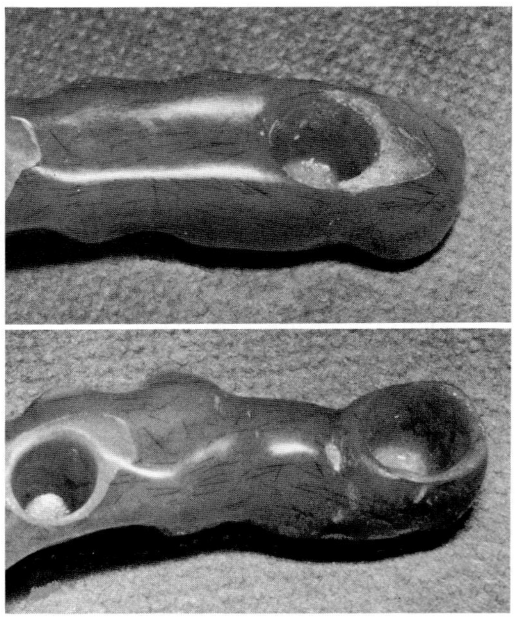

Fig. 5-24. A temporary removable prosthesis may have to be relieved extensively around the implant posts, in order to achieve passive housing of the gingival cuff around the implant post. In this manner, relief of both the base and the contours around the posts prevents impingement on the critical underlying soft tissues.

BIBLIOGRAPHY

Amsterdam, M., and Fox, L.: Provisional splinting—principles and techniques. D. Clin. North America, March, 73-99, 1959.

Beder, O. E., and Eade, G.: An investigation of tissue tolerance to titanium metal implants in dogs. Surgery, *39:*470-473, 1956.

Bernier, J. L., and Canby, C. P.: Histologic studies on the reaction of alveolar bone to Vitallium implants. J. A. D. A., *30:*188-197, 1943.

Bodine, R. L., and de Hernandez, C. J.: Mastication strength with implant dentures as compared with soft-tissue-borne dentures. J. Pros. Dent., *22:*479-486, 1969.

Harris, R.: The reaction of the oral tissues to implants. Australian D. J., *18:*143-151, 1973.

Mack, A. O.: A clinical and histologic assessment of subperiosteal implants. J. Pros. Dent., *30:*516-520, 1973.

Mann, F.: The oral surgeon's role in implant dentures. J. Oral Surg., *29:*799-904, 1972.

Mears, D. C.: Limitations of available prosthetic metals. J. of Metals, *16:*229-231, 1964.

Natiella, J. R., Armitage, J. E., Meenaghan, M. A., and Greene, G. W.: Tissue response to dental implants protruding through mucous membrane. Oral Sc. Rev., *5:*85-105, 1974.

Peters, W. J., and Jackson, R. W.: Reaction of bone to implanted materials. Oral Sc. Rev., *5:*56-67, 1974.

Picton, D. C. A., Johns, R. B., Wills, D. J., and Davies, W. I. R.: The relationship between the mechanisms of tooth and implant support. Oral Sc. Rev., *5:*3-22, 1974.

Ross, I. F.: The relation between periodontal therapy and fixed restorative care. J. Periodont., *42:*13-20, 1971.

Scales, J. T., Winter, G. D., and Shirley, H. T.: Corrosion of orthopaedic implants: screws, plates and femoral nail-plates. J. Bone Joint Surg., *41-B:* 810-820, 1959.

Smith, D. C.: Materials used for construction and fixation of implants. Oral Sc. Rev., *5:*23-55, 1974.

Smith, N. J. D.: Radiographic testing of metal castings for use in dental implants. J. Pros. Dent., *30:*335-338, 1973.

Weinberg, S., and Moncarz, V.: Response of oral tissues to implants totally covered by mucous membrane. Oral Sc. Rev., *5:*68-84, 1974.

Wickstrom, J. K.: Surgical implants—their mechanical and environmental problems. J. of Materials, *1:*366-372, 1966.

6 The Subperiosteal Implant—The Histology of the Hard and Soft Tissues

Roy L. Bodine, D.D.S., and Raymond J. Melrose, D.D.S.

THE NATURE OF THE HISTOLOGIC STUDY

Because subperiosteal implants have been in use for a longer period of time than blade implants, time-tested studies of subperiosteal implants in humans have been possible. Specifically, in 1965 and 1971, mandibles were obtained from two patients with subperiosteal implant dentures that had been in place for 12 and 15 years, respectively; these two patients died from unrelated causes. Prior to these studies, not much was known about the tissues surrounding subperiosteal implant abutment posts and the buried structural frames that had been in place for many years; although, clinically, the oral tissues of many implant denture patients have appeared healthy after 10 or 15 years or more.

Patient X received a cobalt-chromium (Vitallium) subperiosteal implant denture in August, 1953 (Figs. 6-1, 6-2). More than 12 years later, in October, 1965, he died of metastatic carcinoma of the pancreas. Other than slight recession at the left anterior abutment post, his oral tissue was clinically healthy when he died, and there had never been any associated swelling, inflammation, pain, or discomfort (Figs. 6-3, 6-4). (Detailed reports on Patient X have been previously published—Bodine and Mohammed: 1969, 1970, 1971.)

Patient Y received his Vitallium subperiosteal implant denture in May, 1956 (Figs. 6-5, 6-6). Fifteen years later, in Sep-

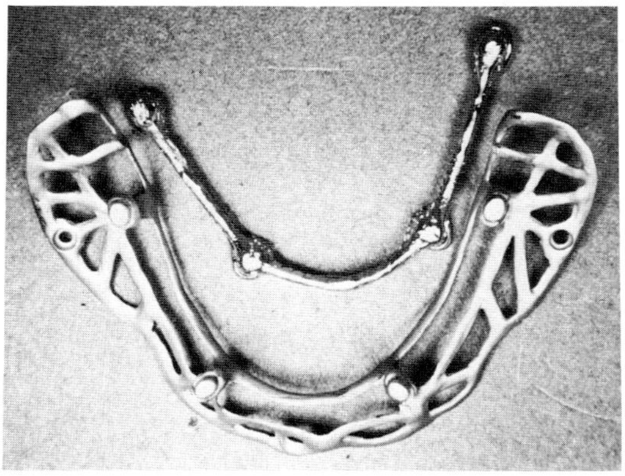

Fig. 6-1. An implant denture that was inserted in August, 1953. According to present standards, it had excessive metal in the mucosa-covered substructure *(bottom.)* (Figs. 6-1 to 6-4 pertain to Patient X.)

tember, 1971, he died suddenly from a massive coronary occlusion. During the first 13 years after insertion of the implant, his oral tissues appeared clinically healthy, and his implant denture was symptom-free (Figs. 6-7, 6-8). During his last 2 years, his general health had deteriorated as a result of several minor heart attacks and because he drank well water that had been polluted with seepage from a barrel of weed killer. Every 2 or 3 months, he experienced periods of discomfort and swelling around the posterior abutments posts, usually on the right side. Sometimes there was also inflammation around one or both

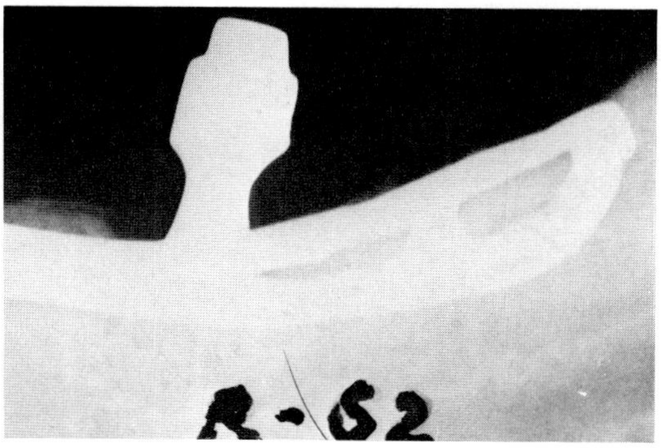

Fig. 6-2. An apical radiograph taken 10 years after implant insertion showed normal bone underlying the implant at one of the distal portions.

Fig. 6-3. One year after implant insertion, the oral tissues around the four implant abutment posts and over the substructure framework were found to be clinically normal.

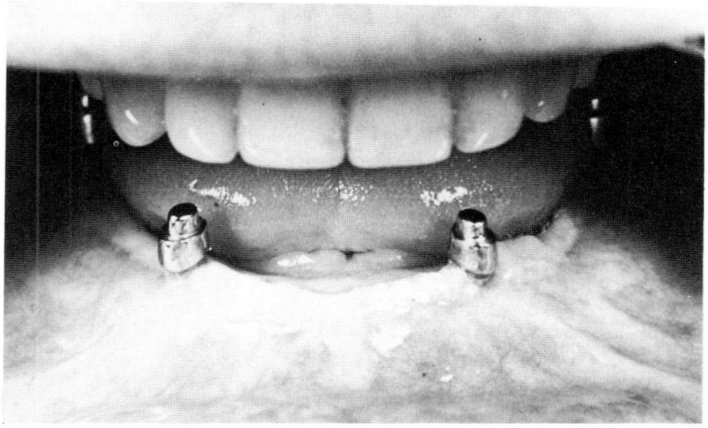

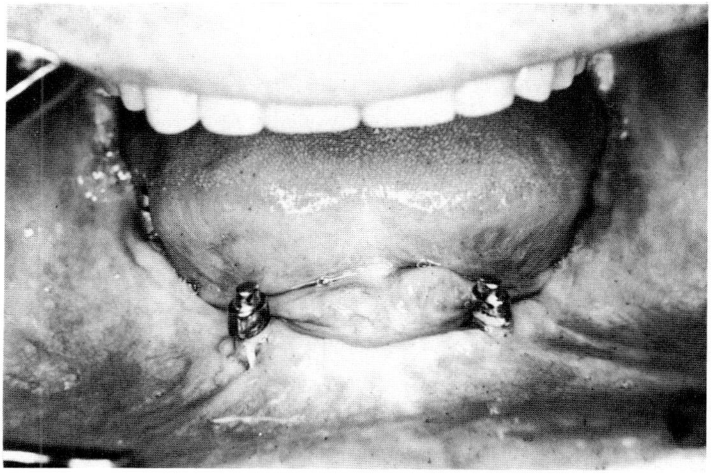

Fig. 6-4. Ten years after implant insertion, the tissues over and around the implant metal were clinically normal, although there was some labial tissue recession at the right anterior abutment post.

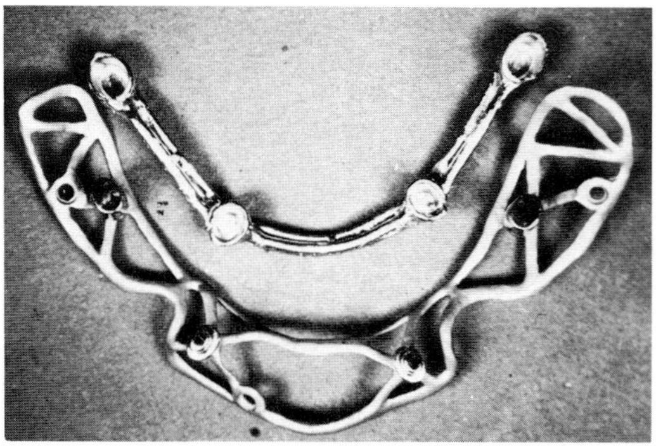

Fig. 6-5. Implant denture inserted in May, 1956, *(bottom),* was similar to a present-day subperiosteal implant frame design. (Figs. 6-5 to 6-8 pertain to Patient Y.)

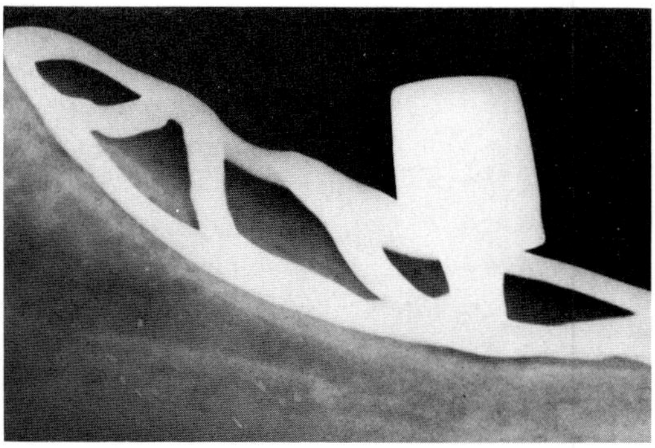

Fig. 6-6. An apical radiograph of a posterior segment of the implant, taken 14 years after insertion, showed normal bone underlying the implant area, and *slight* bone resorption.

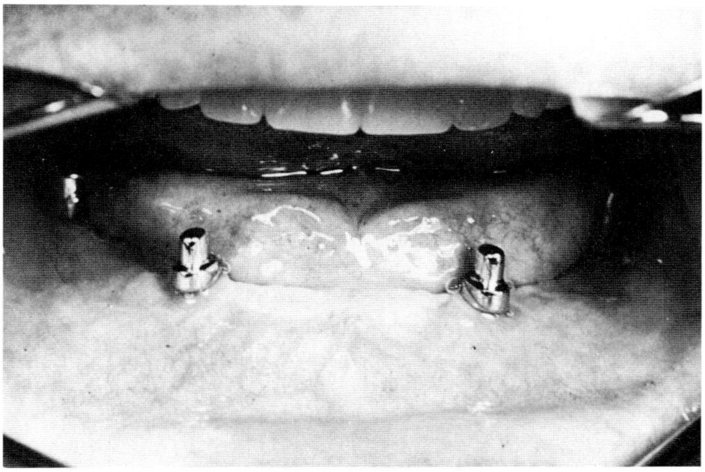

Fig. 6-7. One year after implant insertion, the oral tissues around the four implant abutment posts and over the substructure framework were found to be clinically normal.

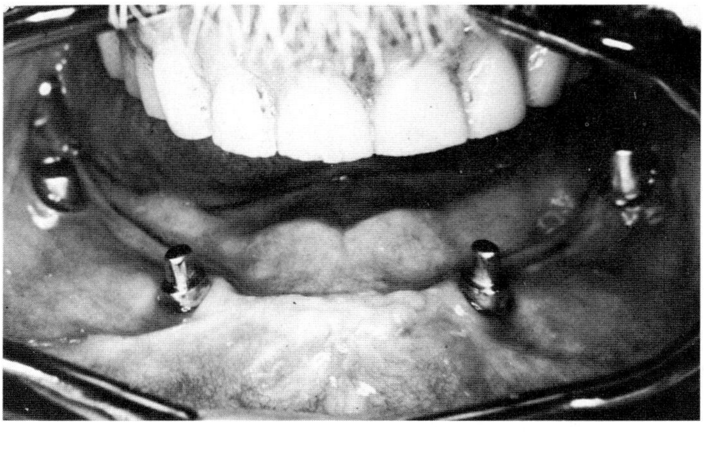

Fig. 6-8. Fourteen years after implant insertion, the oral tissues over and around the implant were clinically normal.

anterior abutment posts. These conditions, which rapidly subsided after a few days of antibiotic treatment, were prevented subsequently by the prophylactic administration of oral antibiotics.

THE METHODOLOGY OF IMPLANT PREPARATION FOR HISTOLOGIC STUDY

The mandible of Patient X was removed a few hours after death, sectioned into quadrants (each containing an implant abutment), and placed in 10 per cent formalin.* Some sections were decalcified for several months in 5 per cent nitric acid and some in 5 per cent formic acid, after which the overlying tissues were cut and the implant metal removed. Smaller sections were then vacuum-embedded in paraffin, serially sectioned at 10 μm., and stained with hematoxylin and eosin.

The mandible of Patient Y was also removed within a few hours after death and was sectioned into halves. The left half of the mandible was prepared.† It was decalcified with Decal, after which the implant metal was traumatically removed. Representative serial sections, stained with hematoxylin and eosin, were done.‡

The right half of the mandible was similarly prepared and studied.§ It was cut into ten 15-mm. sections with a large chrome-cobalt alloy "cut-off" wheel. Every other section was decalcified with Decal. The metal from the decalcified sections was removed. The decalcified sections were then embedded by the usual procedures, sectioned at 6 to 10 μm., and stained with hematoxylin and eosin.

*The mandible of Patient X was studied at the University of Puerto Rico School of Dentistry.
†At Brooke U.S. Army General Hospital in San Antonio, Texas.
‡At the University of Southern California School of Dentistry.
§At the University of Southern California.

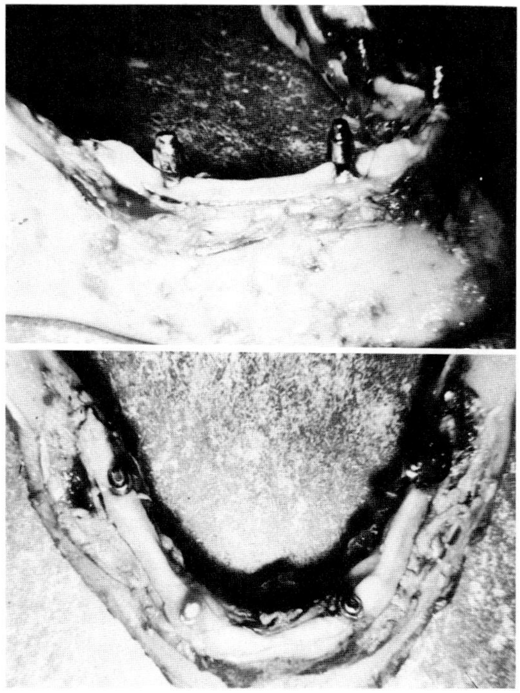

Fig. 6-9. The entire mandible, with implant in place, was removed after the patient died from pancreatic carcinoma in October, 1965; i.e., 12 years and 2 months after insertion. (Figs. 6-9 to 6-22 pertain to Patient X.)

The alternate undecalcified sections, with the implant substructure intact, were dehydrated and were placed in a thin solution of methacrylate monomer activated

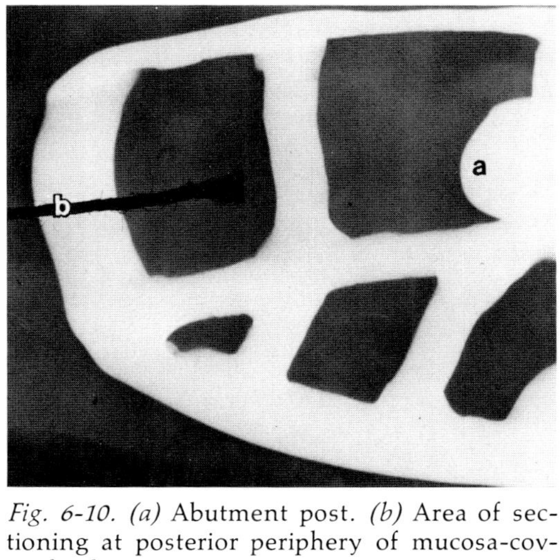

Fig. 6-10. (a) Abutment post. *(b)* Area of sectioning at posterior periphery of mucosa-covered substructure.

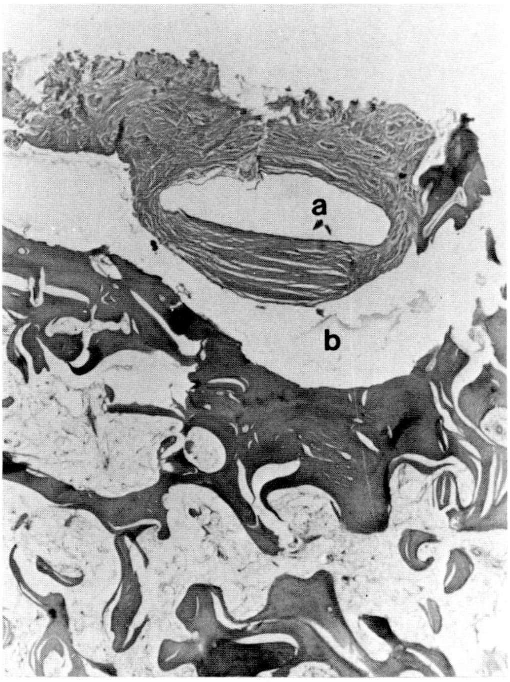

Fig. 6-11. Space *(a),* which had been occupied by implant metal, was surrounded by compressed collagenous fibrous connective tissue. Space *(b)* was an artifact of sectioning; in-vivo normal bone was in contact with fibrous connective tissue. There were no epithelial or inflammatory cells in this area, which was quite a few millimeters away from the mucosa-penetrating abutment posts. (× 25)

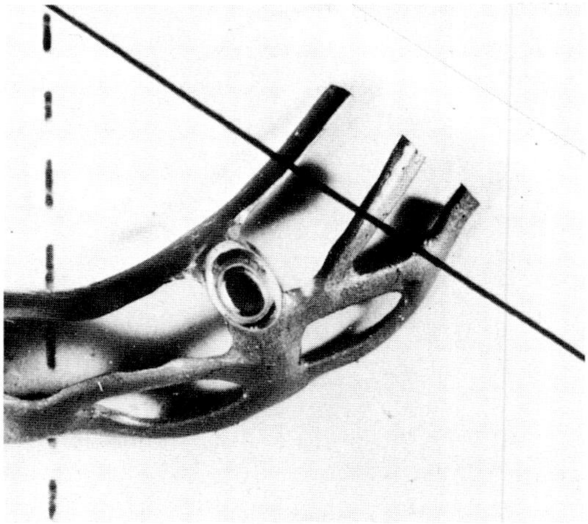

Fig. 6-12. Dotted line shows midline of mandible. Solid line shows direction of sectioning near the mental foramen.

with 0.5 g. of benzoyl peroxide per 100 ml. After 48 hours, the undecalcified sections were embedded in partially polymerized methyl methacrylate and were polymerized slowly at 30 degrees Celsius (° C.). After radiographic study, the exact position of the implant metal and the desired line of sectioning were determined. The plastic blocks were sectioned through soft and hard tissue and implant metal, using a Gillings-Hamco Thin Sectioning Machine with a rotating diamond-edge blade. The 200-μm. sections were stained for from 2 to 3 minutes in Paragon-1301 at 58 degrees Celsius (° C.) and mounted on glass slides with Permount. (Patient X: Figs. 6-9 to 6-22; Patient Y: Figs. 6-23 to 6-33.)
(Text continues on p. 91.)

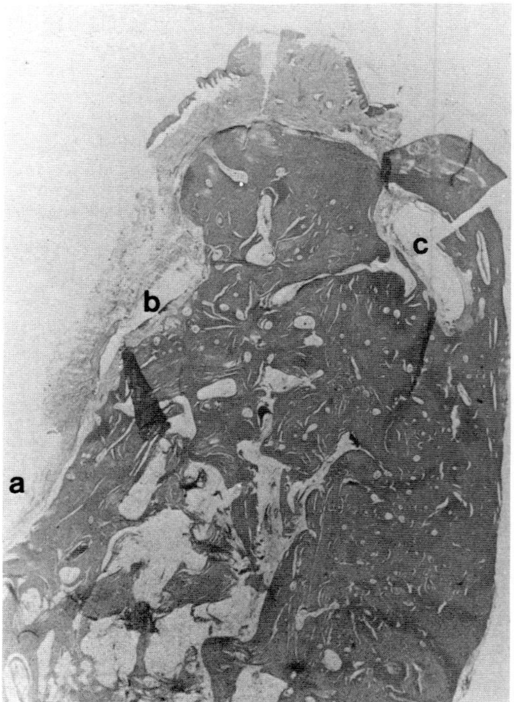

Fig. 6-13. *(a)* Buccal area of the peripheral border of the frame. *(b)* Buccal secondary strut. *(c)* Lingual area of the peripheral border of the frame, which was completely surrounded by normal bone; there were no epithelial or inflammatory cells in these areas. (× 4)

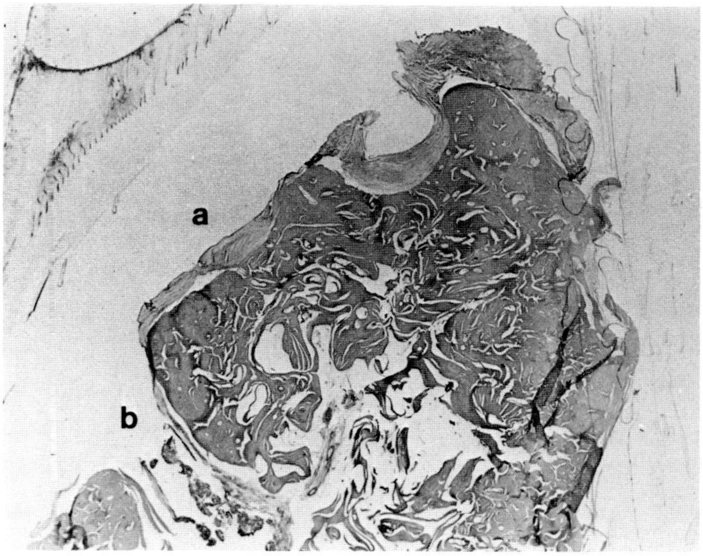

Fig. 6-14. Buccal section of the peripheral border of the frame *(a)* did not change in relation to the mental foramen *(b)* in 12 years. (× 4)

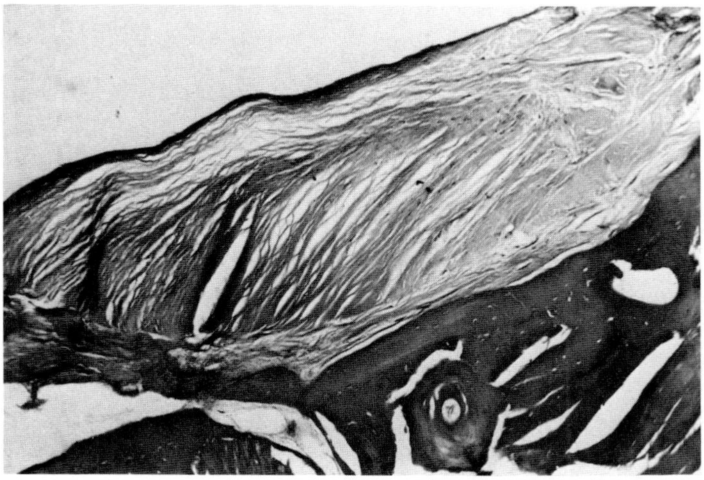

Fig. 6-15. Fibrous tissue under the section of the peripheral border of the frame showed variation in fiber orientation to bone and implant surfaces. (Fig. 6-13 at higher power, × 100)

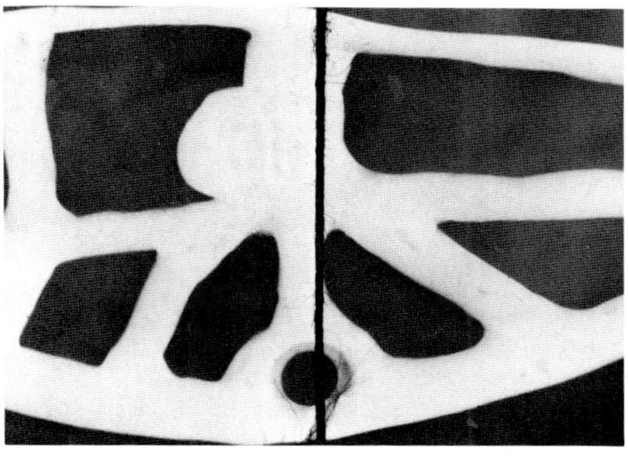

Fig. 6-16. Solid line shows area of sectioning passing directly through the right posterior abutment post, the continuous primary strut, and the unused buccal screw hole.

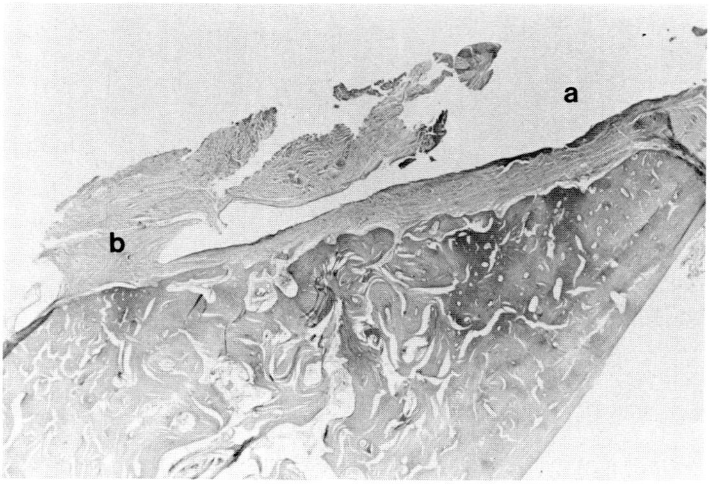

Fig. 6-17. Space that was occupied by implant metal extends from the area of the abutment post *(a)* to beyond the fibrous tissue *(b)* that occupied the unused buccal screw hole. (× 5)

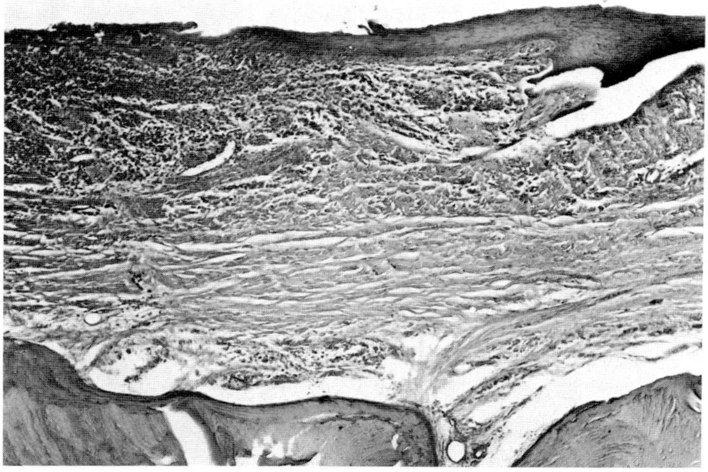

Fig. 6-18. A thin layer of epithelial cells covered the fibrous tissue for a distance of up to 3 mm. beyond the abutment post. Considerable chronic inflammation was found in the part of the fibrous tissue covered by the thin epithelial layer. (× 40)

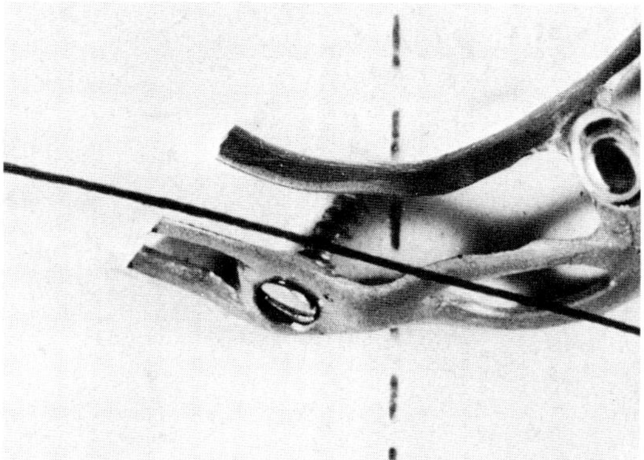

Fig. 6-19. Dotted line shows midline of mandible. Solid line shows direction of serial sectioning through the space occupied by the 7-mm. screw.

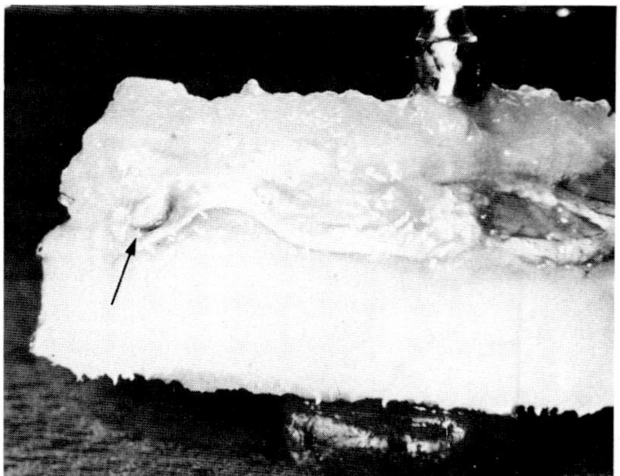

Fig. 6-20. Screw *(arrow)* was raised from its seating and was found to be completely covered by mucosa. It was immobile and free of stress for most of the 12 years it was in place.

Fig. 6-21. Cross section of the area near the surface of the space that was occupied by the screw *(s)* shows that this area was surrounded by normal-appearing cortical bone. (× 10)

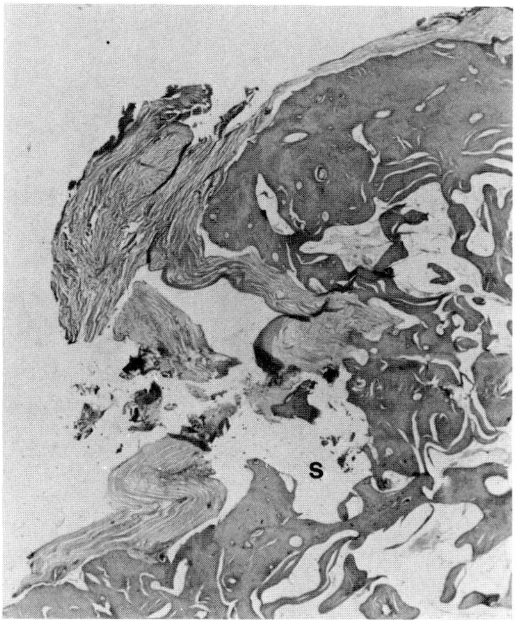

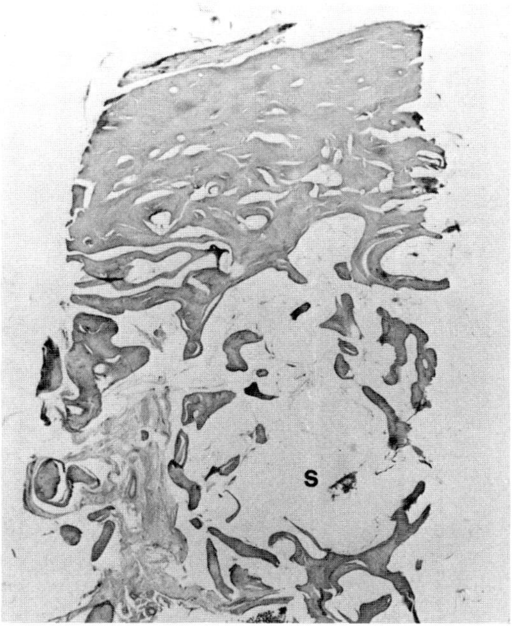

Fig. 6-22. Cross section of the area near the deep end of the space that was occupied by the screw *(s)* shows that this area was surrounded by normal-appearing cancellous bone. (× 10)

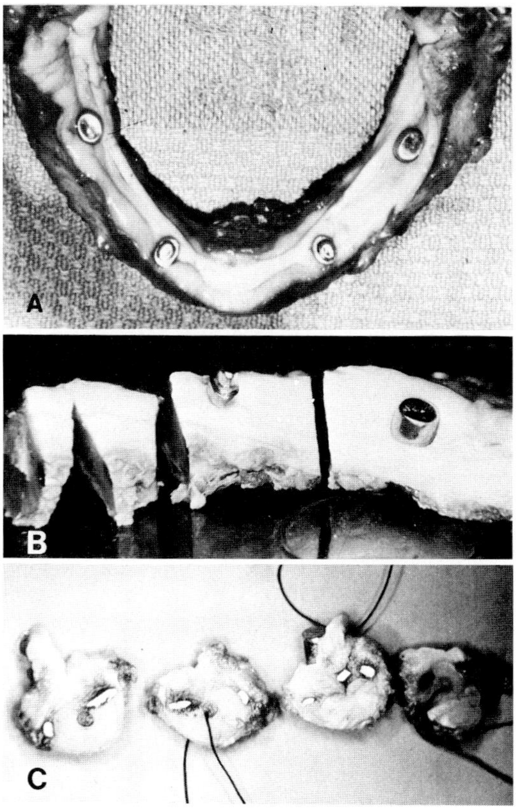

Fig. 6-23. The mandible with the implant in place *(A)* was removed after the patient died; 15 years and 4 months after implant insertion. Each half of the mandible was separated into major portions *(B),* which were further divided into smaller specimens *(C).* (Figs. 6-23 to 6-33 pertain to Patient Y.)

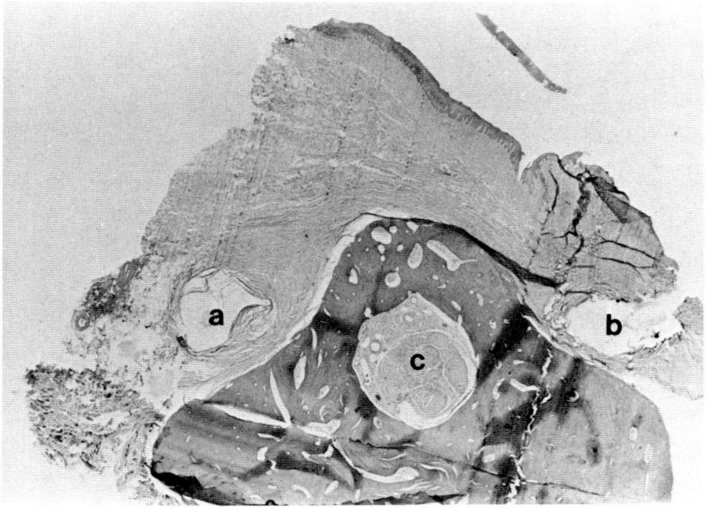

Fig. 6-24. Sections of areas that were quite a few millimeters away from the oral mucosa-penetrating abutment posts showed implant metal spaces covered by normal oral tissues. *(a)* Buccal area of peripheral border of frame. *(b)* lingual area of peripheral border of frame. *(c)* neurovascular canal. (× 3)

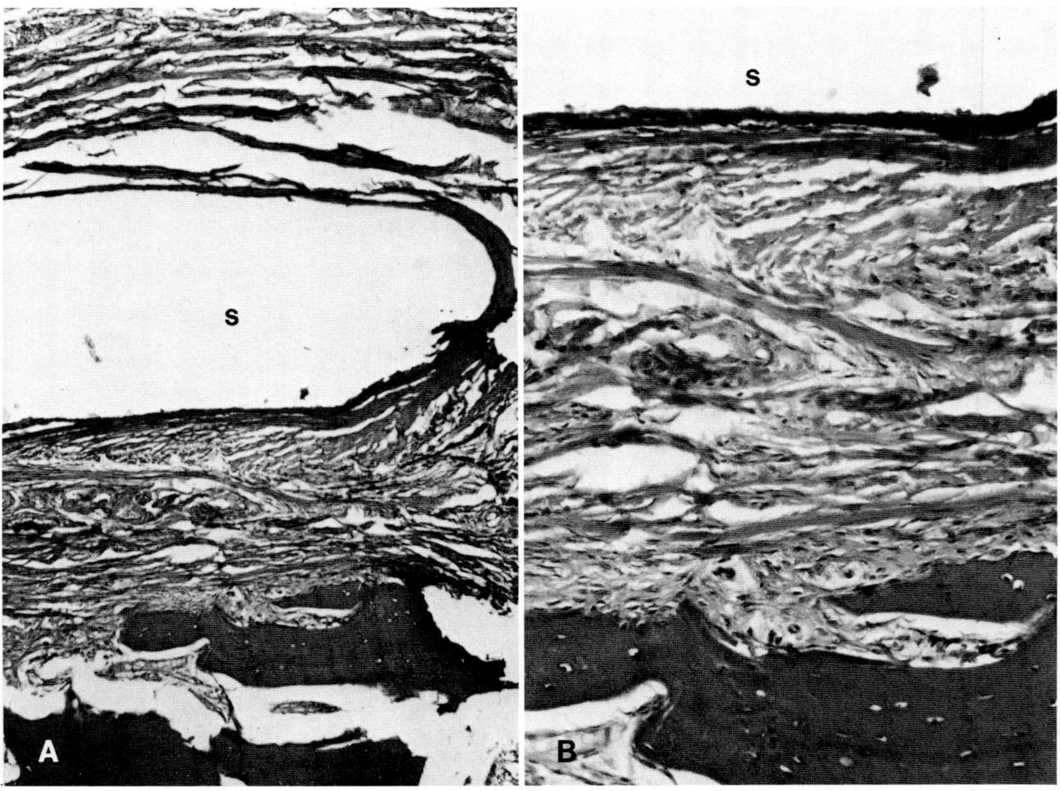

Fig. 6-25. Implant metal space *(S)* was bounded by modified compressed typical implant fibrous connective tissue, with the remaining fibrous connective tissue resting on normal bone. As in Patient X, there were no epithelial or inflammatory cells beyond 3 mm. from any implant abutment post penetration. (A × 40; B × 100)

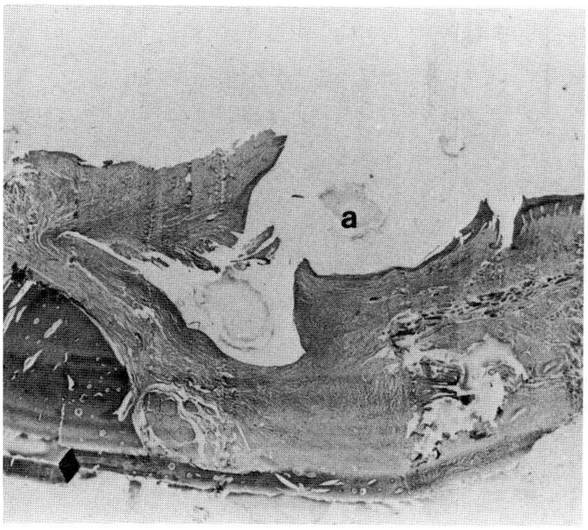

Fig. 6-26. Sections, such as this one, through areas of penetrating implant abutment posts *(a)* showed an epithelial lining extending under the abutment posts and for a few millimeters along the connecting struts. (× 20)

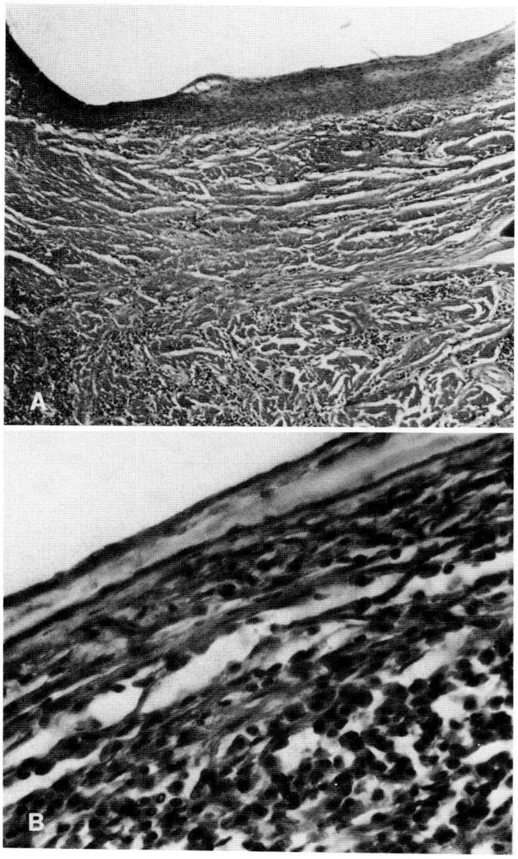

Fig. 6-27. Areas under and near the mucosa-penetrating abutment necks showed flattened squamous epithelium and chronic inflammation in the submucosa. This again was similar to the conditions found near the abutment posts in Patient X. (A × 40; B × 250)

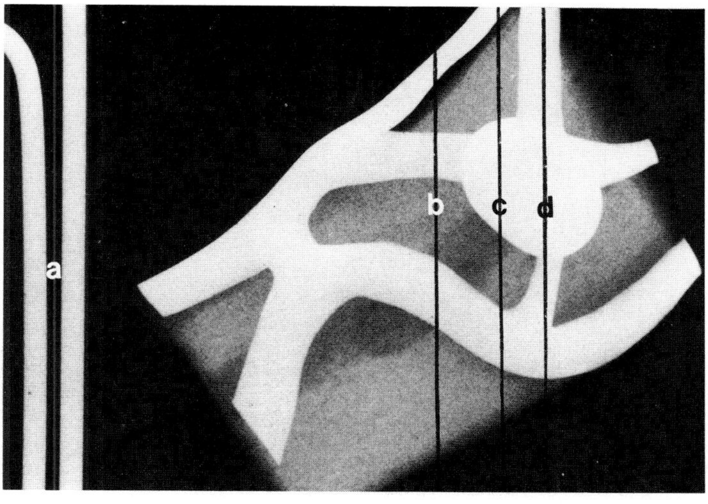

Fig. 6-28. Radiograph of plastic-embedded, undecalcified specimen, with metal implant resting undisturbed on mandibular bone, that was positioned to "diamond-cut" sections parallel to the paper clip *(a)* at left. Vertical lines *(b)*, *(c)*, and *(d)* show location of three sections made. (× 5)

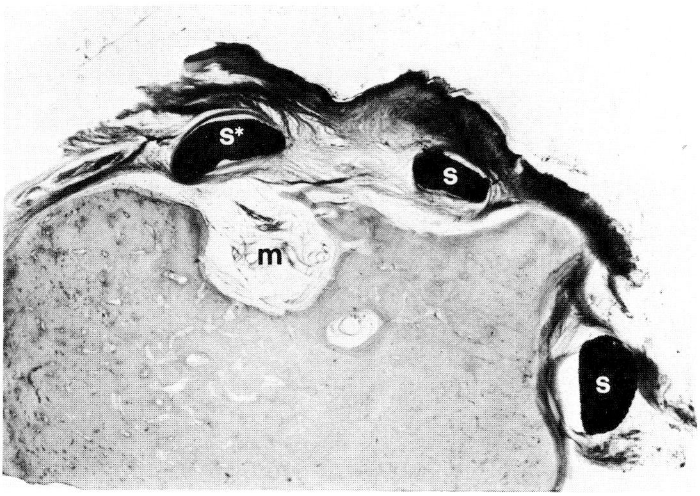

Fig. 6-29. Section through area of line *(b)* in Figure 6-28 showed three sections of metal implant substructure *(s)* surrounded by implant connective tissue. The buccal area of the peripheral border *(s*)* is near the mandibular canal *(m)* near the mental foramen. (× 5)

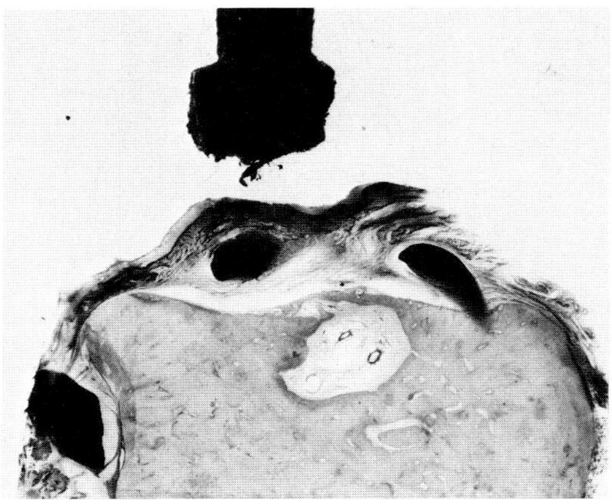

Fig. 6-30. Section through area of line *(c)* in Figure 6-28 at the edge of the abutment post shows three sections of metal substructure and a portion of the implant abutment neck *(top)*.Diamond-cut sections were nearly 200 μm. thick, allowing visualization of tissue-implant relations but not providing high-power microscopic detail of connective tissues. (× 5)

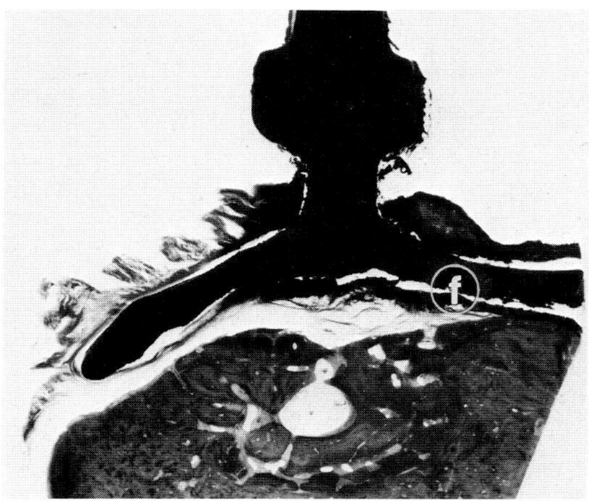

Fig. 6-31. Section through area of line *(d)* in Figure 6-28 showed continuous primary struts extending labially and lingually from the abutment post. Some metal debris was deposited to the right of the abutment post, as the diamond disk rotated from upper left to lower right. The space between the metal and the tissue *(f)* was an artifact caused by fracture of the section after cutting. (× 5)

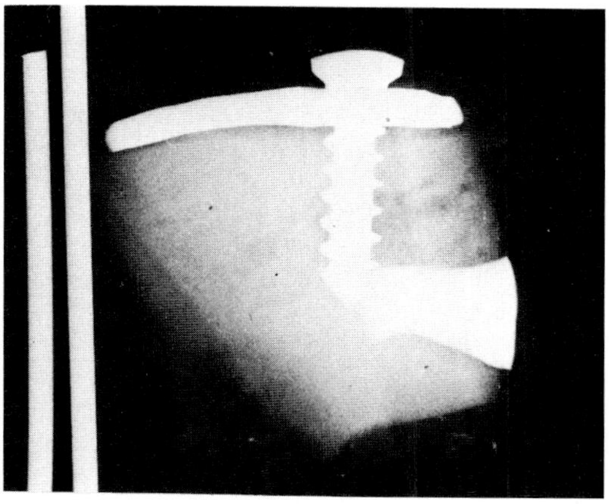

Fig. 6-32. Radiograph of a plastic-embedded specimen, with an undisturbed 7-mm. anterior screw. The screw was positioned for cutting directly through its long axis. (× 10)

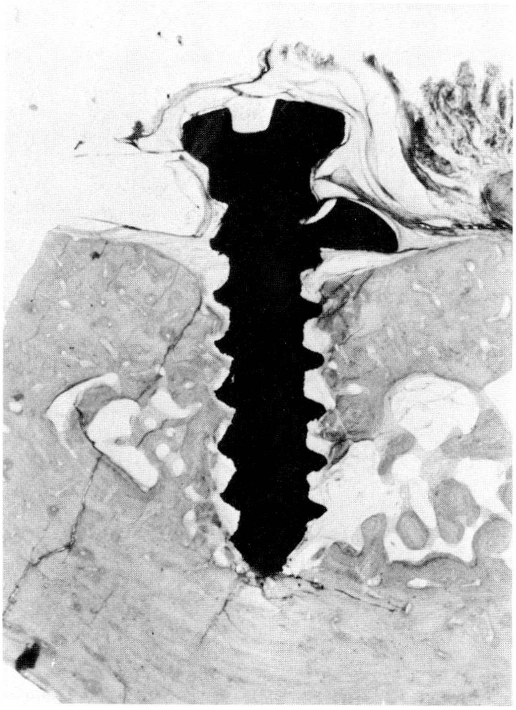

Fig. 6-33. Bone was separated from the threads of the screw by a thin connective-tissue membrane. This differed from Patient X, whose bone seemed to have been in direct contact with the screw threads. (× 25)

HISTOLOGIC OBSERVATIONS

Typical Implant Fibrous Tissue

The tissues surrounding the buried metal frames, in all areas more than 3 mm. from abutment post penetrations, were without epithelial or inflammatory cells. The tissues that were in direct contact over, around, and under buried implant metal were almost always altered fibrous tissues, characterized by flattened, compressed fibers and cells with elongated nuclei. This compressed tissue, only a few cells thick and supported by normal fibrous tissue, may be described as *typical implant fibrous connective tissue* (peri-implant membrane). This tissue certainly was in intimate relationship with the implant metal, and the complete absence of inflammatory cells was an indication of tissue tolerance and adaptability.

Bone Resorption Related to the Subperiosteal Implant ("Settling")

Little significant bone resorption ("settling") occurred. There was 0.5 to 1.0 mm. of bone resorption under the implant abutment posts. The crevice underlying the implant post was lined by squamous epithelium that covered moderately inflamed and thickened fibrous connective tissue. The bone beneath the buried metal frame of the implant substructure generally showed a slight indentation, but there was little or no microscopic evidence of active resorption. This indentation probably represented adaptation to masticatory stress transmitted through the metal substructure. During the 12 and 15 years, respectively, that Patients X and Y wore implant dentures, both patients exerted strong masticatory stress on their implants; however, no appreciable loss of occlusal vertical dimension occurred. This was additional evidence of minimal "settling" of the implant.

Adaptations of the Surrounding Bone

There was a tendency for bone to grow over some struts and portions of the peripheral border of the implant frame in areas of low stress between the abutment posts, especially on the lingual aspect of the bicuspid region. A considerable amount of bone completely surrounded the peripheral border of the implant frame. Although there was generally a thin layer of fibrous tissue (the typical subperiosteal implant fibrous connective tissue) between the bone and the implant metal, movement of the implant under masticatory stress was never noticeable. The bone growth over the lingual aspect of the peripheral border of the frame could not have been caused by the implant sinking into the bone, because the buccal aspect of the peripheral border of the frame had not measurably changed position in relation to the adjacent mental foramen, when compared to the design of the implant substructure drawn on the original cast of the bone surface.

The Implant Abutment Crevice

A normal gingival tooth crevice contains saliva and oral bacteria, and is lined by squamous epithelium that is supported by mildly inflamed fibrous tissue. The implant abutment crevice is similar to, but *not* the same as, a normal tooth crevice. The epithelium of the implant post crevice differs in that it extends around and under the abutment post and terminates 2 to 3 mm. along the primary abutment struts. The implant crevice, as the tooth crevice, is infiltrated by varying amounts of chronic inflammatory cells. It seems that as long as *a tight cuff of relatively immovable tissue* surrounds the penetrating abutment post, a generally effective seal against the ingress of fluids and bacteria is maintained. The structural nature and the mechanical completeness of this seal are not known.

THE SIGNIFICANCE OF HISTOLOGIC EVIDENCE

Based on detailed histologic studies of the previously mentioned two mandibles with clinically healthy implant dentures that were in place for 12 to 15 years, a number of valid conclusions can be drawn.

1. The epithelium did not grow downward along the primary struts to encapsulate the peripheral frame. In all areas that were more than a few millimeters away from abutment post penetrations, there was complete absence of epithelium and no evidence of inflammation.

2. The fibrous tissue that was in contact over, around, and under the buried metal generally was altered, as evidenced by flattened, compressed fibers and cells with elongated nuclei. This compressed tissue—consisting of a few layers of flattened elongated cells and supported by normal fibrous tissue—may be described as "typical implant fibrous connective tissue" (peri-implant membrane).

3. The tissue around the implant abutment post resembled the tissue in a normal gingival tooth crevice, with some important differences. After a number of years, epithelial tissue extended under the abutment post and a few millimeters along the metal struts. This downgrowth of epithelium was slow and had progressed only 2 or 3 mm. from the abutment post penetrations during the 12 to 15 years.

4. Inflammatory cells found in the tissues adjacent to the epithelialized space under and around the implant abutment post were comparable to those found around gingival sulci of natural teeth. The mild degree of chronic inflammation was considered normal and did not, in itself, indicate serious deterioration.

5. The penetrations of implant necks through the soft tissues were sources for the beginning of epithelium extension along the metal of the substructure. (Only four abutment posts, essential to adequately support the implant denture and distribute its stresses to the bone, should be used. Additional exposure of the metal substructure should be avoided.)

6. No significant bone resorption, and therefore minimal sinking of the implant into the bone, occurred in these patients. The amount of "settling" that occurred,

with no measurable loss of occlusal vertical dimension, was minimal, considering the strong masticatory habits of these male patients during 12 to 15 years.

7. There was a tendency for bone to grow over those portions of the peripheral borders of the implant frames that bore the least amount of stress, especially in the second bicuspid–first molar region.

8. These subperiosteal implant dentures were remarkably well-tolerated by the patients' tissues during the 12 to 15 years before these patients died. There was no histologic evidence of damage to the approximating and adjacent tissues.

SUBSTRUCTURE METAL EXPOSURES

Every penetration of the oral mucosa by implant metal should be regarded as a potential source of inflammation and epithelial extension. Therefore, in a good implant denture, the only metal exposures should be the four essential penetrating abutment posts. However, an undesirable, small, secondary metal exposure, in an area of relatively immovable tissue that can be kept clean, detracts only slightly—if at all —from the long-term prognosis.

ORAL HYGIENE

Proper oral hygiene for implant dentures is essential. The thoroughness of oral-hygiene measures, the amount of calculus formation, and individual systemic factors all affect the resistance to inflammation of the tissues around the abutment post. These factors appear to also affect the rate and extent of undesired overextension of the epithelial crevice. Individual patient differences can be expected. Oral fluids and debris must infiltrate, to some extent, the epithelialized tract that forms over the healthy tissues that are under the implant abutment posts. Home use of a water-spray device *may* be indicated for cleaning around an implant abutment post, but it is only secondary to the mandatory use of a toothbrush. The jet of pulsating water of the water-spray device should irrigate the surface around the abutment post efficiently, but the water-spray device must be used *in conjunction with* brushing and mouth rinsing. Excessive water pressure must be avoided because it might lacerate epithelium, initiate inflammation, and actually stimulate epithelial growth. The safest method of cleaning and of plaque removal is direct massage with a soft toothbrush (see Chap. 12, Home Care).

BIBLIOGRAPHY

Benson, D., Reisbick, M. H., and Furstman, L. L.: Ceramic-coated subperiosteal implants. Part II. Clinical and histologic evaluations. J. Pros. Dent., *31:*323-328, 1974.

Bodine, R. L., and Mohammed, C. I.: Histologic studies of a human mandible supporting an implant denture. J. Pros. Dent., *21:*203-215, 1969.

———: Implant denture histology: gross and microscopic studies of a human mandible with a 12-year implant denture. D. Clin. North America, *14:*145-159, 1970.

———: Histologic studies of a human mandible supporting an implant denture. Part II. J. Pros. Dent., *26:*415-423, 1971.

Gershkoff, A.: Implant dentistry, problems and progress. D. Survey, *47:*24-26, 1971.

Mentag, P. J.: Subperiosteal prosthesis after skin graft into the oral cavity. D. Clin. North America, *14:*169-172, 1970.

Weinman, J. P.: Biological factors influencing implant denture success. J. Implant Dent., *2:*12-15, 1956.

7 The Endosteal Blade-Vent Implant

Charles A. Babbush, D.D.S., M.Sc.D.

RATIONALE AND DESIGN

The endosteal blade-vent implant provides the dentist with another dimension in the placement of artificial abutment teeth in an edentulous ridge. Whereas the subperiosteal implant should be placed only on cortical bone, the blade-vent implant allows the operator to make use of bony support that may be completely alveolar or may be partly alveolar and partly compact.

The blade-vent implant is most often used in areas where teeth should probably not have been extracted in the first place. Specifically, (a) the tooth was extracted from a periodontally sound environment; (b) the tooth was extracted prematurely, without the benefit of periodontal treatment; (c) the tooth was indiscriminately removed, without the possibly beneficial use of endodontic treatment; and (d) any and all were premature extractions, without recourse to any attendant dental treatment. Naturally, a situation may have existed in which it was impossible to treat the remaining tooth by means of root-canal therapy. Any of these situations may have been precursors of edentulous ridges that have varying amounts of alveolar bone remaining.

In the completely edentulous arch containing substantial amounts of remaining alveolar bone, the use of blade-vent implants may be precluded in favor of well-executed procedures for complete dentures. As mentioned in Chapters 1 and 2, however, patients with psychological adversities with respect to complete removable prostheses may be candidates for complete-arch blade-vent implants. More often than not, the blade implant is indicated in edentulous areas that are bounded by natural teeth that may serve as either intermediary or terminal abutments for a fixed prosthesis.

Because alveolar bone could not sustain the pressures placed upon it under the frame of a subperiosteal implant, an intraosseous type of implant, the endosteal blade-vent implant, was eventually designed. The very nature of establishing a channel within bone, for the blade-vent implant, precludes the use of an impression technique and allows for the use of prefabricated implants of various designs in anatomical areas different from those areas that are acceptable for the insertion of subperiosteal implants. The implant described in this chapter (manufactured by Implants International) is an endosteal blade implant that was designed and has been fabricated since late 1971. In order to fabricate such implants that would conform to anatomic variations, the scientific efforts of dentists, laboratory analysts, metallurgists, and mathematical frequency statisticians were coordinated. This analysis included the measurement of numerous panoramic radiographs. The data that derived from this analysis was plotted on graphs. The study of the graphs led to implant designs that took into account anatomic entities such as the borders of the maxillary sinus, the inferior alveolar canal, the mental foramina, the roots of adjacent teeth, and the crestal variations of the alveolar ridges. Sharp angles within the frame design of an intra-osseous implant may cause adverse stresses to be placed within the confines of the supportive bone. Therefore, these angles have been modified in the design, to conform to the gentle curves and blunted angles of the anatomic structures. The blade implant, like the subperiosteal implant, is designed to accommodate the soft tissues and to ensure the proper vertical distribution of occlusal forces.

Aside from criteria previously established for all implant case selections (see Chap. 2), the elective use of blade-vent implants has additional specific guidelines:

1. Endosteal blade-vent implants should not be used as abutments for a removable prosthesis. The exception to this rule is the complete-arch overdenture.
2. Endosteal blade-vent implants should not be used as a single-tooth replacement unless these implants are splinted to at least one adjacent natural-tooth abutment.
3. Blade implants are well suited for any distal extension case that has sufficient depth of bone to avoid the sinus in the maxilla and the inferior alveolar canal in the mandible. These implants are especially useful for the long intertooth span that otherwise would not support a rigid fixed prosthesis.
4. In completely edentulous arches, a prosthesis should be supported by a minimum of four implants.

NOMENCLATURE OF AN ENDOSTEAL BLADE-VENT IMPLANT

The following terms relate to a specific, prefabricated blade implant (Fig. 7-1). This in no way precludes the use of other prefabricated blade implants, as long as they are consistent with the goals of sound oral implantology. It is for the sake of clarity, universality, and consistency with the technique of insertion subscribed to herein that the following terms are described.

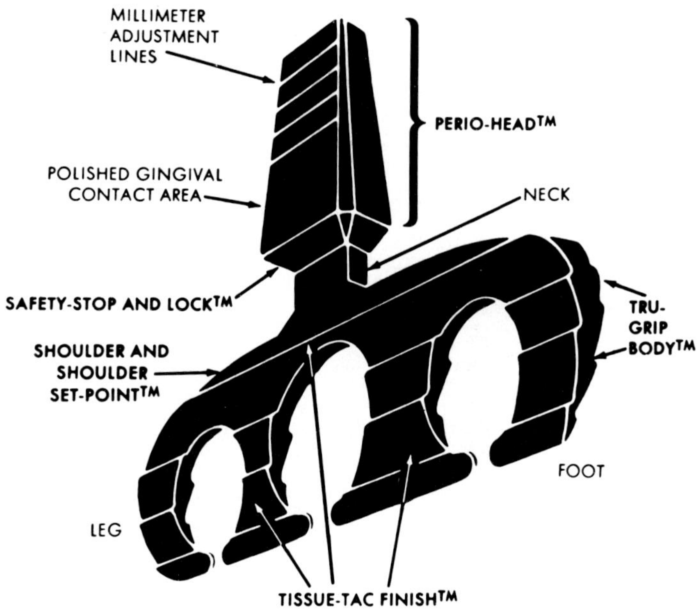

Fig. 7-1. A blade-vent implant. The basic entities are the post (Perio-Head), the neck, and the frame (body). This particular design includes a nomenclature that is endemic to the manufacturer (Implants International, Division of Oratronics Inc., New York, New York).

The Implant Post and Neck

The implant post (Perio-Head) and neck originate at the crest of the residual osseous ridge. The neck is designed to allow for as short and as uneventful a healing period as possible after insertion. It is also designed to facilitate plaque control, by the elimination of as many undercuts as possible. The length, taper, and faceting of the post (head) are designed for proper retention and cementation of the crown. The specific posts (heads) described herein have score marks that are 1 mm. apart and that serve as guides for the removal of any excess occlusal length. This allowance is for clearance to accommodate the anatomic occlusal carvings of the superimposed crown retainer.

The Base of the Implant Post

The base (automatic Safety-Stop and Lock) of the implant post is designed to prevent the overseating of the implant base within the encompassing bone. It is also designed to position the shoulder of the implant under the crest of the alveolar ridge. When wedged within the buccal and lingual confines of bone, the base of the intra-osseous implant post should aid in providing adequate stabilization and lack of mobility.

The Implant Frame

The implant frame (Tru-Grip Body) is designed to give as much contact as possible with bone. The frame has multiplaned configurations. The frame is also designed to provide immediate retention within the intra-osseous housing at the time of insertion. This is in addition to the stability that is achieved by the gentle wedging of the implant base within the confines of the buccal and lingual plates of bone. The slim, 1.2-mm. width at the shoulder affords a margin of safety even in narrow ridges, because this width can prevent excessive encroachment on the buccal and lingual bony plates.

The Shoulder Set-Points aid in the correct placement and seating of the implant below the crest of the ridge. They are readily engaged by a pointed instrument and serve as positive seats for the Titanium-Tipped Shoulder Set-Point Instrument. Thus, the implant can be placed in its predetermined position with exactness, without damaging the crestal bone by slippage of a seating instrument on the shoulder of the frame.

INSTRUMENTATION FOR THE INSERTION OF THE ENDOSTEAL BLADE-VENT IMPLANT

In order to prevent the possible contamination of the implant by incompatible metals, it is suggested that inserting instruments with titanium tips be used. These instruments, along with those usually necessary for mucoperiosteal and osseous surgery, constitute the complete endosteal blade-vent implant armamentarium (Fig. 7-2):

1. Local Anesthetic Syringe with Anesthesia. The standard Carpules of anesthesia with epinephrine are used as infiltration and blocks where necessary. Also, in healthy individuals, such anesthesia used in the site of surgery, even during the procedures, can aid in hemostasis. A surgical bite-block may also be used intra-orally in order to maintain the mouth in an open position.

2. Fine-Line Tissue Marker is used to mark the line of initial incision, as well as the outline of the channel on the exposed ridge.

3. Scalpel and Handle. The standard handle and No. 15 blade should be used.

4. Periosteal Elevators. The standard sized elevator is used for the reflection of a full-thickness flap of mucoperiosteum. The heavy-duty elevator is more ideally utilized in the maxilla, where the tissues are of a thicker and denser nature. Both elevators are blunted on the edges to prevent the laceration of the flap, and both are curved to follow the osseous curvatures.

5. Shaping and Trimming Rongeurs. The bayonet design of the rongeurs permits clearance of the natural teeth. The rongeurs are used to remove the thin spinous spurs of bone that are so often found on the crest of the residual alveolar ridge.

6. Multi-Access Tissue Scissors are used to trim the irregular tissue tags that may, but should *not,* result from the incisions. Removal of these tags prevents clogging of the bur during the channeling procedure and allows a finer approximation of the tissues during suturing, which is conducive to uneventful healing.

7. Manual and Automatic Tissue Retractors. The curved and blunted fingers of the tissue retractors gently yet securely engage the mucoperiosteal flaps. The manual retractors are usually used in pairs. On the lingual flap, the flat area of the retractor adjacent to the fingers helps to protect and restrain the tongue and sublingual tissues. The bayonet feature of the automatic retractor provides clearance around the anterior teeth. The bayonet feature of the retractor is most efficiently used in the mandible.

8. Implant Channeling Burs. The 700 XL and 700 XXL carbide surgical burs are used. The 700 XL bur is used for initial entry into the bone, and the 700 XXL bur is used for the preparation of the deeper aspects of the intra-osseous groove. The dimensions of each bur match the buccolingual dimension of the frame (body) of the implant.

9. Channel Curette and Depth Gauge. The Channel Curette is used to remove debris from the prepared intra-osseous channel. The markings on the curette are identical to those on the implant frame, in order to facilitate measurement comparisons.

10. Implant Carrier. This instrument is used to carry the implant to the channel, and, although not necessary, it is especially useful in the posterior aspect of the mouth. It is preferable, however, if accessibility allows, to carry the implant to and into the seating site between the thumb and index finger. This allows the operator to better feel the implant in place at various stages of insertion.

11. The Single-Headed Seating Instru-

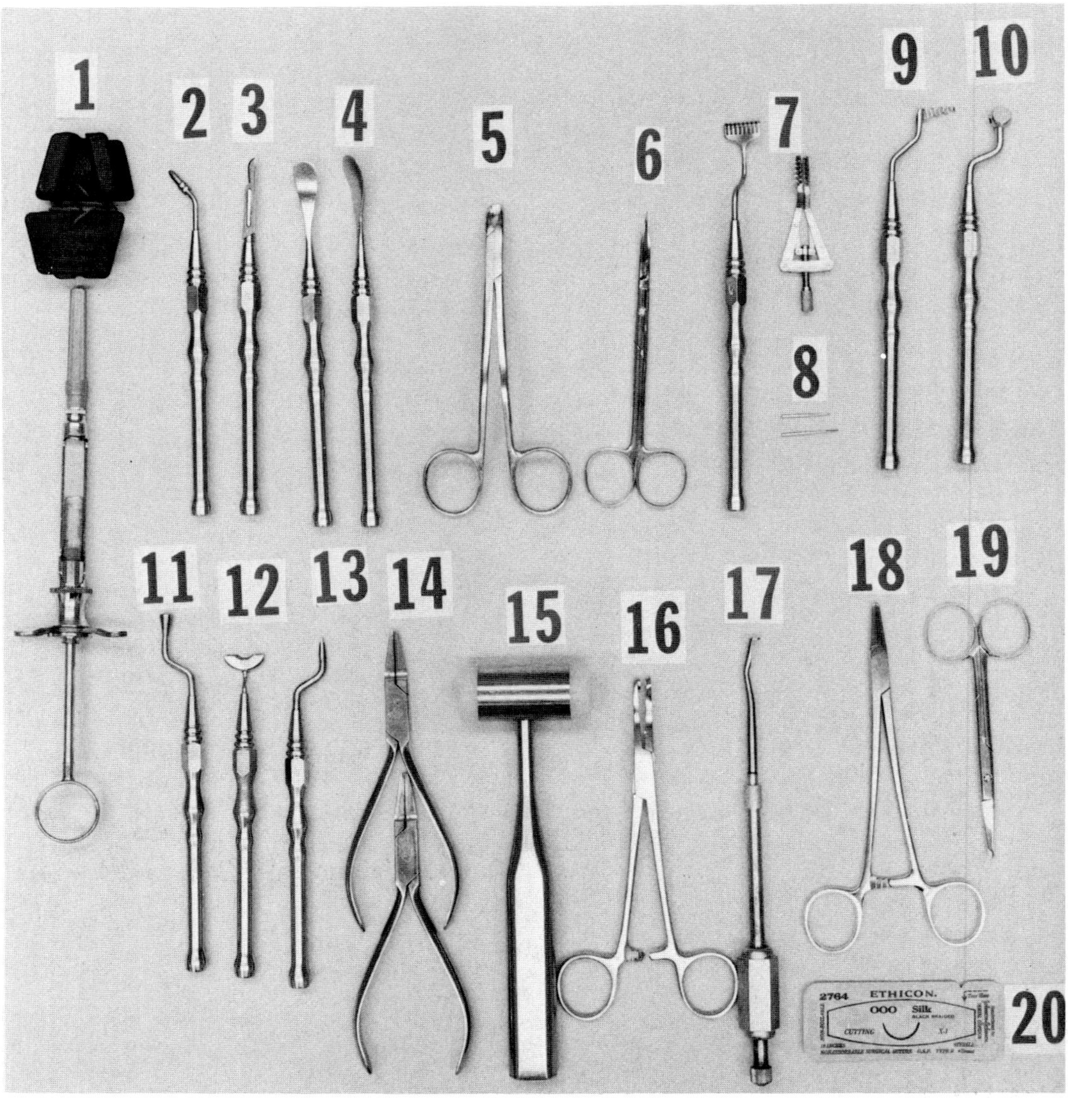

Fig. 7-2. The suggested endosteal blade-vent implant armamentarium: *(1)* Local anesthetic syringe, with anesthesia Carpule and surgical bite-block. *(2)* Fine-line tissue marker. *(3)* Scalpel and handle. *(4)* Periosteal elevators. *(5)* Shaping and trimming rongeurs. *(6)* Multi-access tissue scissors. *(7)* Manual and automatic tissue retractors. *(8)* Implant channeling burs. *(9)* Channel curette and depth gauge. *(10)* Implant carrier. *(11)* Single-Headed Seating Instrument. *(12)* Double-Headed Seating Instrument. *(13)* Shoulder Set-Point Instrument. *(14)* Contouring pliers. *(15)* Tapping mallet. *(16)* Semilunar tissue punch. *(17)* Implant remover. *(18)* Needle holder. *(19)* Suture scissors. *(20)* Suture silk.

ment is used to direct a force on the single-post implant, for even, horizontal seating. It may also be used on one head of a double-headed implant.

12. The Double-Headed Seating Instrument directs an equal force on both posts of a double-headed blade; however, a slight tipping in a mesiodistal direction can direct unequal insertion forces. Therefore, better finite seating can be established by using the single-headed instrument on any one post.

13. The Titanium-Tipped Shoulder Set-Point Seating Instrument is used as a final seating tool, primarily with single-headed implants. It does not damage the crestal bone, because the width of its functional end is narrower than both the channel and the implant shoulder. This instrument neatly engages the depressions in the implant shoulder.

14. Contouring Pliers. It may be necessary to shape an implant frame so that it conforms to the architecture of the arch, especially in the cuspid–bicuspid area, and in the anterior narrow-arch curvatures. The pliers are always used in pairs.

15. The Tapping Mallet is used in conjunction with a seating instrument, which is used as an intermediary. The blows are gentle and direct, to ensure final seating. No more than three strokes are necessary at any given point.

16. The Semilunar Tissue Punch creates a neat, semilunar contour of gingival tissue around an implant neck. It may be used to prevent bunching and straining of the soft tissue during suturing. This instrument should be used *only* if there is a substantial buccolingual width of attached-type gingival tissue. It should *never* be used to eliminate this important cuff of gingival tissue.

17. The Implant Remover is used only if the implant must be disengaged from the channel in order to alter the channel or to recontour the implant. The prongs of the remover fit under the base of the implant post.

18. Needle Holder. The choice of the type of needle holder to use is a personal decision, based on the proper dimension, balance, and comfort for the operator for intra-oral use.

19. The Suture Scissors are used in conjunction with the needle holder and the suture material of choice.

20. Suture Silk. Ethicon* 3-0 or 4-0 Cuticular Silk Atraumatic Sutures are generally used, with a delicate semilunar needle such as the J-1.

PRE-INSERTION PRECAUTIONS

Proper Use of Insertion Instrumentation

The insertion armamentarium is designed to help the operator insert an implant as efficiently and predictably as possible. Improper instrument utilization, such as incompatible metallic instruments, can certainly contribute to implant failure. The use of undersized burs would cause over-compression of the bone on either side of the groove. The implant would then have to be forcefully malleted into position, and osseous fractures may result. An oversized bur would create too large a groove, and the implant would then be mobile.

The use of the high-speed bur without copious amounts of water can cause burning of the bone, with consequent sequestrations. If the improper inserting instrument is used, slippage may occur; this may result in fracture of the adjacent bone, or in the eccentric seating of the implant. The Titanium-Tipped Shoulder Set-Point Seating Instrument is an example of a properly designed inserting instrument; it is specifically oriented to fit between the walls of the groove without damaging the crestal bone.

Blade Implant Mobility

If, upon the final seating of the blade-vent implant, there is any mobility, the implant should not be left in the groove. The implant remover should be employed to withdraw the implant. Two pairs of contouring pliers should then be used to contour the body of the blade in a bowed fashion or to alternate the legs of the implant

*Somerville, New Jersey.

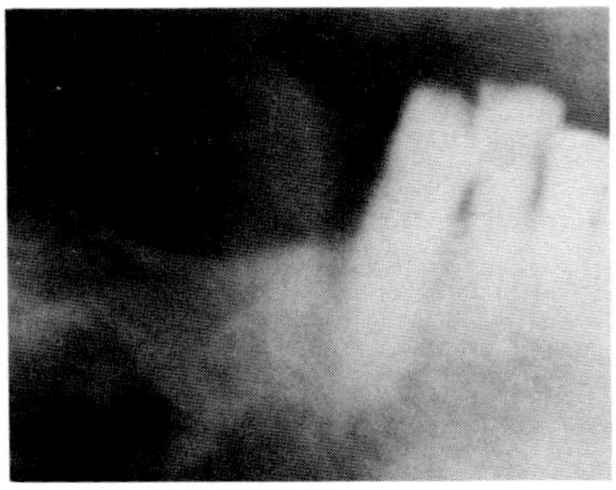

Fig. 7-3. Presurgical radiograph of the mandibular right posterior edentulous segment, where a blade-vent implant is to be inserted.

in a slight buccolingual variation. Then the implant should be reseated and checked for stability. In addition, the buccal and lingual cortical plates of bone should be examined to eliminate the possibility of any visible bony fracture. If a fracture of any degree exists, the implant should be removed and the procedure terminated. If it is desired to insert a new implant, a waiting period of about 6 to 9 months is mandatory; this figure has been attained strictly through clinical observation.

The Knife-Edged Ridge

In many instances, when the mucoperiosteal flaps are reflected, a knife-edged bony ridge is revealed. This situation appears to be more frequently encountered in the maxilla than in the mandible. To improve this anatomic topography, a high-speed drill is held perpendicular to the bony crest. Then the ridge should be reduced until a flat surface, approximately 1.5 mm. in width, is achieved. This architecture and dimension should allow room for the thickest portion of the blade, which is 1.2 mm. wide at the shoulder. The bony groove can then be prepared and the procedure carried to completion. It is safer and advisable to wait the mandatory 6 to 9 months (see Blade Implant Mobility) before the implant is reinserted. This will ensure as uneventful a healing period as possible, as well as a greater degree of predictability of crestal healing, because of the reduced amount of manipulation of osseous structures at any subsequent operation.

INSERTION TECHNIQUE AND SEQUENCE OF PROCEDURES

The implant and instruments must be autoclaved prior to surgery. The prefabricated blade-vent implant that is selected must meet the specific requirements of the area under treatment with respect to mesiodistal length, vertical depth, and the number of abutment posts (heads). The selection should be made according to clinical and radiographic measurements, in addition to the blade guide (Figs. 7-3 to 7-5).

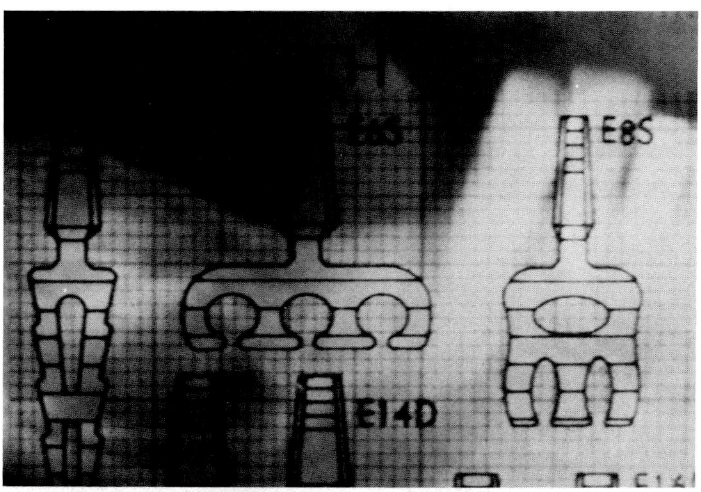

Fig. 7-4. A millimeter grid has been superimposed over a segment of a panoramic radiograph. This procedure can aid in proper implant selection. (Implants International, Division of Oratronics Inc., New York, New York)

The blade guide is superimposed over the available bone portrayed in the radiograph. It is important to use as much available bone as possible without encroaching on such anatomical sites as the inferior alveolar canal, the mental foramen, the floor of the nasal cavity, or the floor and walls of the maxillary sinus. Within these limitations, still using as much supportive bone as possible, the proper implant size should be obvious. On the other hand, the operator may use the grid marks of any millimeter grid, which is superimposed on the radiograph, to measure both the implant and the available bone depth and length. In the partially edentulous arch, a reliable guide to the depth of the body of the implant would be to compare it to the apices of the adjacent natural teeth. Once the appropriate implant has been selected, it should be held over the mucosa in the area of implantation. Probe-point or indelible markings may be made, in the mucosa, which correspond to the mesiodistal length of the implant or to the area of extrusion of the implant neck (Fig. 7-6).

Preparation of the Intra-Osseous Channel

A single, definite, long, mesiodistal incision is made through the midpoint of the gingival band of attached-type soft tissue, about 0.5 cm. longer than the probe-point markings at both the mesial and distal terminal points (Fig. 7-7). The mucoperiosteum is reflected in both the buccal and lingual directions with a periosteal elevator, so that the entire buccolingual dimension of the bone may be viewed (Fig. 7-8).

The groove in the bone must be placed midway between the cortical plates of bone, so that the implant neck may eventually extrude through a band of gingival tissue. The angulation of the groove must be such as to avoid perforating either the buccal or the lingual plates of bone that parallel the intra-osseous channel. Prior to any drilling, the implant is held against the alveolar ridge to determine the exact mesiodistal length of the groove that is to be cut in the bone (Fig. 7-9). Using a 700 XL bur, in a high-speed handpiece, with copious water irrigation, a groove is prepared in the bone (Fig. 7-10). This groove is normally perpendicular to the

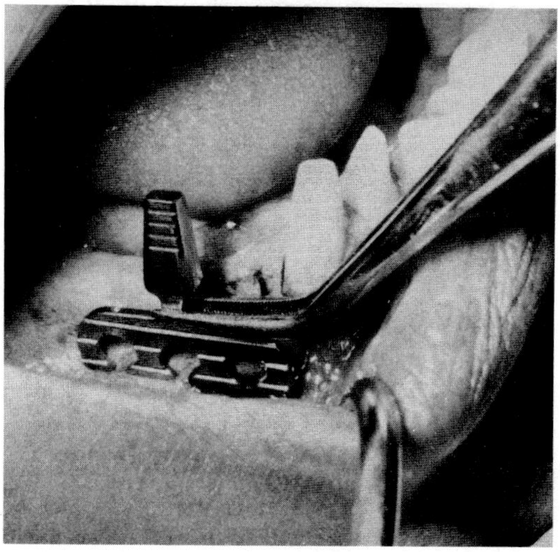

Fig. 7-5. To recheck implant selection, a blade-vent endosseous implant is being held in the area of insertion. Two anterior mesial natural-abutment teeth have already been prepared.

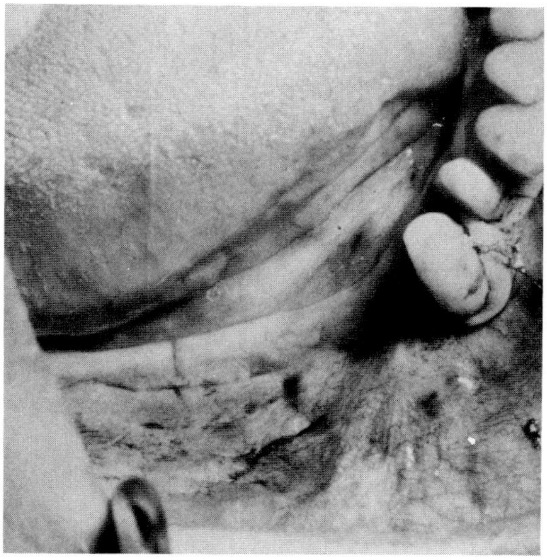

Fig. 7-6. Occlusobuccal view of the implant site. The buccal gingiva has been marked with an indelible pencil. The attached band of gingival tissue lingual to this mark is the point at which the implant neck will be located.

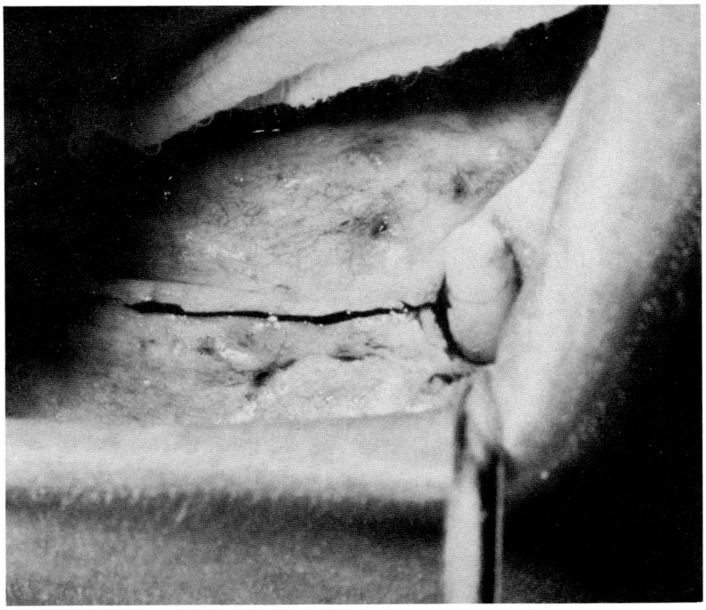

Fig. 7-7. This incision through the mucoperiosteum is approximately 1 1/2 times longer than the length of the implant. It is *not* necessary to surgically infringe upon the gingival unit of the anterior abutment tooth, as is shown here. Some operators, however, prefer such surgical access. As long as the surgery is minimal, and the postsurgical suturing taut, such an initial incision may not be harmful to the marginal gingiva of the natural-abutment tooth.

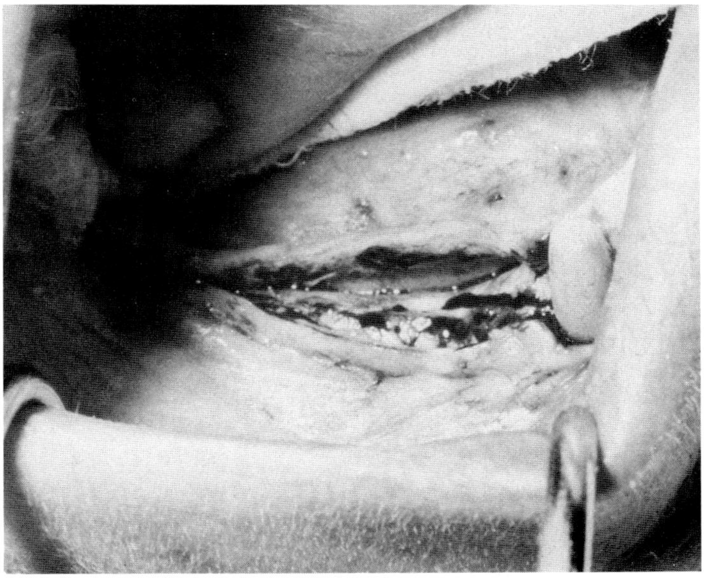

Fig. 7-8. The mucoperiosteal flaps have been reflected toward the buccal and the lingual aspects in order to expose the full width of the alveolar ridge. This has been accomplished by blunt dissection only.

crest of the alveolar ridge and may be initiated by one of two techniques:

1. Numerous puncture points, approximately 5 mm. apart, may be made along the crest of the ridge. These are subsequently connected to form a single channel.

2. The operator may prefer to use the bur with a paintbrush motion and gently stroke back and forth in a mesiodistal direction until the groove is started.

Regardless of the technique chosen, the drilling should be completed to the full required depth. This depth can be predeter-

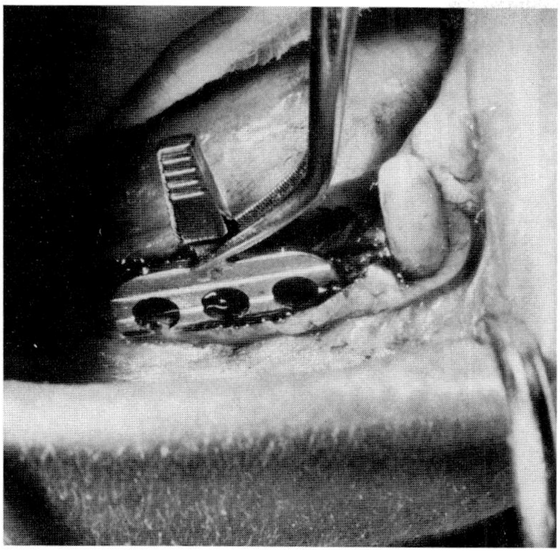

Fig. 7-9. The selected implant, which has been sterilized, is being held against the alveolar ridge. This checking is done in order to anticipate the mesiodistal length of the bony channel.

mined by matching the implant frame (body) plus the implant neck against the correct bur length. This channel is then cleansed by saline irrigation and the channel curette.

Placement of the Blade Implant in the Prepared Channel

The implant is placed in the channel with finger pressure only (Fig. 7-11). The implant should be seated to the level of the shoulder at this time. Also, the mesiodistal and buccolingual alignments with the adjacent natural-abutment teeth should be checked, and the occlusal clearance with the opposing dentition should be verified. The implant is then removed with the implant remover. If reduction of the implant post (head) is necessary, an end-cutting disc or a heatless stone with water spray may be used extra-orally. The final polishing of the implant may be done with a metal polishing wheel of choice. The implant is then placed in an ultrasonic cleaner. Then the implant is resterilized in

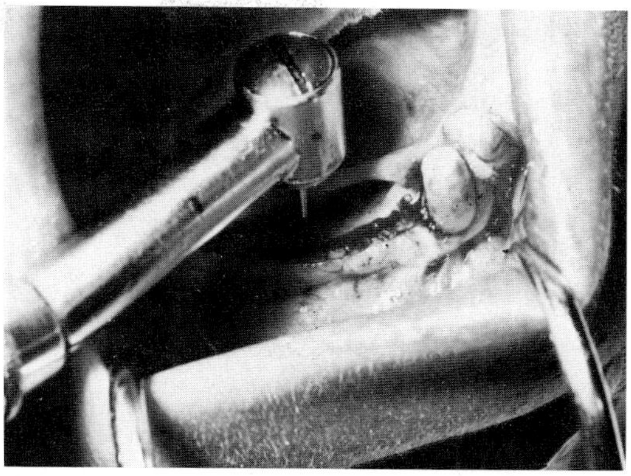

Fig. 7-10. The intra-osseous channel is created by a gentle sweeping motion. The bur is positioned perpendicular to the crest of the alveolar ridge.

a bead sterilizer, which is commonly used during endodontic treatment.

During the preparation of the channel, several apical radiographs should be taken

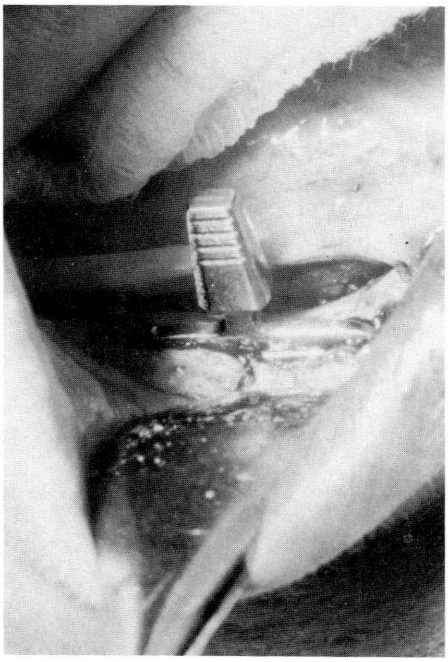

Fig. 7-11. The implant has been inserted with finger pressure only, in order to check the depth of the channel, the buccolingual alignment, and the path of insertion with the adjacent natural-abutment teeth.

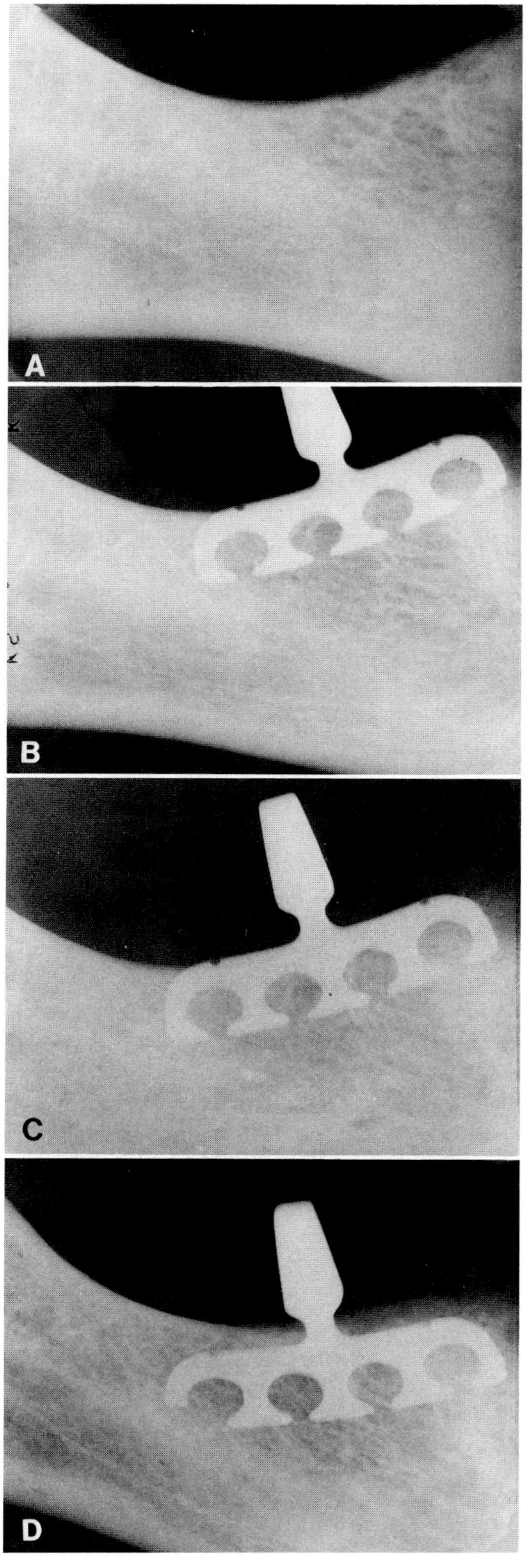

Fig. 7-12. Example of a series of apical radiographs that is used during the insertion of a blade-vent implant. These radiographs have been taken by the long-cone technique. The superior clarity, definition, and dimensional accuracy aid the implantologist, as does a similar series for the endodontist. In this case, a portion of the distal leg of the implant frame has been removed in order to prevent impingement of the inferior alveolar canal *(D).*

with the implant in place (Fig. 7-12). This procedure is similar to the series of radiographs that accompany endodontic filing and filling techniques. The use of multiple apical films assures and reassures the operator of his relative intra-osseous positioning (Fig. 7-13). In this manner, more precise channeling can be accomplished without overpreparation, and without impingement of such vital structures as the mandibular canal. At times, the evaluation of such radiographs indicate the necessity of the chair-side modification of an implant frame in order to circumvent major, radiographically visible landmarks. In light of this, it is not uncommon to remove one of the leg-extensions of the implant frame, to avoid encroachment of a structure such as the mandibular canal. (Fig. 7-12D).

The implant is repositioned in the channel with the implant carrier and firm, but gentle, finger pressure (Figs. 7-14 to 7-17). The inserting instrument should then be placed over the abutment post (head) and tapped gently with a mallet into a final seating position (Fig. 7-18). A guide to the definite seating of the implant is to view the engagement of the base of the post (Safety-Stop Lock) at the crestal bone, to make sure that the shoulder is well below the crest of the alveolar ridge. If the mesiodistal alignment requires some further minor adjustment, the Shoulder Set-Points may be engaged with the Titanium-Tipped Shoulder Set-Point Seating Instrument without traumatizing the crestal bone (Figs. 7-19, 7-20).

Once the implant is in its final position, the channel should be irrigated above the

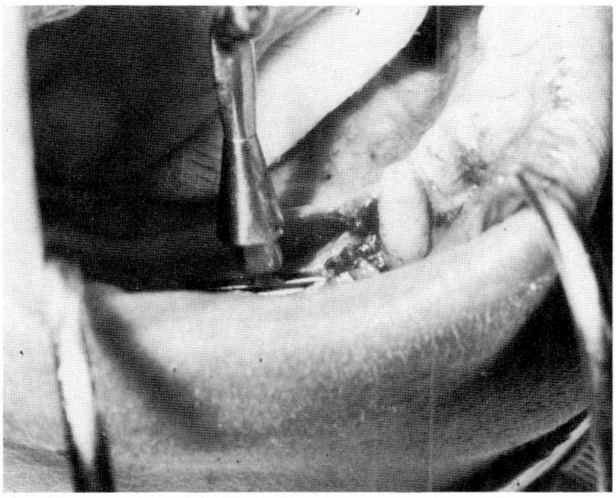

Fig. 7-18. A single-headed inserting instrument placed over the post of the implant. With this instrument acting as the intermediary, a surgical mallet is used. The instrument is gently tapped three times. The implant is properly seated when the base of the abutment post is engaged within the crestal bone.

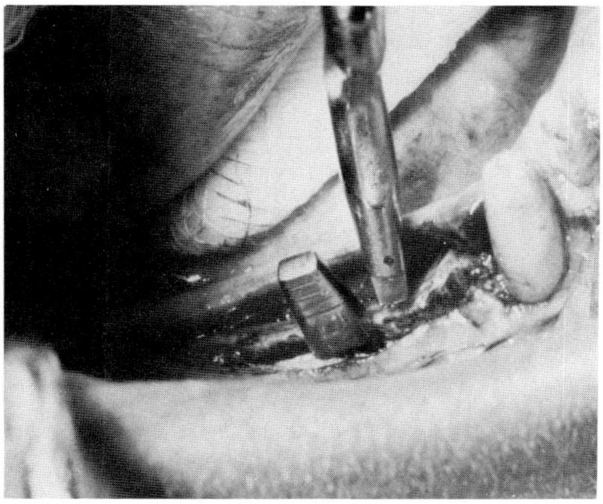

Fig. 7-19. The Shoulder Set-Point Instrument engaged in the mesial aspect of the shoulder of the implant. The tapping of this instrument is especially helpful in modifying the mesial or distal seating of the implant shoulder below the crest of bone.

Fig. 7-20. A blade-vent implant finally and completely seated within the intra-osseous channel. The final position is apparent when the base of the implant post engages the buccal and lingual aspects of the crest of the alveolar ridge. A slight resorption of this crestal bone is to be anticipated as a result of surgical manipulation; it is for this reason that the implant neck is sunk within these confines Eventually, after complete healing, the soft-tissue cuff will engage the base of the post and the implant neck circumferentially.

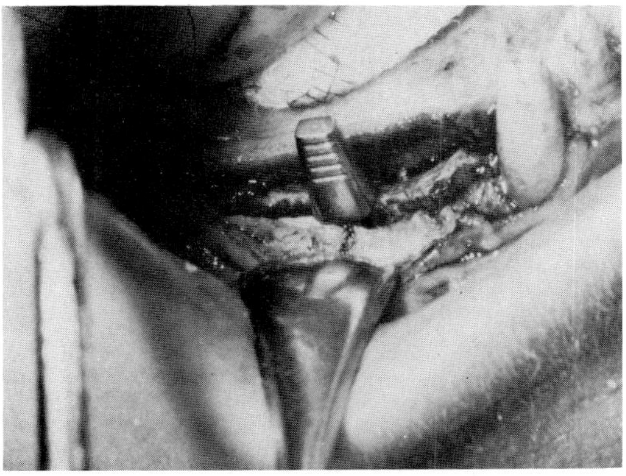

Fig. 7-21. The full-thickness mucoperiosteal flaps have been approximated. Their positioning has been secured by means of interrupted, individual silk sutures. There is a lack of attached gingiva at the labial aspect of the cuspid *(arrow)*. In this particular case, periodontal treatment *must* be instituted to correct this defect *prior* to prosthetic restorative procedures.

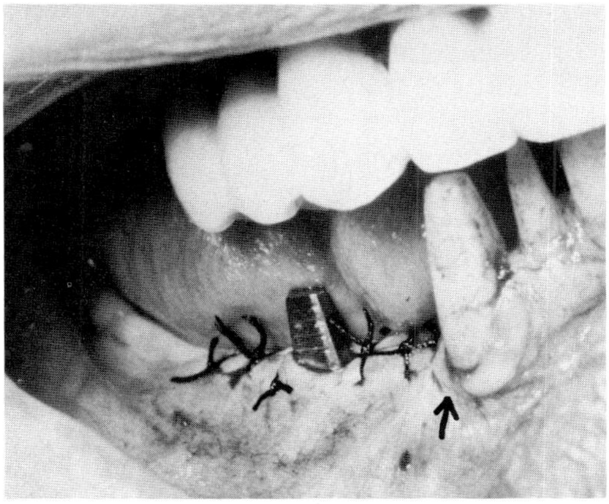

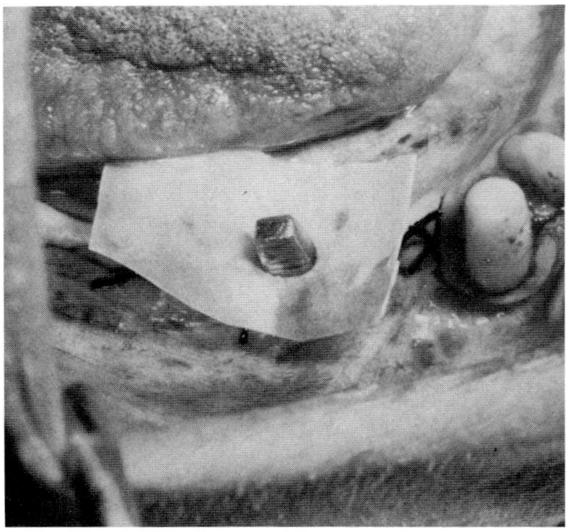

Fig. 7-22. Occlusal view of a freshly inserted mandibular posterior blade-vent implant. A small square of rubber dam material has been placed over the implant post. This material prevents the ingress of cement below the post and into the incision, and prevents the disturbance of the sutures. After the insertion of the temporary acrylic-resin prosthesis, the rubber dam material is cut and removed, prior to the dismissal of the patient.

alveolar ridges higher than the buccal portions. Often, when the final seating of the implant is attempted, the shoulder or the base of the post may engage the lingual aspect of the ridge first. Thus, the buccal portion of the implant would not be sunk below the crest of bone. This situation can be easily remedied by preparing a notch in the lingual bone that is slightly wider than the base of the post (Perio-Head). The implant will then seat in its final position within the confines of osseous structure.

In any case, a slight amount of crestal bone loss should be anticipated after any intra-osseous implant insertion, which involves the exposure and manipulation of bone. This should not, however, cause exposure of the shoulder of the frame. Because minor crestal resorption is anticipated, the entire implant body should be seated well below and within the confines of its osseous supportive walls.

THE TEMPORARY PROSTHESIS

The placement of a temporary bridge is important (see Chaps. 5 and 9). Whenever bone is traumatized, whether it be accidental or surgical in etiology, the bone resorbs. This applies to the surgical trauma that is caused by the cutting of the channel for the placement of the implant. Therefore, the implant must be splinted, to help in its stabilization during this catabolic phase. Aside from this physiologic factor, the placement of a temporary bridge is important for its psychological benefits. The patient can thus be discharged from the office with an esthetically acceptable and functional prosthesis.

A temporary prosthesis may be prefabricated prior to the insertion appointment. Once the implant is inserted and the flaps sutured, a small piece of rubber dam material may be placed over the abutment posts (Fig. 7-22). This procedure will prevent the ingress of either acrylic-resin reline material or temporary cement into the incision; such an iatrogenic factor can retard and upset the normal healing process. It is preferable to use a non-eugenol temporary cement, to prevent the deterioration of the acrylic resin by any free eugenol. When the prosthesis is in position and cemented, the rubber dam may be removed. The occlusion is then checked for proper centric holds and freedom from any potential traumatic prematurities in lateral and protrusive excursions.

The only medication that the patient is given upon discharge is an analgesic, to alleviate postoperative discomfort. The patient may eat and drink as he desires; the only limitation at this preliminary healing stage is hard foods. The reason for any such limitation, only at this phase, is to prevent the flexure of the temporary acrylic-resin splint. Such flexure may create a pumping effect that is transmitted through the implant-bone interface and may preclude proper initial healing.

The patient should return to the office

7 days after insertion. At that time the temporary prosthesis is removed first, providing better access for suture removal and a better visual field for the inspection of wound healing. Then, the proper standards for prosthetic reconstruction may be followed (see Chap. 9).

THE PLACEMENT OF BLADE-VENT IMPLANTS IN DIFFERENT CLINICAL SITUATIONS

As has been alluded to, the blade-type implant may be used as an intermediary or terminal abutment in conjunction with natural teeth; or blades may be used in a series, for a complete-arch implant. The following cases are presented in order to illustrate six variations of blade implants, using the aforementioned technique of implant insertion.

The Intermediary Implant Abutment

A 52-year-old female presented for the insertion of an endosteal blade-vent implant, which was to aid in the support of a long-span fixed prosthesis in the mandibular right quadrant. The patient's past medical history was essentially negative. She had mild hypertension that was controlled with antihypertensive medication. A double-headed endosteal blade-vent implant was inserted while the patient was under intravenous sedation and local anesthesia (Fig. 7-23). A postoperative radiograph (Fig. 7-24) revealed that the implant was in good position, with no impingement on the adjacent structures. This radiograph included the lower right posterior quadrant that was temporized, and an old upper fixed prosthesis.

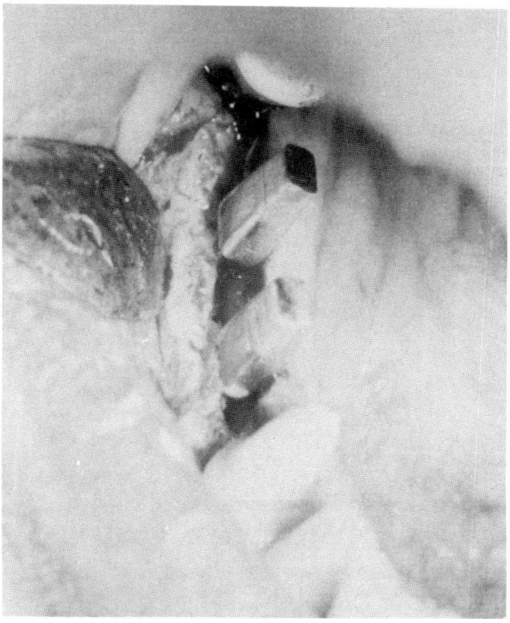

Fig. 7-23. A double-headed blade-vent implant in final position. The bases of the posts are in contact with the crest of the alveolar ridge. The posts lie within the path of insertion of the prepared natural-abutment teeth.

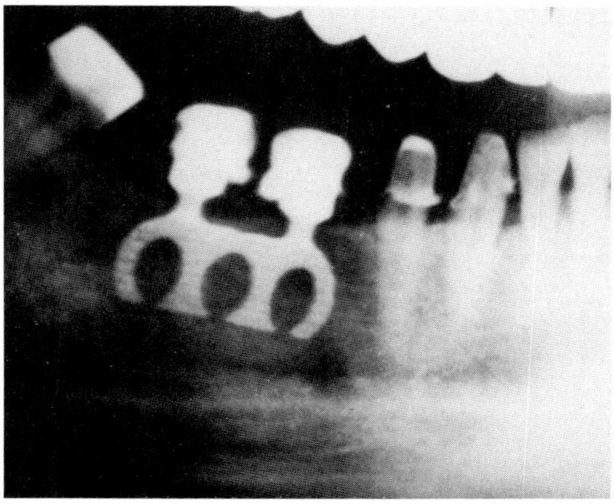

Fig. 7-24. Radiograph taken after insertion shows the final seating of the implant, with an acrylic-resin temporary splint superimposed on it.

The Terminal or Distal Free-End Extension Implant

A 48-year-old female presented for placement of two endosteal blade-vent implants: a right posterior maxillary implant and a right posterior mandibular implant. The patient's past medical history was negative.

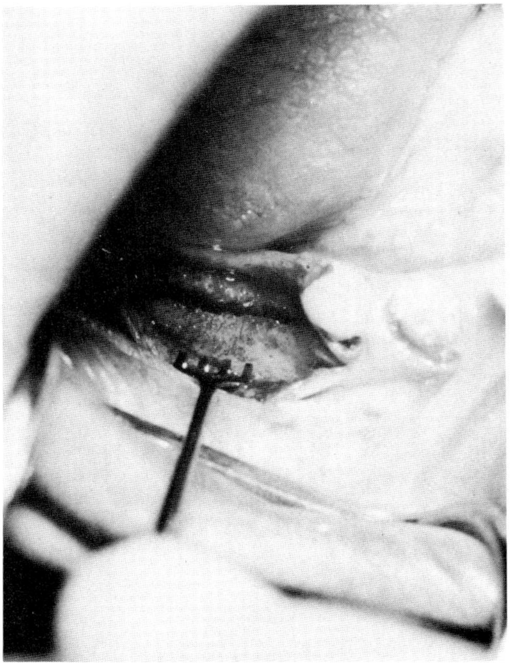

Fig. 7-25. Occlusobuccal view of the mandibular posterior ridge area. The reflection of the full-thickness mucoperiosteal flap reveals the preparation of the intra-osseous channel.

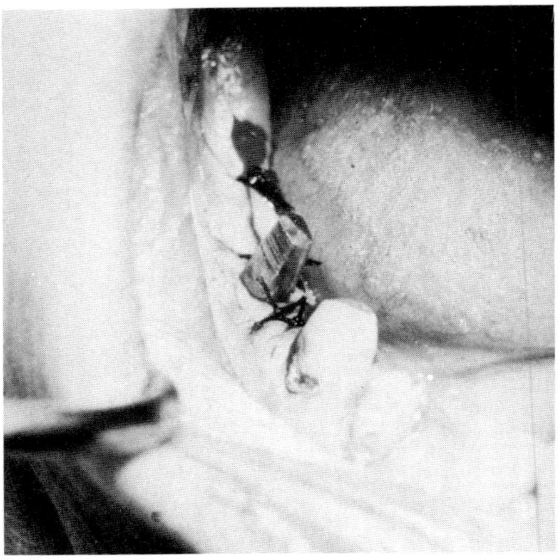

Fig. 7-26. Mesiobuccal view of the mandibular posterior area immediately after insertion of a blade-vent implant. Individual sutures approximate the full-thickness flaps around the implant neck and post base.

While the patient was under intravenous medication and local anesthesia, a blade-vent implant was inserted in the posterior section of the mandible (Figs. 7-25, 7-26). A temporary acrylic-resin prosthesis was placed for the duration of the healing period. A four-unit fixed bridge was later fabricated and inserted.

One month later, the patient returned for the placement of the maxillary implant; the same techniques were used as for the mandibular implant (Figs. 7-27, 7-28). A fixed prosthesis was later fabricated and inserted.

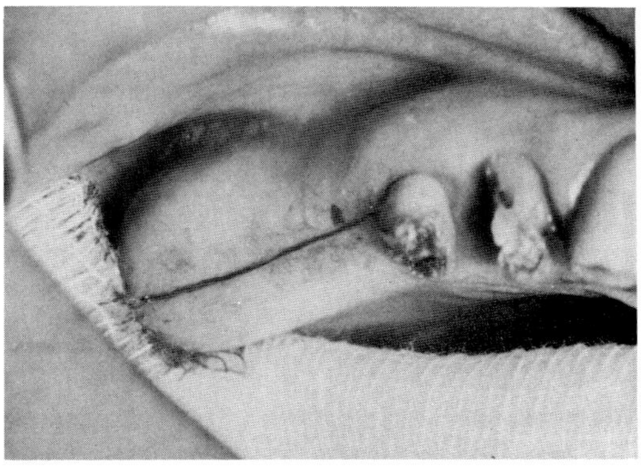

Fig. 7-27. Occlusobuccal view of an upper right posterior ridge. A clean initial incision has been made at the height of the ridge. This will be followed by blunt dissection.

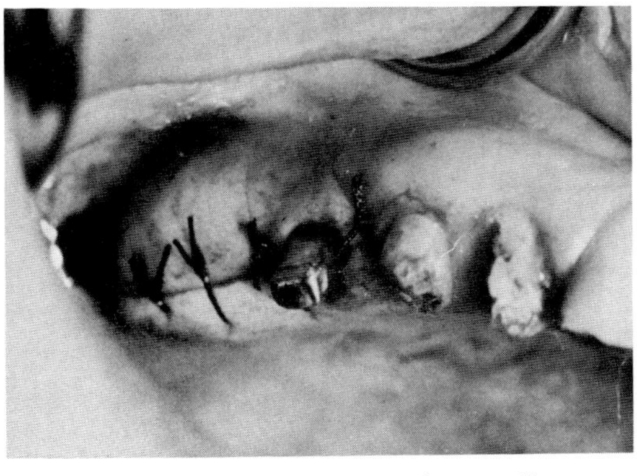

Fig. 7-28. Occlusobuccal view of a maxillary terminal blade-vent implant immediately after insertion. The post has been aligned with the prepared natural-abutment teeth.

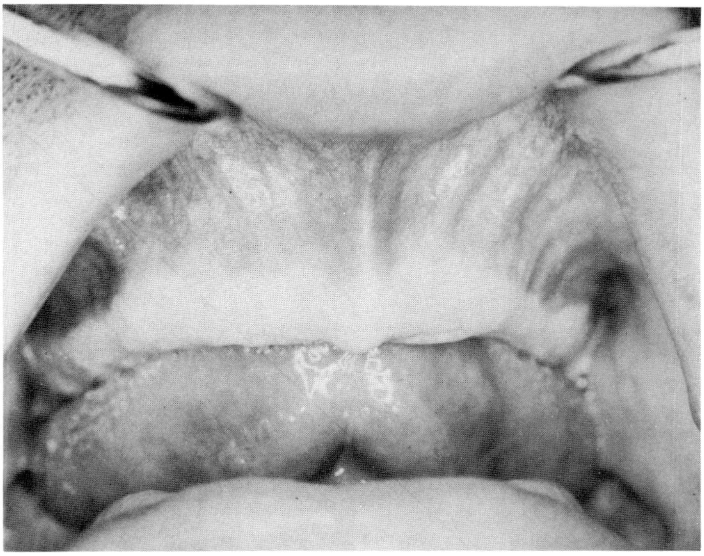

Fig. 7-29. Labial view of a completely edentulous maxillary ridge. In a case such as this, implants should only be used as a last resort. If a well-fabricated complete upper denture fails to satisfy the patient's needs, then an implant, or implants, may be used. Note the broad expanse of the attached gingival soft-tissue band.

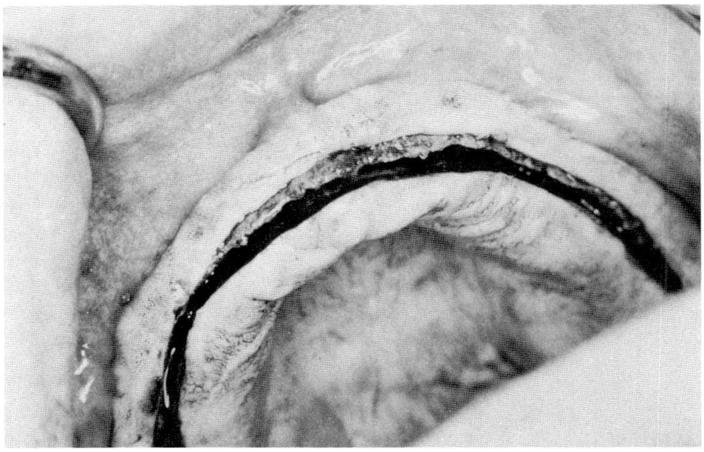

Fig. 7-30. Occlusal view of a portion of the edentulous ridge that has been prepared for multiple implant insertion. The initial incision, the reflection of the full-thickness flaps, and the preparation of an intra-osseous channel have been accomplished.

The Maxillary Complete-Arch Implant with Multiple Blades

The patient who presented for this form of treatment was a 37-year-old male with a negative medical history. The patient had a severe gagging reflex, which had caused him to have had five sets of dentures fabricated during the past several years. Although the patient had a good, clinically and anatomically healthy ridge, conventional dentures were useless for him (Fig. 7-29). His last denture had been constructed without palatal coverage.

While the patient received intravenous medication and local anesthesia, four endosteal blade-vent implants were inserted in the maxillary arch (Figs. 7-30 to 7-32). The patient's last denture was contoured to serve as a temporary appliance. A post-insertion radiograph revealed the complete-arch implants in position (Fig. 7-33). After adequate healing (Fig. 7-34), cast-gold telescope copings were soldered to a cast bar and cemented to the implant posts (Fig. 7-35). A new denture without palatal coverage was then fabricated. Clips were placed in the prosthesis to increase reten-

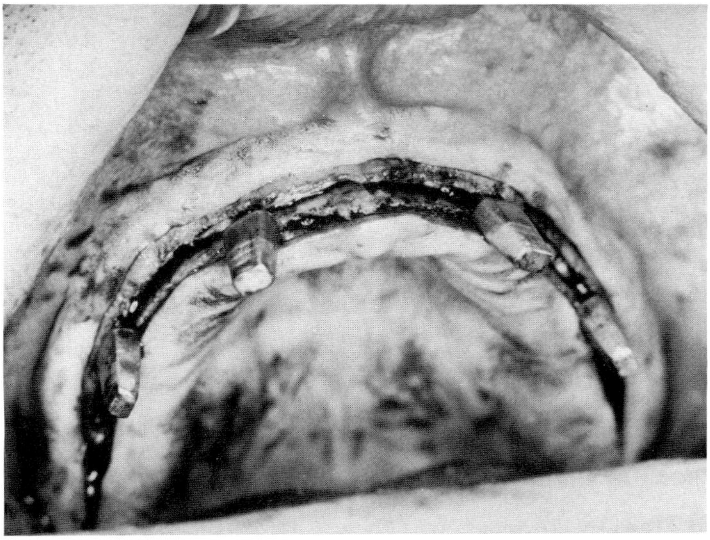

Fig. 7-31. Four individual blade-vent implants inserted in a completely edentulous maxillary arch.

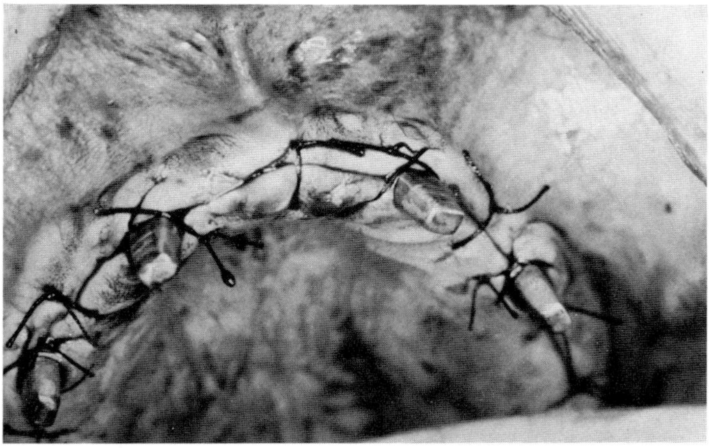

Fig. 7-32. The mucoperiosteal flaps have been approximated and adapted around each implant with individual sutures.

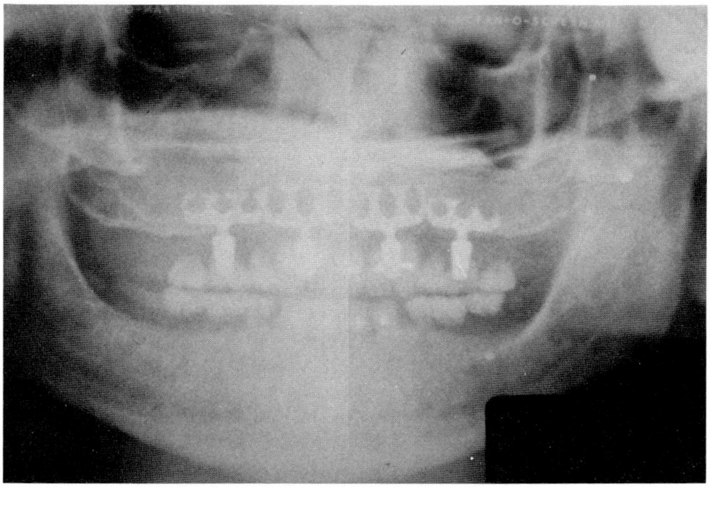

Fig. 7-33. Panoramic radiograph showing four maxillary blade-vent implants supporting a temporary prosthesis. The left posterior implant was recontoured in order to circumvent the maxillary sinus. The right posterior implant is buccal to the sinus on the right side.

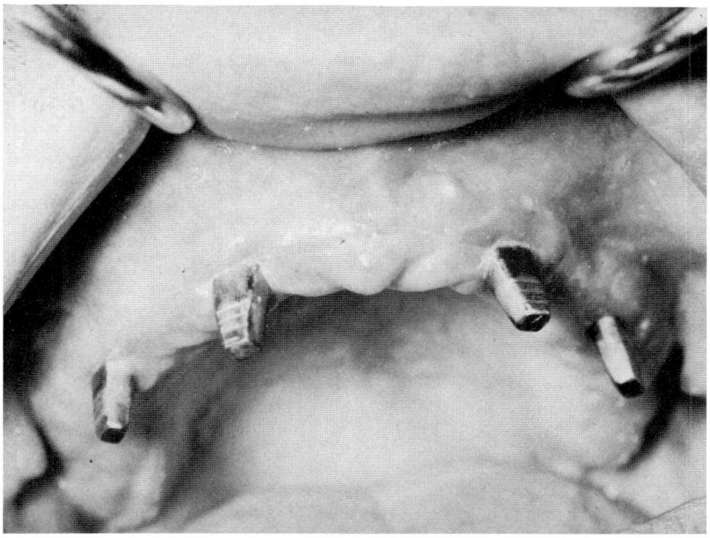

Fig. 7-34. Occlusolabial view of the four maxillary blade-vent implants 2 weeks after insertion.

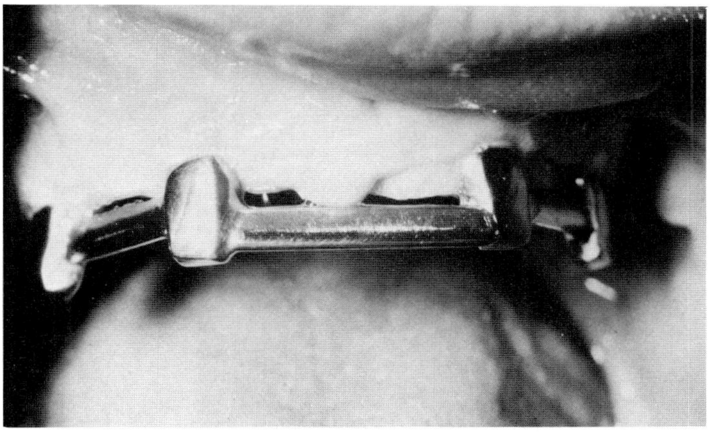

Fig. 7-35. A fixed-splint cast superstructure has been cemented to the four implant posts. This will serve as an intermediary structure for the support of a removable prosthesis.

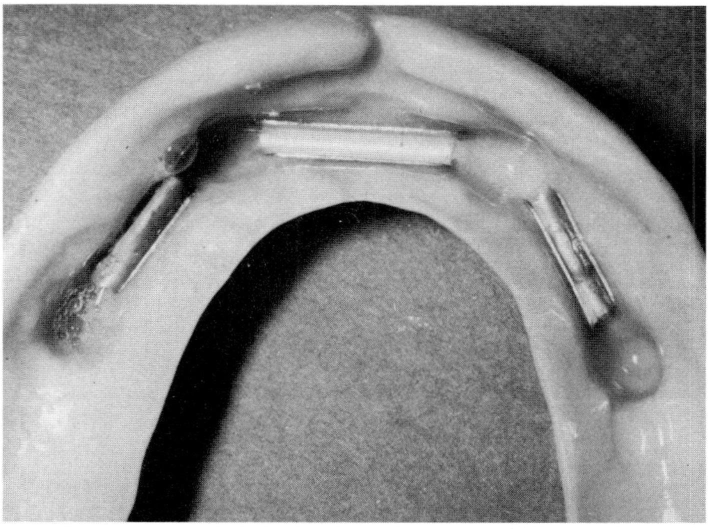

Fig. 7-36. Inner aspect of the final maxillary prosthesis that is to be superimposed on the intermediary cast superstructure. Retentive clips are in position. The palatal segment has been omitted because of the patient's gag reflex.

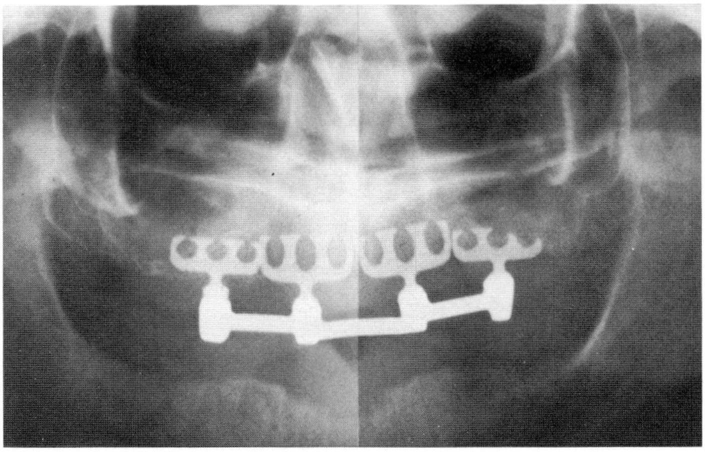

Fig. 7-37. An 18-month follow-up panoramic radiograph demonstrates the relative positions of the implants with an intermediary superstructure cemented on the posts.

tion (Fig. 7-36). Eighteen months later, a radiograph revealed that the implants were in good position (Fig. 7-37).

Bilateral Terminal or Distal Free-End Implant Abutments

In order to avoid the use of bilateral free-end removable prosthesis, a 28-year-old female, with a noncontributory negative medical history, presented for the consideration of implants to support fixed prostheses. After the patient was given a local anesthetic, bilateral posterior mandibular blade-vent implants were inserted (Fig. 7-38). The routine follow-through consisted of acrylic-resin temporary prostheses placed bilaterally. Later, the sutures were removed, and the final fixed prostheses were fabricated and inserted. A 1-year post-insertion evaluation demonstrated no abnormal pathological findings (Fig. 7-39).

Mandibular Complete-Arch Multiple-Blade Implants to Support a Fixed Prosthesis

A 58-year-old male with a negative medical history presented for the consideration of mandibular implants because of a general inability to adapt to a conventional removable mandibular complete-arch prosthesis (Figs. 7-40, 7-41).

While the patient was under intravenous sedation and local block and infiltration anesthesia, four blade-vent implants were inserted. When the mucoperiosteal flaps were reflected, a severe knife-edged ridge was seen. The sharp crest of the ridge was reduced *slightly* to accommodate the diameter of the bur for the preparation of the intra-osseous groove (Fig. 7-42). After the implants were inserted and the flaps sutured, a temporary prosthesis was placed (Fig. 7-43). Later, a full-cast porcelain-fused-to-metal fixed bridge was fabricated and cemented in position. Post-prosthetic radiographs demonstrated the successful positions of the implants and the prosthesis (Fig. 7-44).

Mandibular Complete-Arch Multiple-Blade Implants to Support a Removable Prosthesis

The following procedures were performed for a 51-year-old male with a negative medical history:

After the patient was given intravenous medication and local block and infiltration anesthesia, four endosteal blade-vent implants were inserted in the mandibular arch (Figs. 7-45 to 7-49). A temporary removable prosthesis was inserted immediately after implant insertion (see Chap. 5). Later, an intermediary superstructure,

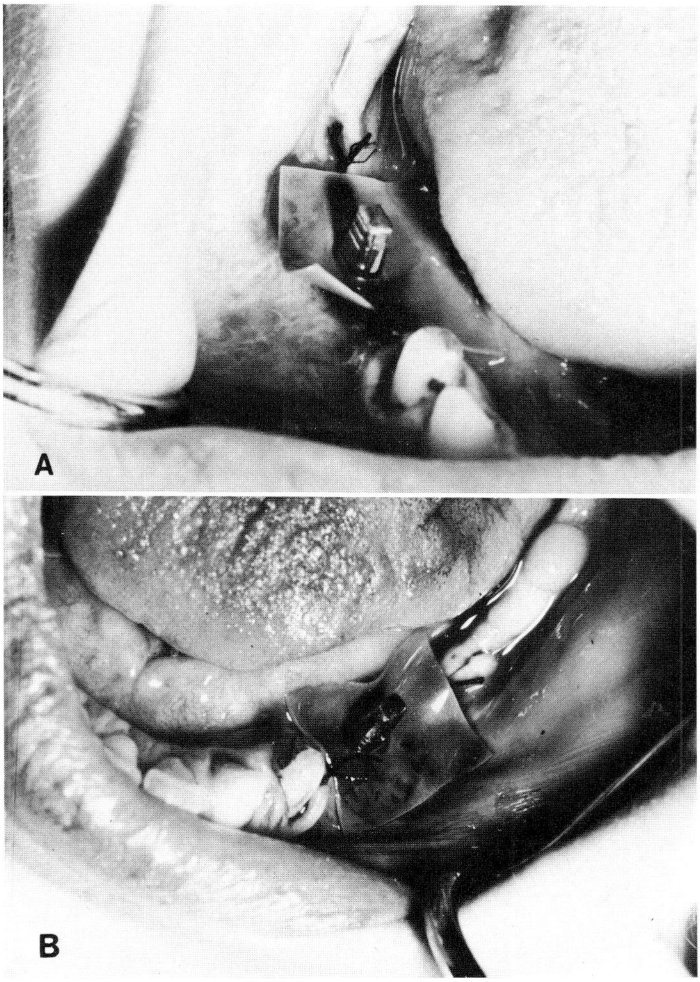

Fig. 7-38. Right *(A)* and left *(B)* terminal blade-vent implants have been inserted. Rubber dam material has been temporarily superimposed on the approximated suture lines in order to prevent the ingress of cement. Such protection is necessary because of the immediate insertion of a temporary acrylic-resin fixed splint.

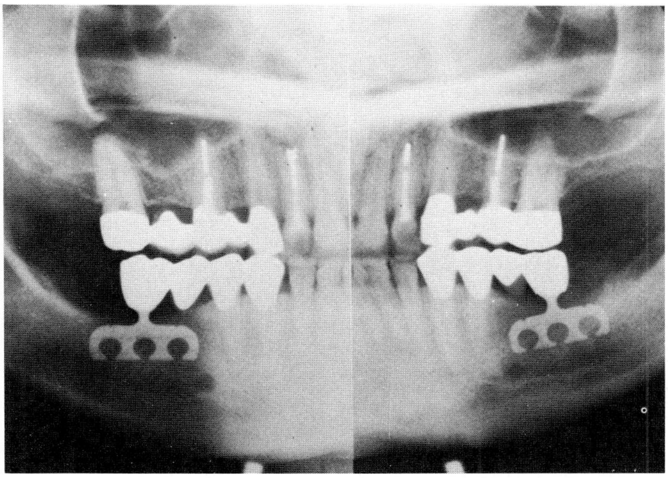

Fig. 7-39. Panoramic radiograph showing bilateral blade-vent implants 1 year after insertion. Both implants serve as distal abutments for a four-unit fixed bridge.

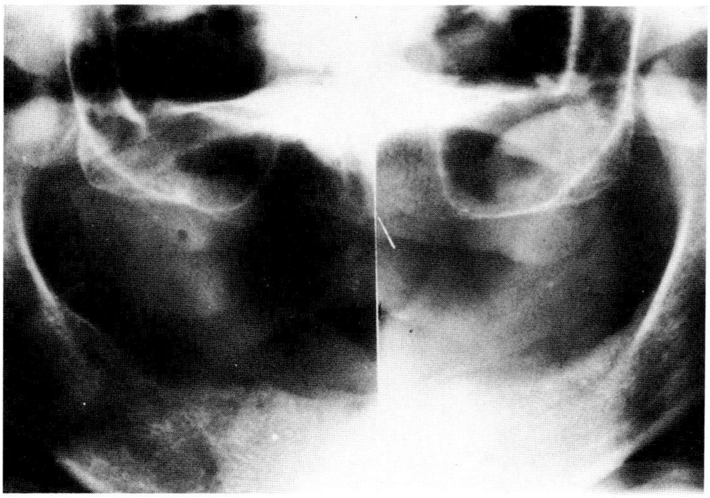

Fig. 7-40. Pre-operative panoramic radiograph of an edentulous mandible, revealing the bony consistency of the residual ridge. The presence of alveolar bone is an indication for the use of intraosseous implants. If alveolar bone is not obvious on such a radiograph, it is advisable to supplement this with a series of individual apical long-cone radiographs.

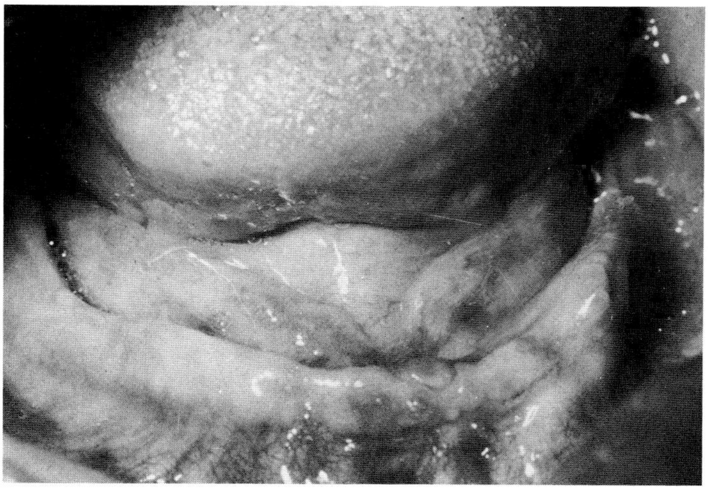

Fig, 7-41. Occlusolabial view of an edentulous mandible that is to receive multiple blade-vent implants. Note the band of attached gingival tissue.

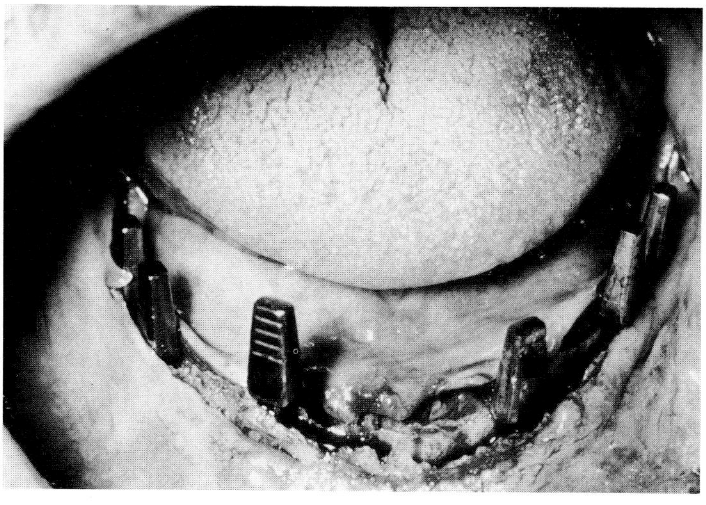

Fig. 7-42. Four individual blade-vent implants have been placed within intra-osseous channels. Both of the posterior implants are double-headed (i.e., two posts on each single frame).

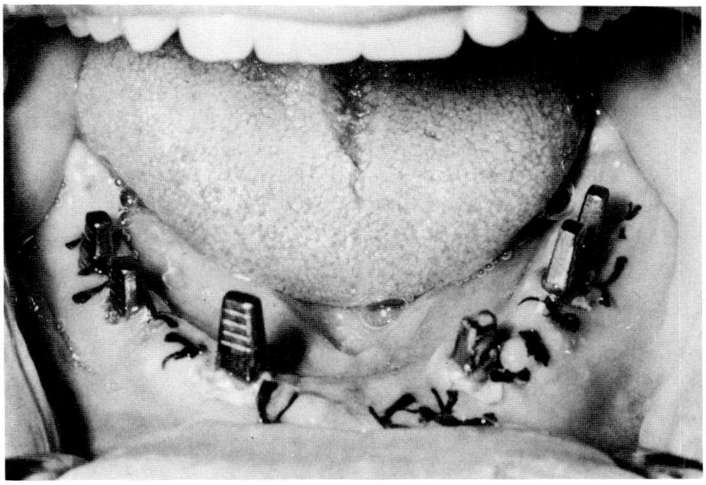

Fig. 7-43. Multiple mandibular implants 1 week after insertion. This photograph was taken just prior to the removal of the sutures. As is often the case within the first week after implant insertion, home care has been difficult, but it will be more easily tended to after the removal of the sutures.

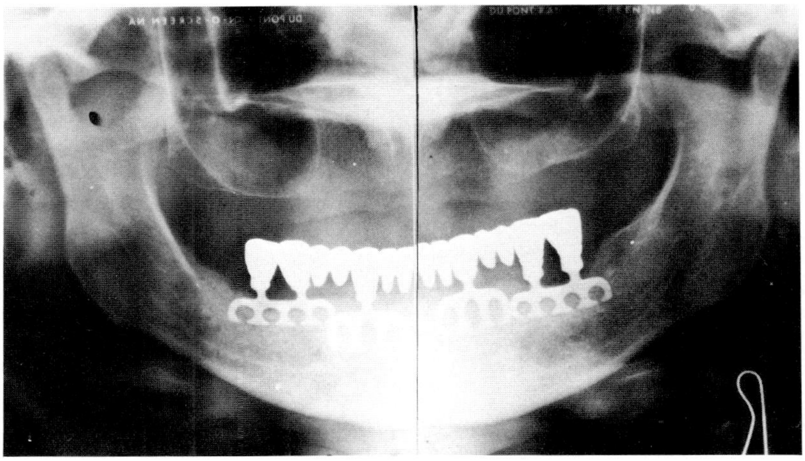

Fig. 7-44. Panoramic radiograph taken 1 year after the insertion of multiple mandibular blade-vent implants that serve as abutment posts for a fixed prosthesis.

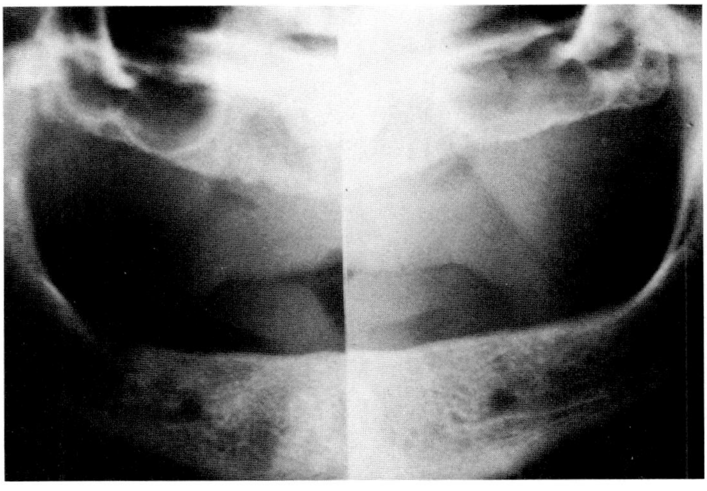

Fig. 7-45. Pre-operative panoramic radiograph of an edentulous mandible.

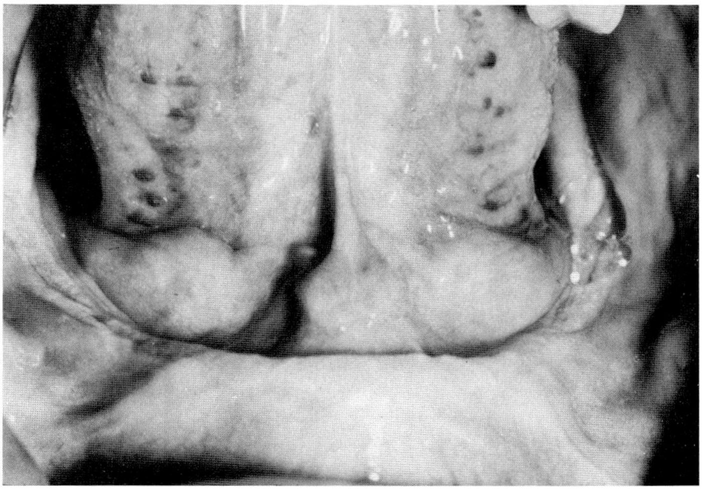

Fig. 7-46. Photograph of the same edentulous mandible in Figure 7-45, prior to surgical procedures.

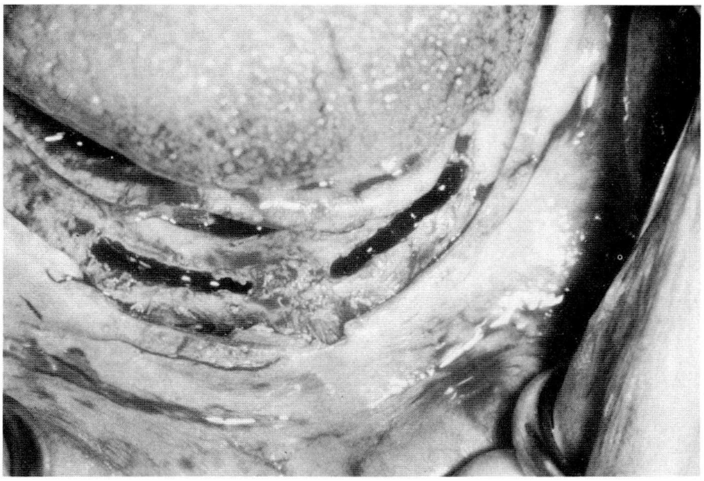

Fig. 7-47. Occlusal view of the surgically exposed edentulous ridge. Individual intra-osseous channels have been prepared for the two anterior blade-vent implants.

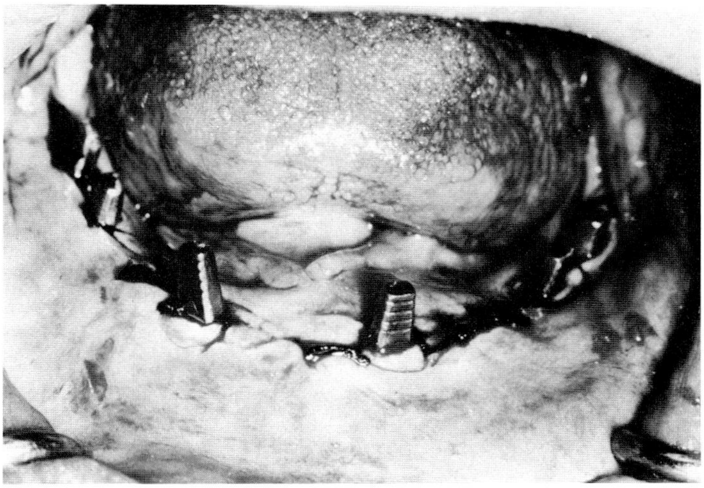

Fig. 7-48. Four blade-vent implants have been inserted, and the full-thickness flaps have been approximated with individual sutures.

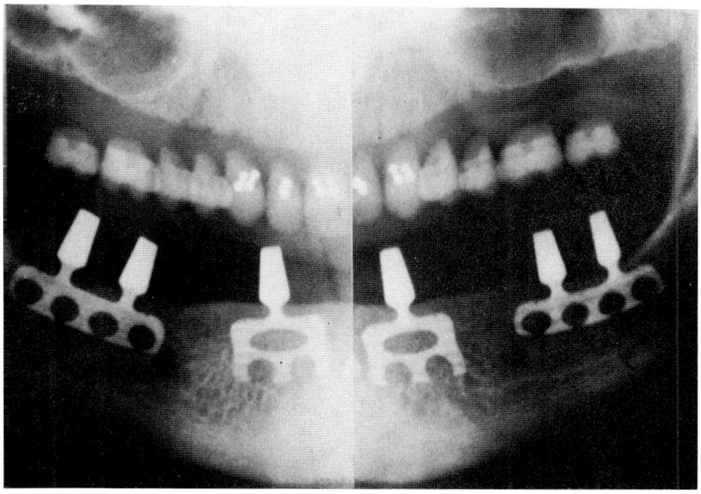

Fig. 7-49. The use of different types of blade-vent implants is revealed in this panoramic radiograph taken within 1 week of insertion. Without impinging on vital intra-osseous channels—such as the inferior mandibular canal—all of these implants are contained within as much alveolar bone as possible. Also, each of the implant frames is well contained within the bony confines.

consisting of cast-gold telescope copings soldered to cast-gold connecting bars, was fabricated and cemented to the implant abutments (Fig. 7-50). An overlay denture with internal clip fixation was fabricated to seat as a removable appliance over the cast-gold frame. A radiograph taken $2^1/_2$ years after implant insertion demonstrated the successful appearance of the implants (Fig. 7-51).

IMPLANT FOLLOW-THROUGH

Patients with blade implants should be recalled to the office every 6 months for examination and evaluation of home care. During every recall appointment, the dentist should routinely follow a checklist (see Chap. 12):

1. Clinical evaluation must include (a) periodontal probing; (b) visual inspection of the soft tissues; (c) visual inspection of the patient's control of plaque; (d) digital inspection for any mobility; and (e) digital inspection for any swelling.
2. Radiographic examination should be made.
3. It is wise to ask the patient if there are any problems. Despite other negative findings, the patient may have discomfort. As with natural teeth, it is best to treat dis-

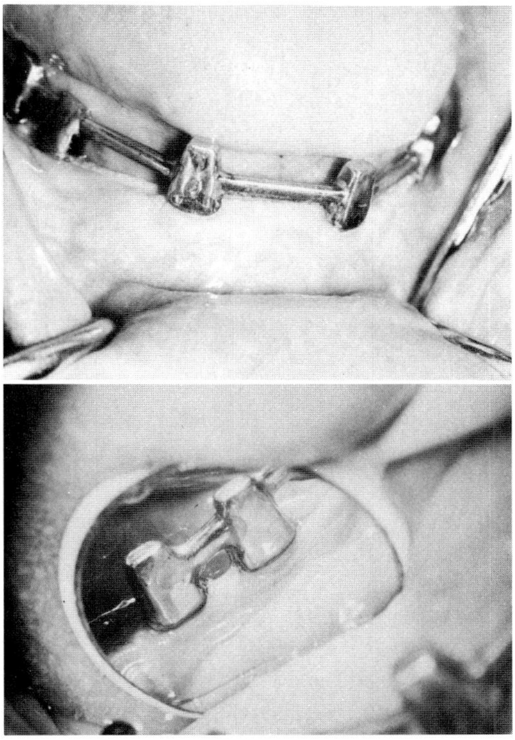

Fig. 7-50. It is preferable to splint the posts of complete-arch blade-vent implants with an intermediary cast superstructure. This serves a purpose similar to the frame of a complete subperiosteal implant (i.e., to dissipate, distribute, and share forces). The superimposed removable prosthesis shoud be supported by all the posts and should not be specifically stressful on any one implant.

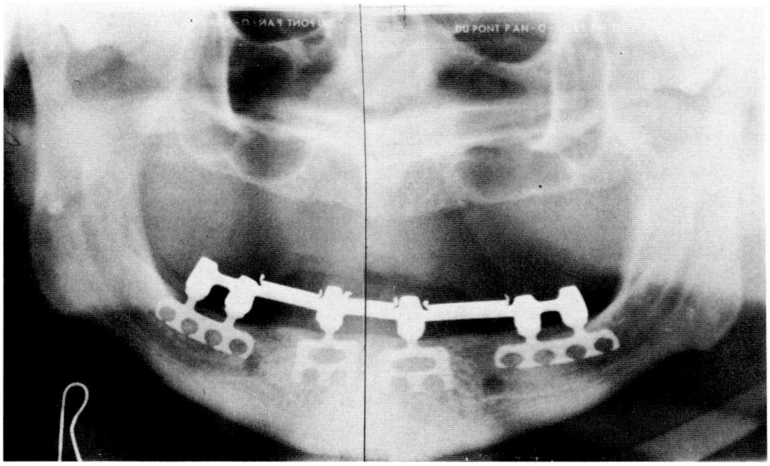

Fig. 7-51. This panoramic radiograph was taken 2 1/2 years after the insertion of multiple blades in the mandible. It is interesting to note the uneventful comparison to Figure 7-49 of the same case. Although no bone loss is present at this time, such is not necessarily the rule. At times, some osseous resorption that causes a saucer-shaped depression may be present around the blade-implant neck; however, such resorption is of itself not indicative of implant failure.

comfort or note and observe it. If necessary, prompt removal of an implant may prevent an anticipated emergency—such as an acute inflammation—from occurring.

In summary, careful insertion techniques and responsible recall follow-throughs constitute essential parts of the implantologist's total treatment.

BIBLIOGRAPHY

Baumhammers, A.: Custom modifications and specifications for blade-vent implant designs to increase their biologic compatibility. J. Oral Implantol., *2:*276-296, 1972.

Beck, P. M.: Versatility of endosseous blade implants. J. Ontario D. A., *48:*110-112, 1971.

Bicoll, N.: Preparation, the keyword for implant dentistry. Oral Implantol., *3:*354-385, 1973.

Cranin, A. N.: Oral Implantology. Springfield, Illinois, Charles C Thomas, 1970.

———: Some comments on the endosseous implant, including operative and postoperative care and observations. D. Clin. North America, *14:*117-123, 1970.

Grafelmann, H. L.: Modern concepts of implant prosthetics for reconstruction with removable superstructures. Telescopic swing-lock system. Oral Implantol., *4:*386-402, Spring, 1974.

James, R. A.: Periodontal considerations in implant dentistry. J. Pros. Dent., *30:*202-209, 1973.

James, R. A., Woods, W., and Kurti, R.: "Blade-vent" implant resulting in an oro-antral fistula. Report of a case. Oral Surg., *37:*350-354, 1974.

Linkow, L. I., and Chercheve, R.: Theories and Techniques of Oral Implantology. St. Louis, C. V. Mosby, 1970.

Smithloff, M., and Fritz, M. E.: The use of blade implants in a selected population of partially edentulous patients: a preliminary report. J. Periodont., *43:*723-736, 1972.

Starshak, T. J.: Preprosthetic Oral Surgery. St. Louis, C. V. Mosby, 1971.

Weiss, C. M., Judy, K. W. M., and Chiarenza, A. R.: Precompacted, coined titanium endosteal blade implants. J. Oral Implantol., *3:*237-257, 1973.

Zola, M. B.: Methods of designing, elevating, and suturing the intra-oral flap. J. Oral Implantol., *3:*5-18, 1972.

8 The Endosteal Blade-Vent Implant—The Histology of Animal Studies and Scanning Electron-Microscope Observations

Charles A. Babbush, D.D.S., M.Sc.D.

HISTOLOGIC STUDIES OF SOFT AND HARD TISSUES IN ANIMALS

During today's renaissance of implantology, the greatest degree of attention and research is being directed to the "attachment" of the implant to the surrounding bone.

According to Bhaskar, the periodontal ligament serves numerous functions. The ligament attaches the natural tooth to the surrounding tissue. After development, the ligament takes over the function of dental follicle and produces cementum and alveolar bone. The nerve endings in the ligament give proprioceptive capabilities to the dental apparatus. These nerve endings contain pain fibers. Therefore, it may be said that the functions of the ligament are supportive, formative, proprioceptive, and sensory.

In the natural dento-alveolar complex, as soon as the forces of mastication and functional stresses are applied, the periodontal ligament widens to its normal size from its developmental phase. This widening of the ligament occurs when there is rapid, yet transitory, resorption of the bone of the socket due to these functional stresses; the periodontal ligament then acts as a suspensory apparatus for the tooth. The fibers of the ligament aid in the dissipation of occlusal forces from the tooth to the surrounding alveolus, in a manner that is analogous to a well-functioning shock absorber. The fibers of the periodontal ligament are ar-

In conducting the research described in this chapter, the investigator followed the *Guide for Laboratory Animal Facilities and Care*, as promulgated by the *Committee on the Guide for Laboratory Animal Facilities and Care* of the Institute of Laboratory Animal Resources, National Academy of Sciences, National Research Council.

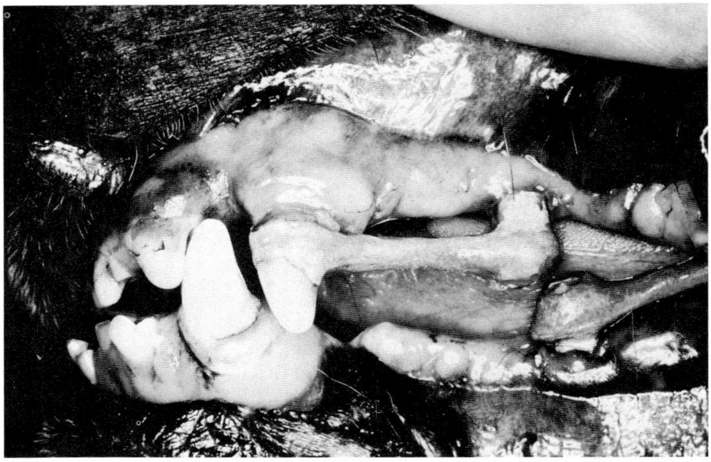

Fig. 8-1. Buccal view of prosthetic appliances in the dog mandible and maxilla 24 months after insertion. Note the occlusal wear.

ranged in a wavy configuration. When forces of tension are applied, the fibers straighten. This causes a slight movement of the tooth, within physiologic limits, when it is in function. If these functional forces exceed the physiologic limits of the ligament, the fibers of the ligament, as well as the surrounding bone, are destroyed.

In addition to the periodontal ligament, the surrounding bone plays an equally important role. The alveolar portion of the maxilla and of the mandible constitutes the wall of the tooth socket and is the bone to which the terminal end of the periodontal ligament is attached.

The design and requirements of the dental implant create a communication between the oral cavity and the bone. The dental implant disrupts the soft-tissue covering of the bone. This disruption becomes an avenue for invasion by bacteria, which becomes more evident when the integrity of the base of the gingival sulcus is not maintained. The research described in this chapter was designed to demonstrate the nature of the soft tissues and osseous structures in relation to the endosteal blade-vent implant.

Implant Insertion in Animals

Three male mongrel dogs, approximately 8 to 10 years of age, were studied in this project. The dogs were anesthetized intravenously with 1 ml. of 1 per cent veterinary sodium pentobarbital per 5 lbs. (2.27 kg.) of body weight. Stage III, Plane I of surgical anesthesia was obtained in 5 to 10 minutes.

The second and third premolars were removed from all quadrants, and the extraction sites were allowed to heal for 120 days. After this postoperative period, the dogs were similarly anesthetized.

A blade-vent implant of proper length and width was selected according to clinical and radiographic measurements. The same procedures, described in Chapter 7, concerning the clinical application of endosteal blade-vent implants, were utilized for the insertion of the implants in this project.

After each implant had been completely seated and the mucoperiosteal flaps sutured, a prefabricated plastic coping was placed over each post. A hole was drilled buccolingually in the mesial cusp of the adjacent molar. A 0.020 stainless-steel wire was brought through the hole and was wrapped around the plastic coping. Cold-cured acrylic resin was painted over the entire structure, simulating a rigid fixed prosthesis (Fig. 8-1).

Implant Removal

None of the animals was sacrificed. After 12, 18, 24, and 30 months, the animals were anesthetized, and the pros-

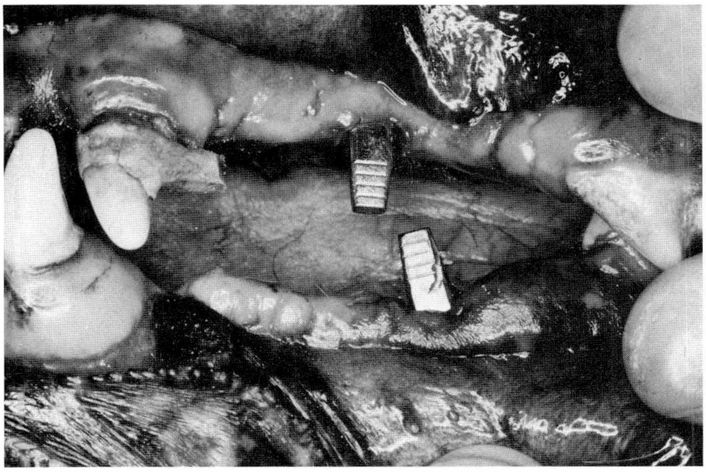

Fig. 8-2. The maxillary and mandibular acrylic-resin prostheses were cut through the pontic area with a carbide bur and removed. The gingival tissues adjacent to the implant neck were hypertrophic, and an accumulation of debris was noted.

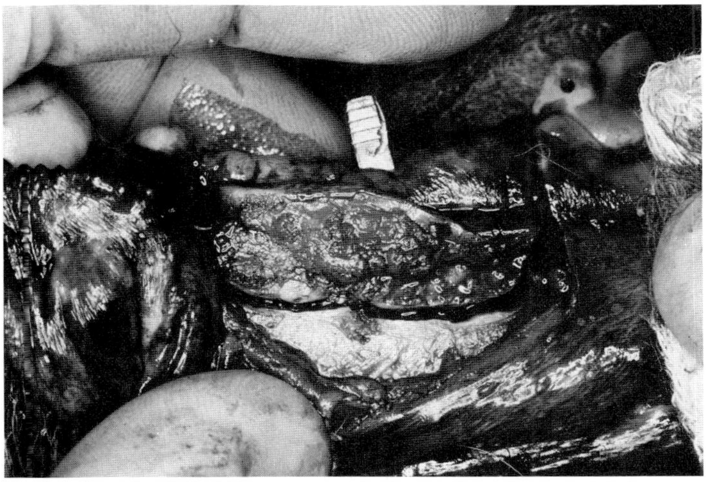

Fig. 8-3. An incision through the mucoperiosteum was made over a wide area that circumscribed the entire implant.

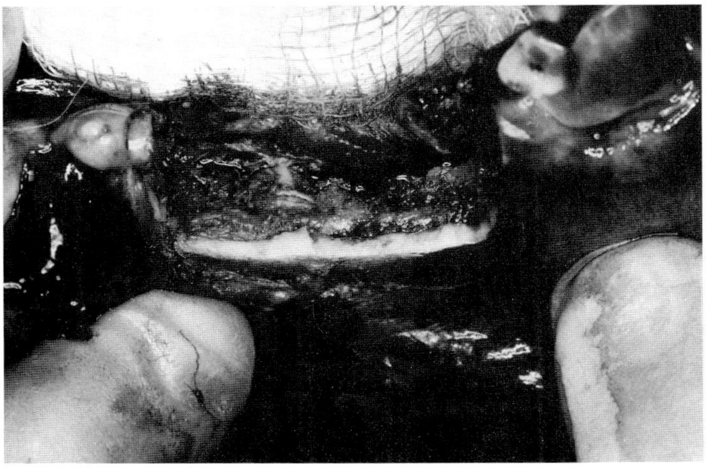

Fig. 8-4. Block section of the bone, including the implant, was removed with a high-speed drill.

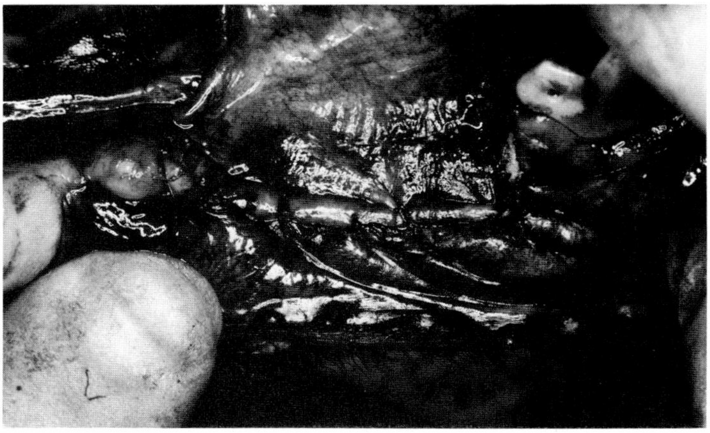

Fig. 8-5. Soft-tissue flaps were elevated and sutured to facilitate healing by primary intention.

theses were removed by cutting through the pontic with a carbide bur. Once these superstructure prostheses were cut, they were easily removed from the implant posts. The gingival tissues adjacent to the implant necks were hypertrophic, and an accumulation of debris was noted (Fig. 8-2). No clinical mobility of the implants was noted.

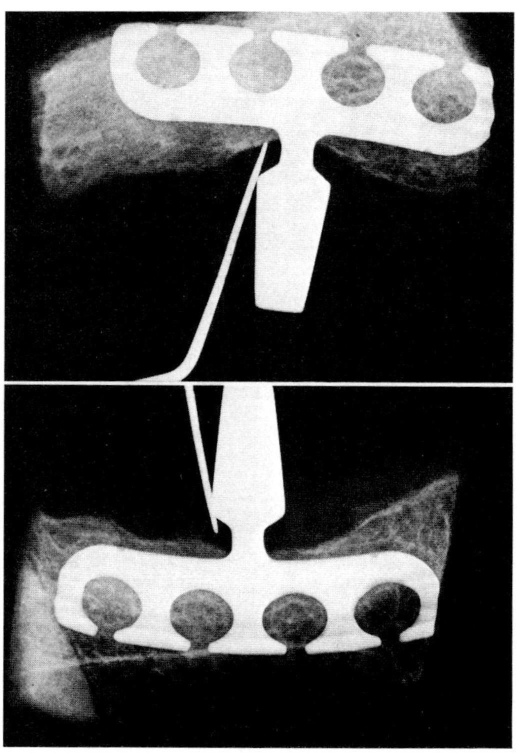

Fig. 8-6. Radiographs of periodontal probing of the sulcular area revealed no pathology.

An incision through the mucoperiosteum of each dog was made over a wide area that circumscribed the entire implant. A block section of the bone, including the implant, was removed with a high-speed drill. Soft-tissue flaps were elevated and sutured to facilitate healing by primary intention. (Figs. 8-3 to 8-5). Radiographs of periodontal probes in the sulcular areas of the block sections revealed no pathology (Fig. 8-6). The specimens were then fixed in 10 per cent formalin and were decalcified with RDO.*

Visual Examination of Removed Implants

After the bone had been decalcified, the entire buccal bone was removed from the surface of the implant (Fig. 8-7). Each implant was then examined visually in its bony crypt. The four compartments between the vents of the implants were occupied with a calcified tissue. The tissues over the shoulder of the implant also appeared to be calcified. The tissues adjacent to the neck of the implant were very closely adapted. The implant was then dissected from its surrounding tissues. Four distinct

*Dupage Kenetic Laboratories, Inc., Downers Grove, Illinois.

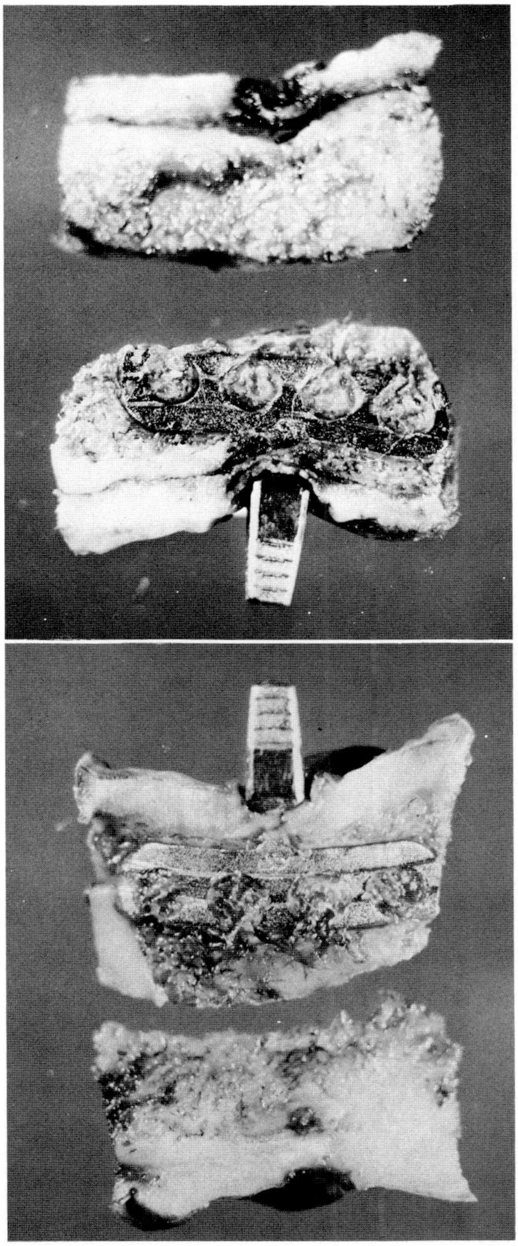

Fig. 8-7. After the bone had been decalcified, the buccal bone was removed from the surface of each implant. The four compartments between the vents of the implants were occupied with a calcified tissue. The tissue over the shoulder of the implant also appeared to be calcified. The tissues adjacent to the neck of the implant were very closely adapted to the neck.

cores of tissue were observed. The horizontal notching of the implant body (frame) was duplicated in the adjacent tissue (Fig. 8-8).

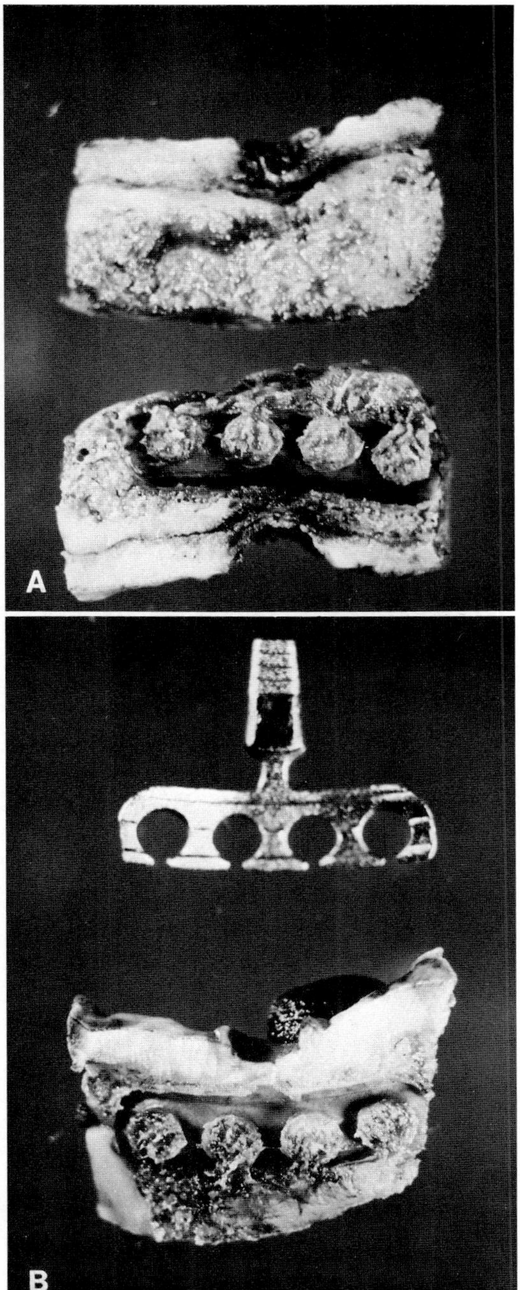

Fig. 8-8. The implants were dissected from the surrounding tissues. Four distinct cores of tissue were observed. The horizontal notching of the implant body was duplicated in the adjacent tissue.

Histologic Observations in Animals

The specimens were then prepared for histologic examination. Sections were cut

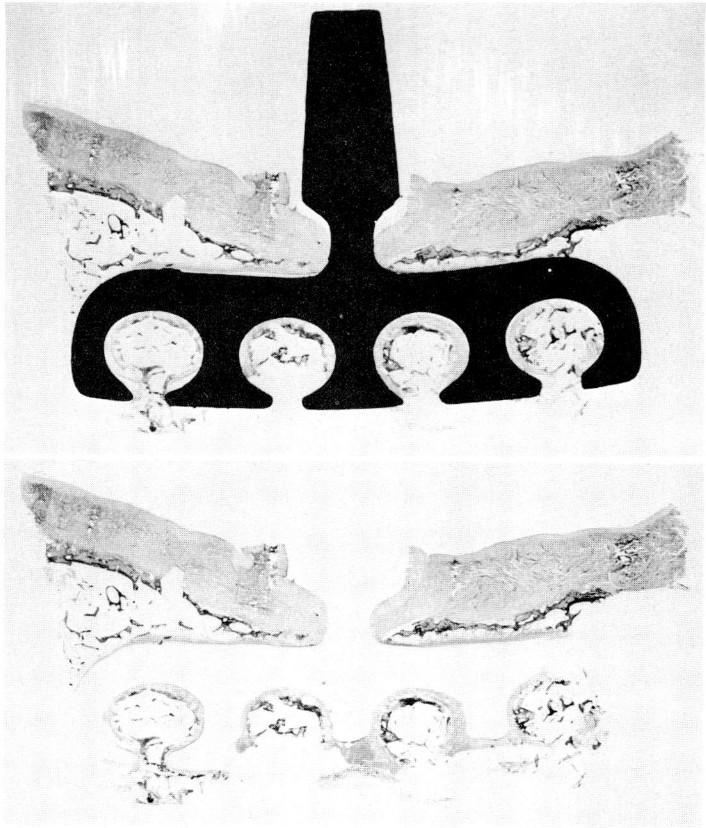

Fig. 8-9. The specimens were prepared for histologic examination. The outline of the implant has been superimposed for clarity. Sections were alternately cut. Some sections were stained with hematoxylin and eosin and some with azocarmine connective-tissue stain. (× 2)

and stained with hematoxylin and eosin and with azocarmine connective-tissue stain (Fig. 8-9). The histologic maxillary and mandibular specimens were reviewed:

1. The surface of the histologic specimens consisted of a relatively thick, stratified, squamous epithelium (Fig. 8-10).
2. A defect approximately 2-mm. wide

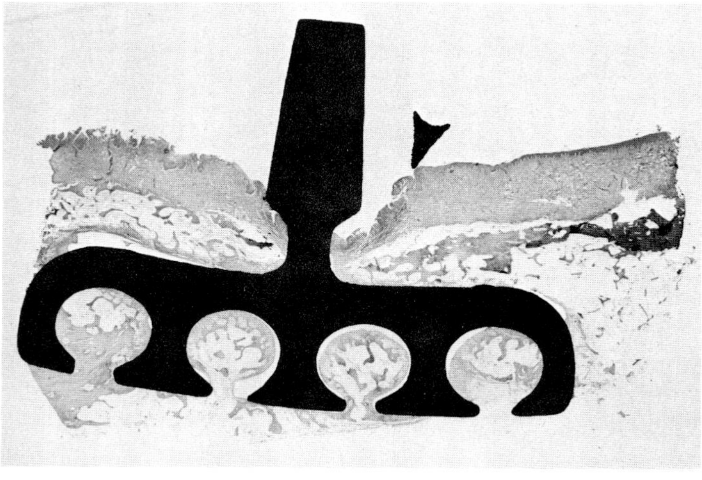

Fig. 8-10. The surface of the histologic specimens was covered by a relatively thick, stratified, squamous epithelium (*arrow*). (Hematoxylin and eosin; × 2)

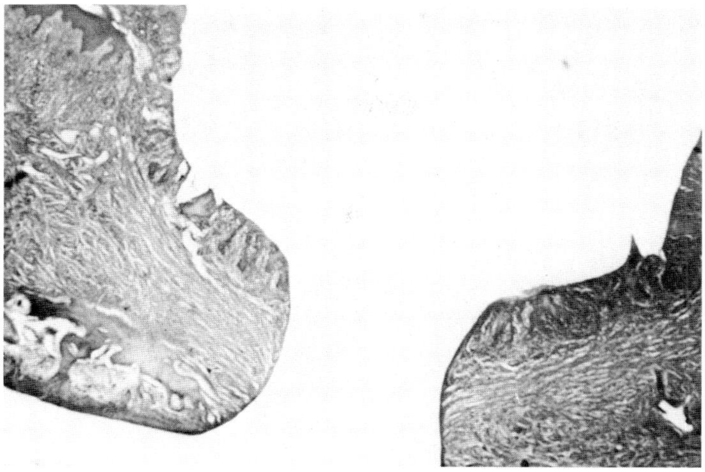

Fig. 8-11. A defect (opening) approximately 2 mm. wide was located in the mid-portion of the specimen, through which the neck of the implant extruded. (Hematoxylin and eosin; × 20)

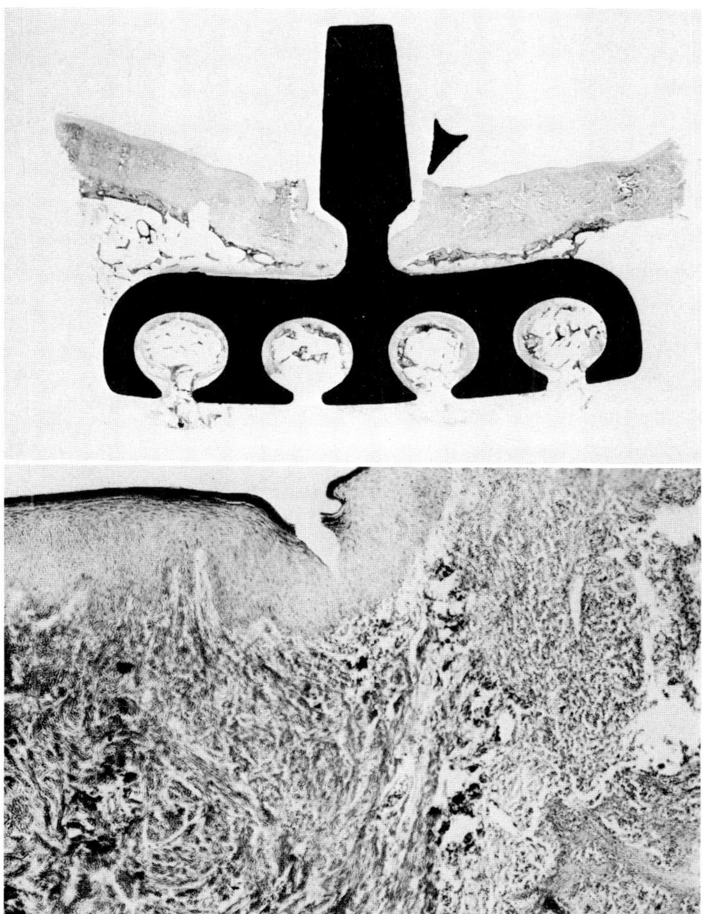

Fig. 8-12. The stratified squamous epithelium (*arrow*) showed no significant abnormalities; but in some specimens, the subepithelial connective tissue adjacent to the neck area was densely infiltrated with lymphocytes. (Azocarmine; × 2, × 50)

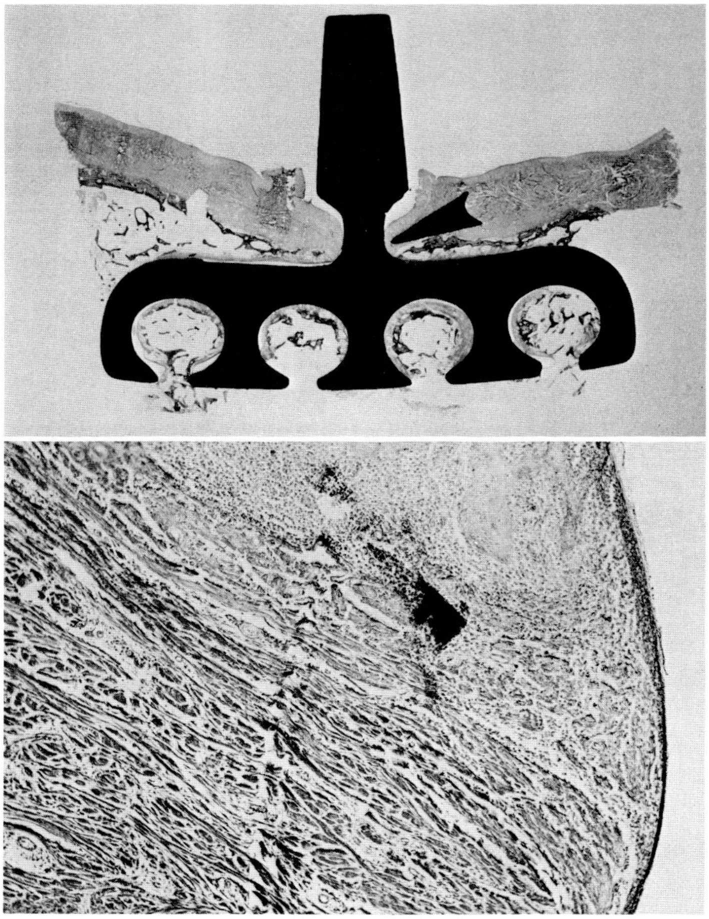

Fig. 8-13. At a short distance from the defect, there was no inflammatory infiltrate. The epithelial layer turned inferiorly and followed the course of the defect, becoming thinner as it approached the base of the implant neck (*arrow*). (Azocarmine; × 2, × 50)

was located in the mid-portion of the specimen, through which the neck of the implant extruded (Fig. 8-11).

3. The tissue on both sides of the defect was densely collagenous, sparsely nucleated, and almost completely hyalinized.

4. The stratified squamous epithelium showed no significant abnormalities; but in some specimens, the subepithelial connective tissue adjacent to the neck area was densely infiltrated with lymphocytes (Fig. 8-12).

5. At a short distance from the defect, there was no inflammatory infiltrate. The epithelial layer turned inferiorly and followed the course of the defect, becoming thinner as it approached the base of the implant neck (Fig. 8-13).

6. In both the maxillary and mandibular specimens, the calcified tissues in the regions over the shoulder and in the vented portions of the implant were surrounded by a band of densely collagenous, sparsely nucleated, partly hyalinized, fibrous connective tissue (Fig. 8-14).

7. The bony trabeculae were well calcified and were covered by low cuboidal or flattened osteoblasts, with layers of osteoid tissue beneath the osteoblasts (Fig. 8-15).

8. The remainder of the area surrounding the implant consisted of a clear space in which there were four separate and distinct circular areas that were filled with an ingrowth of tissue (Fig. 8-16). In both the mandibular and maxillary specimens, these circular areas represented cross sec-

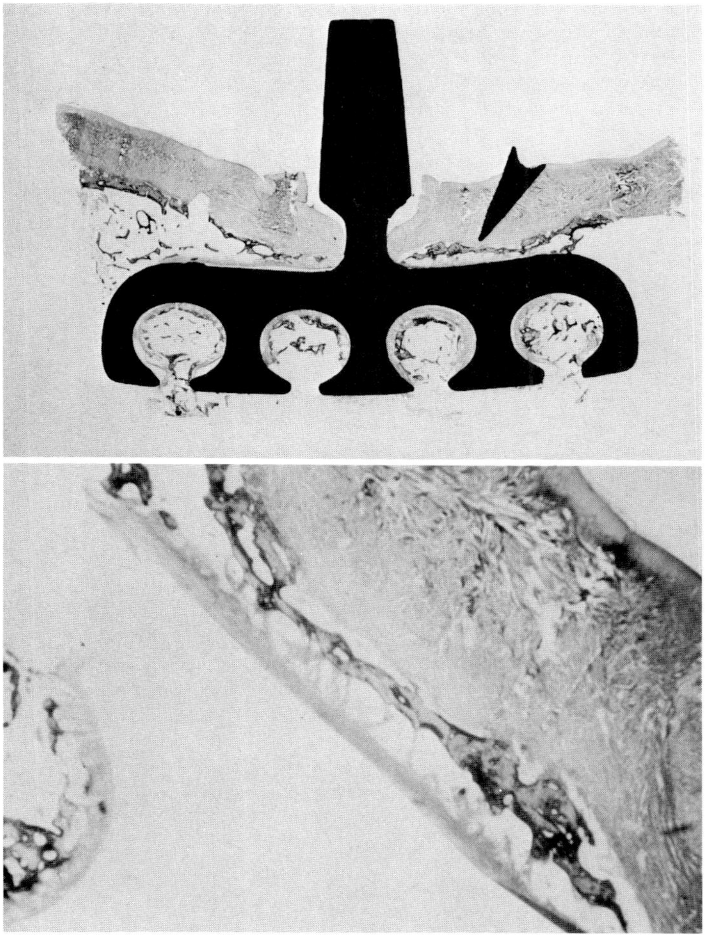

Fig. 8-14. In both the maxillary and mandibular specimens, the calcified tissues in the regions over the shoulder (*arrow*) and in the vented portions of the implant were surrounded by a band of densely collagenous, sparsely nucleated, partly hyalinized, fibrous connective tissue. (Hematoxylin and eosin, azocarmine; × 2, × 50)

tions of bony tissue, consisting of a central core of trabeculated bone that was surrounded by a thick band of densely collagenous, sparsely nucleated, partly hyalinized connective tissue. The bony trabeculae seemed well calcified and were surrounded by a single layer of flat cuboidal osteoblasts.

All the specimens were histologically similar. There were no signs of rejection or foreign body giant cells reaction.

Evaluation of Clinical and Histologic Animal Observations

The implants were in a functional or in a modified functional state, as was noted from the amount of occlusal wear of the acrylic prostheses. When the prosthetic appliances were removed, all implants were clinically supportive and functional, asymptomatic, nonpathologic, and immobile. Localized edema and accumulation of debris occurred in the gingival area of several specimens, apparently because of the lack of any form of oral hygiene. The pontics had been designed for self-cleansing; to a limited degree, the soft-tissue response (the soft tissue was healthier under the pontic areas than around the natural tooth or the implant crown) reflected the sanitary nature of these pontics.

In all specimens, the sulcular areas maintained their integrity; this finding was supported by histologic examination and by periodontal probing. If a sulcus were to

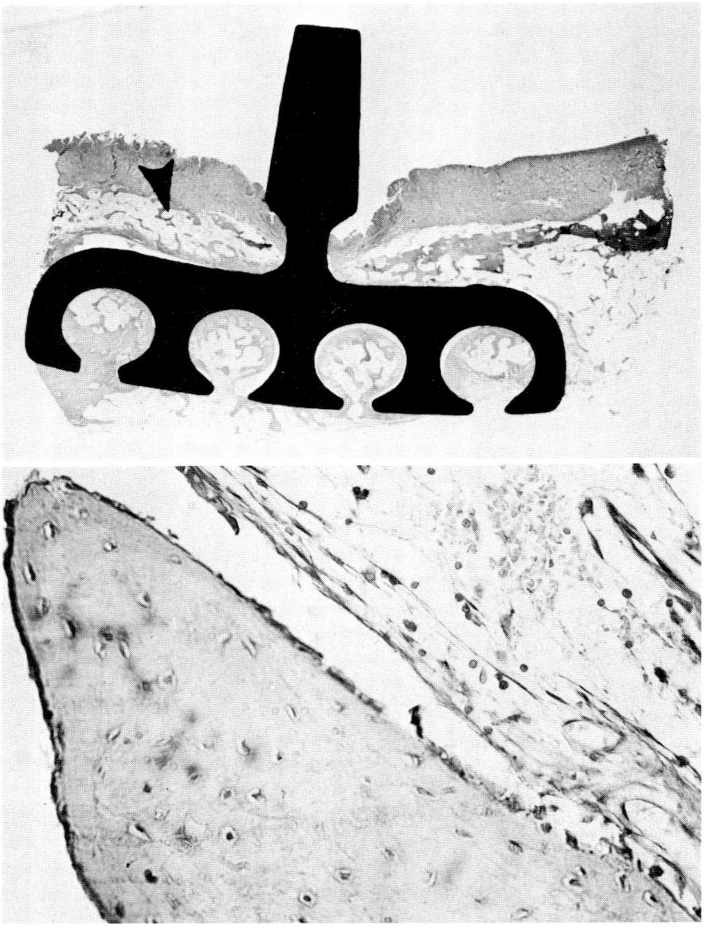

Fig. 8-15. The bony trabeculae (*arrow*) were well calcified and were covered by low cuboidal or flattened osteoblasts, with layers of osteoid tissue beneath the osteoblasts. Osteocytes filled the lacunae. (Hematoxylin and eosin; × 2, × 200)

become pathologic, bacteria might then infiltrate the tissues beyond the base of the sulcus, perhaps surrounding the entire implant. Thus, mobility and supportive failure might eventually occur.

The study of the histologic sections revealed an "implant periodontal ligament." This is a fibrous connective-tissue membrane that occupies the space between the implant and the surrounding bone. In the natural dentition, the fibers of the periodontal ligament are oriented obliquely or perpendicularly to the teeth; these fibers are usually aligned and realigned in the direction of the forces of occlusion or the lack of same. In an arch that has an implant, the fibers of the ligament are parallel to the implant; however, in the core that occupies the vent, in the area adjacent to the membrane, perpendicular fibers are present, apparently in response to the forces of occlusion.

It was concluded that the thickness of the ligamentous sheaths, the direction of the fibers, and the nature of the cribriform plate to which the fibers are attached were determined by design and function of the implant.

SCANNING ELECTRON-MICROSCOPE OBSERVATIONS

Another method of examining the blade-vent implant is the use of the scanning electron microscope. This instrument makes possible the study of the topography of a given specimen by a magnification

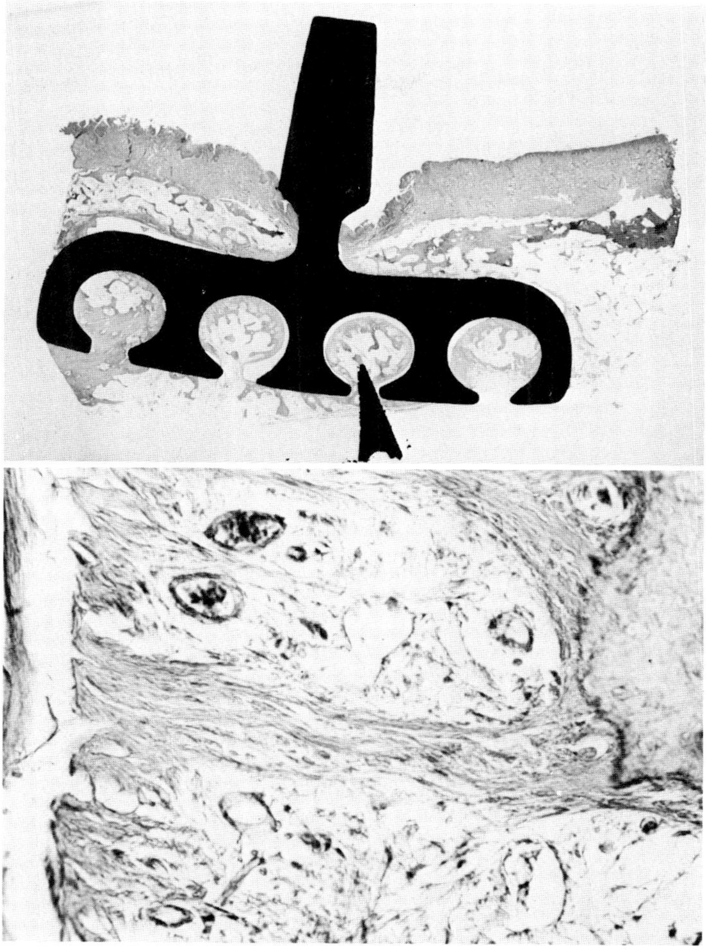

Fig. 8-16. The remainder of the area surrounding the implant consisted of tissue-bearing spaces of which there were four separate and distinct circular areas (*arrow*) that were filled with an ingrowth of tissue. In both the mandibular and maxillary specimens, this tissue consisted of a central core of trabeculated bone, surrounded by a thick band of densely collagenous, sparsely nucleated, partly hyalinized connective tissue. (Hematoxylin and eosin; × 2, × 200)

of from 12 to 100,000 times. It also enables a large specimen to be studied in its entirety.

Two endosteal blade-vent implants were inserted in the dog mandible according to techniques described in Chapter 7. One implant was maintained under usual procedures for 12 months. The second implant was continuously traumatized during the same period of time.

At the termination of the 12 months, the implants were removed with a block section of surrounding tissue. The nontraumatized implant was clinically and radiographically successful at the time of removal. Periodontal probing could only be extended to the base of the "implant periodontal sulcus"; the implant was found to

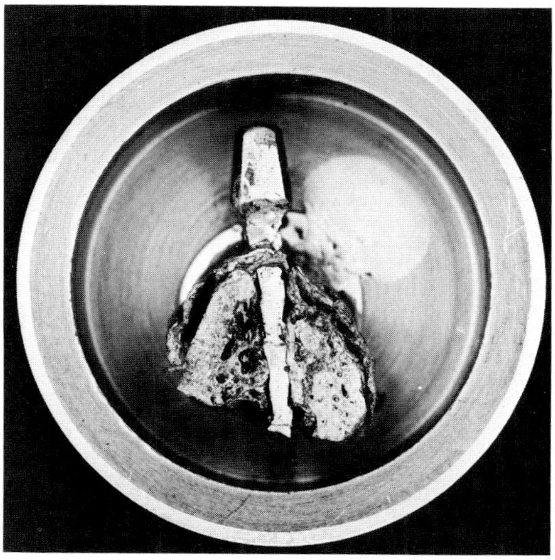

Fig. 8-17. Block section cemented to aluminum and coated with gold-palladium alloy.

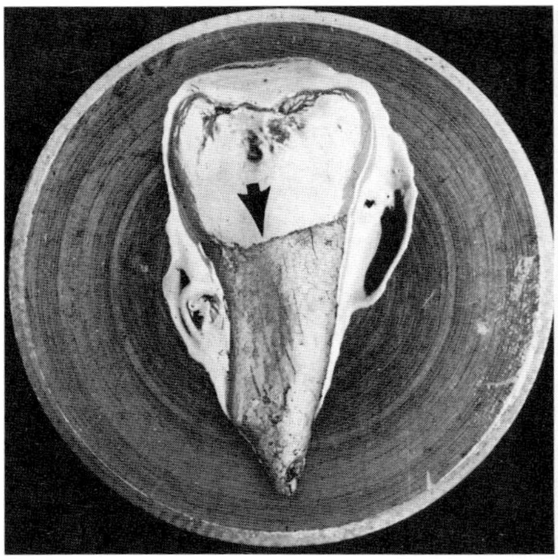

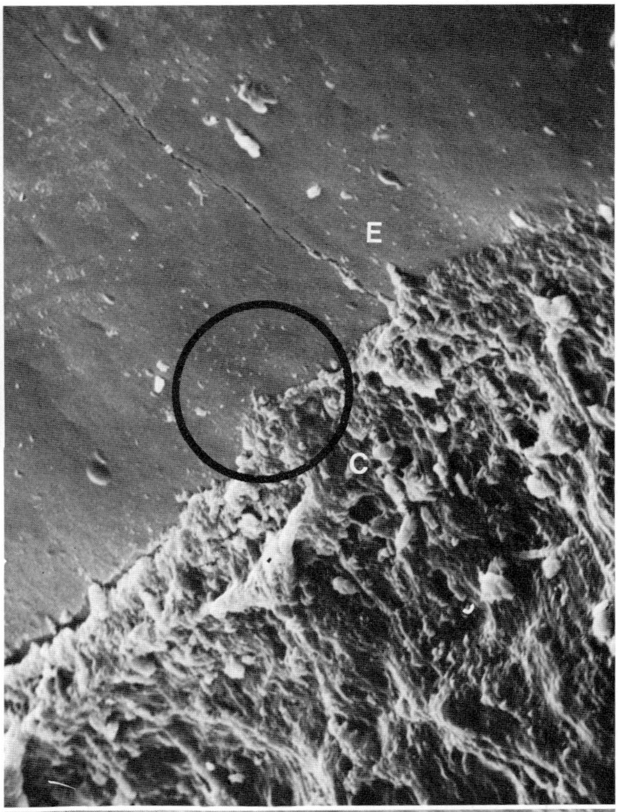

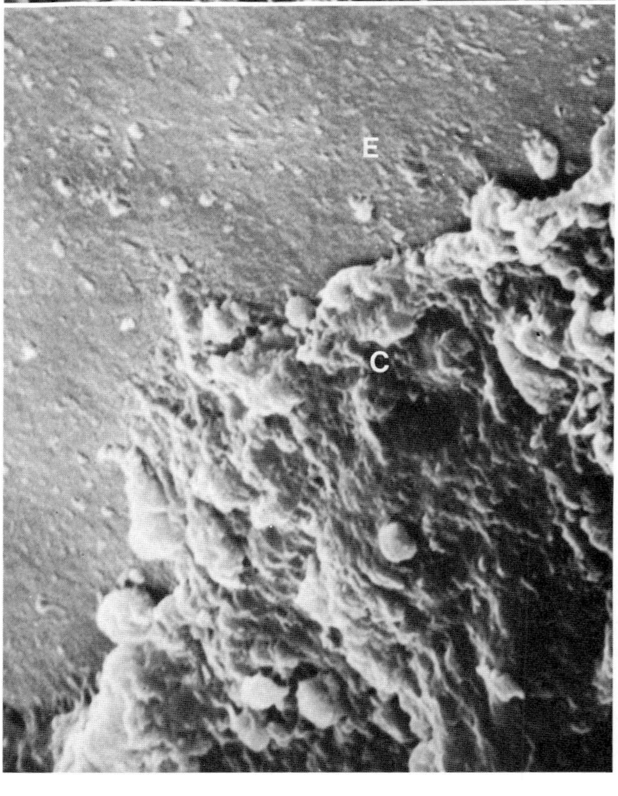

Fig. 8-18. (*Top left*) Human molar tooth. (*Bottom right;* × 5,000) Smooth coated with gold-palladium alloy (arrow shows cemento-enamel junction). (*Top right*) Scanning electron micrograph (× 1,000) of cemento-enamel (C-E) junction of human molar tooth.(*Bottom right;* × 5,000) Smooth surface above is enamel (E); rough, irregular surface below is cementum (C).

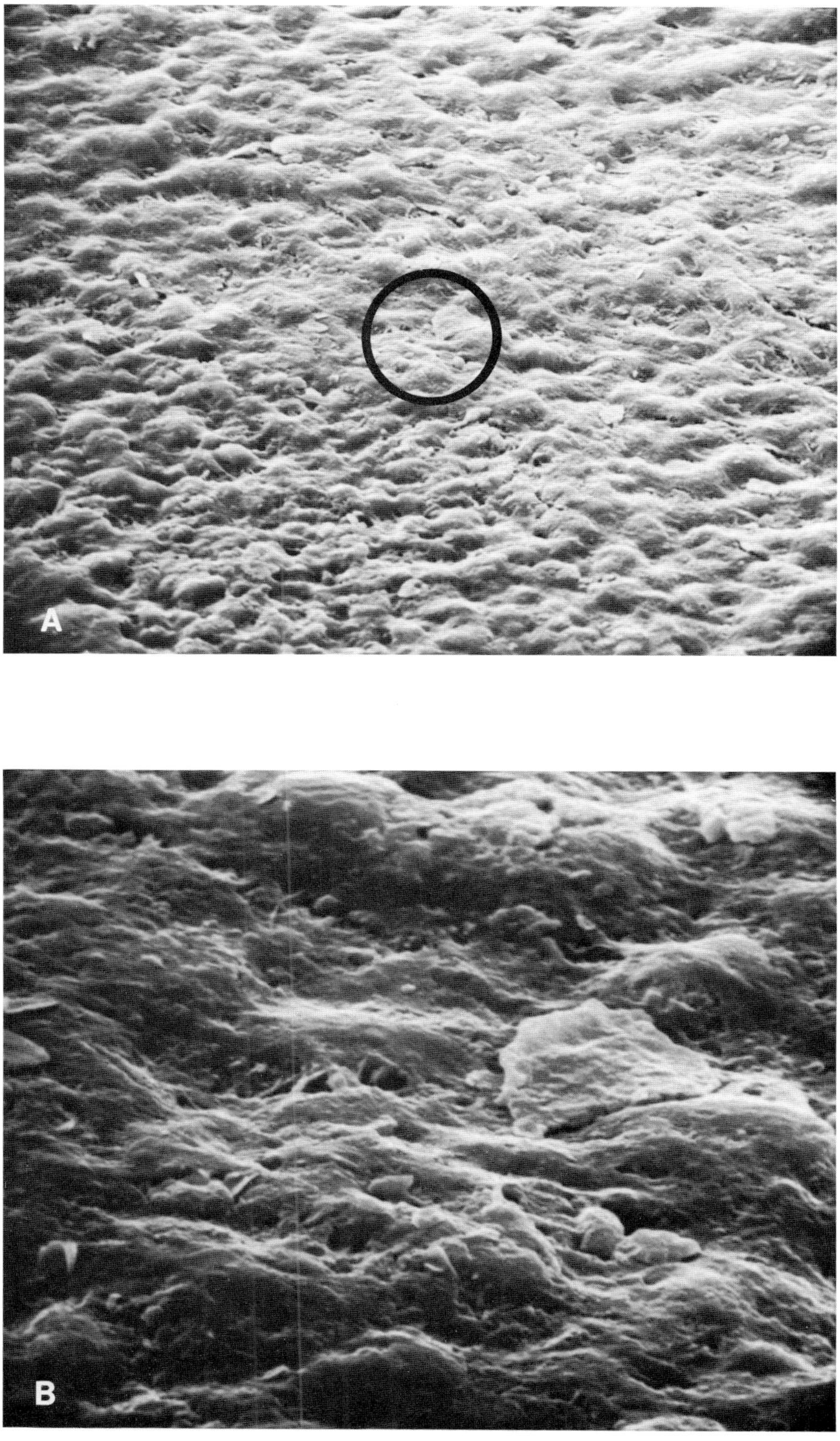

Fig. 8-19. Scanning electron micrographs of surface of root of human molar tooth, showing the irregular surface of the cementum. *B* (× 5,000) shows detail of circled area in *A* (× 1,000).

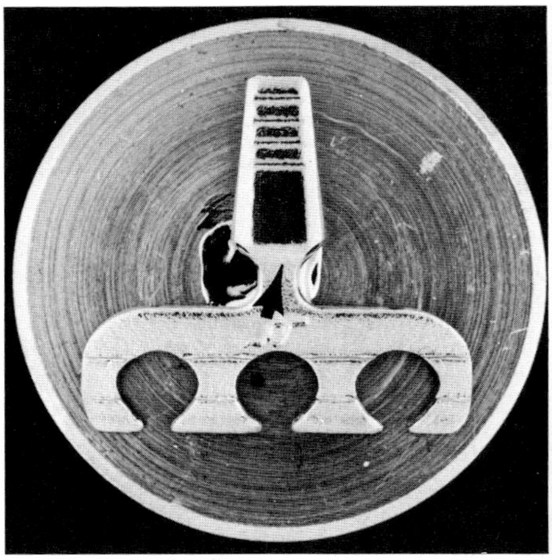

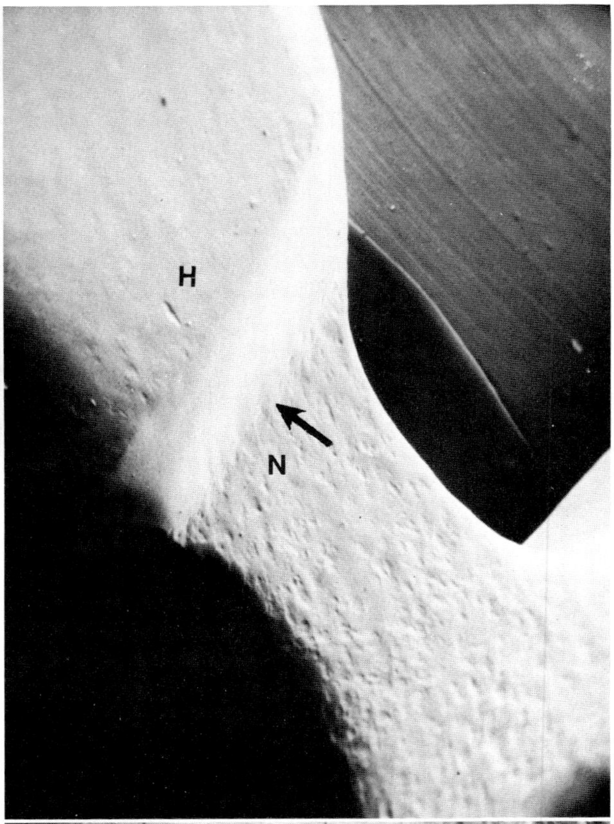

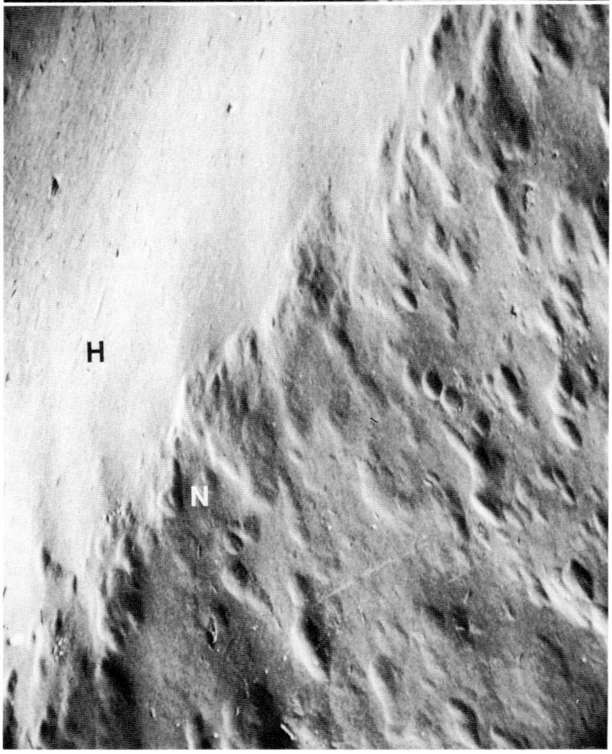

Fig. 8-20. Gross (*top left*) and scanning electron microscopic (*top right,* × 20; *bottom right,* × 100) views of a control endosteal blade-vent implant mounted on aluminum disc and coated with gold-palladium alloy. The arrows show the corresponding junction of abutment head (H) and neck (N) of the implant in the gross and microscopic views. The area of the junction of the abutment head with the neck of the implant simulates *but does not duplicate* the cemento-enamel junction of human teeth.

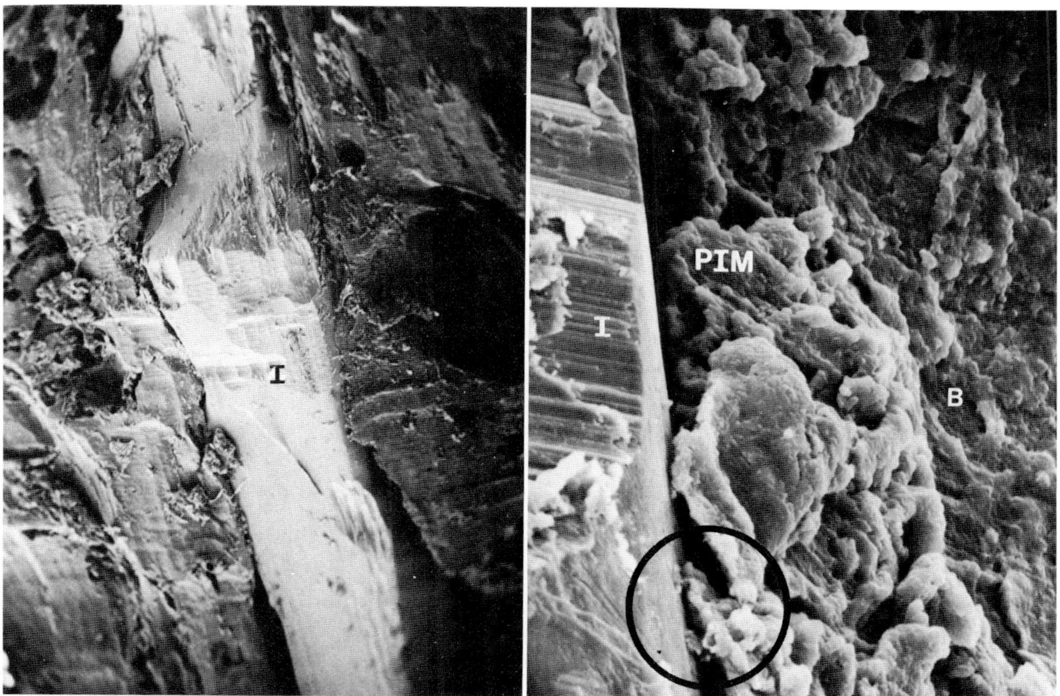

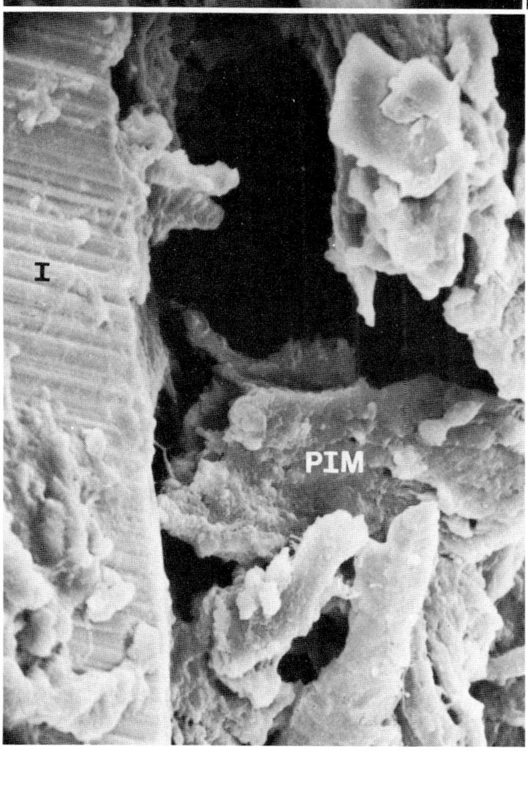

Fig. 8-21. Scanning electron micrographs of a block section of the clinically successful endosteal blade-vent implant in a dog mandible, 12 months after insertion. The implant (I) was surrounded by a zone of well-organized "peri-implant tissue" (PIM) that simulates *but does not duplicate* the periodontal ligament in natural dentition. This zone of tissue was surrounded by another type of tissue (B) that appeared to be calcified and resembled bone. (*Top left,* × 20; *top right,* × 1,000; *bottom left,* × 5,000)

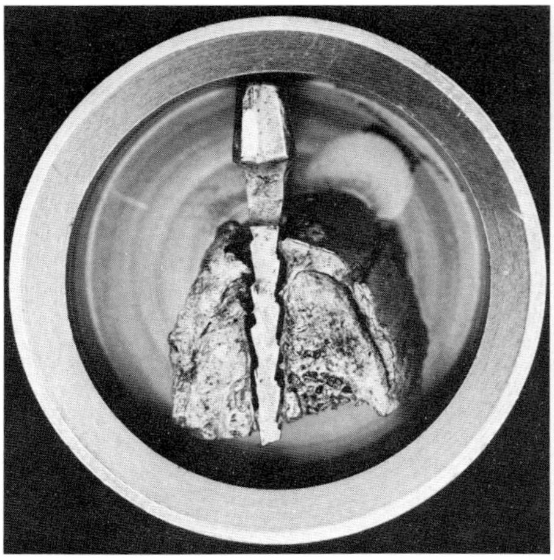

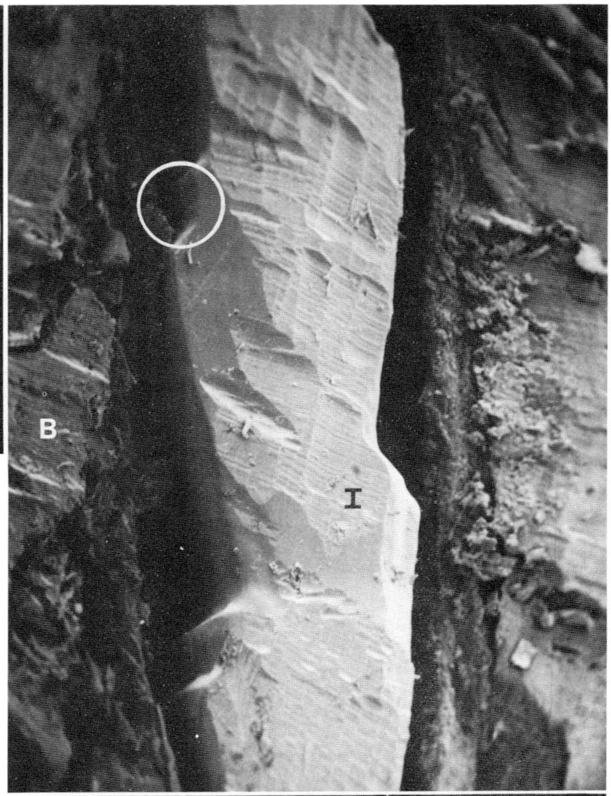

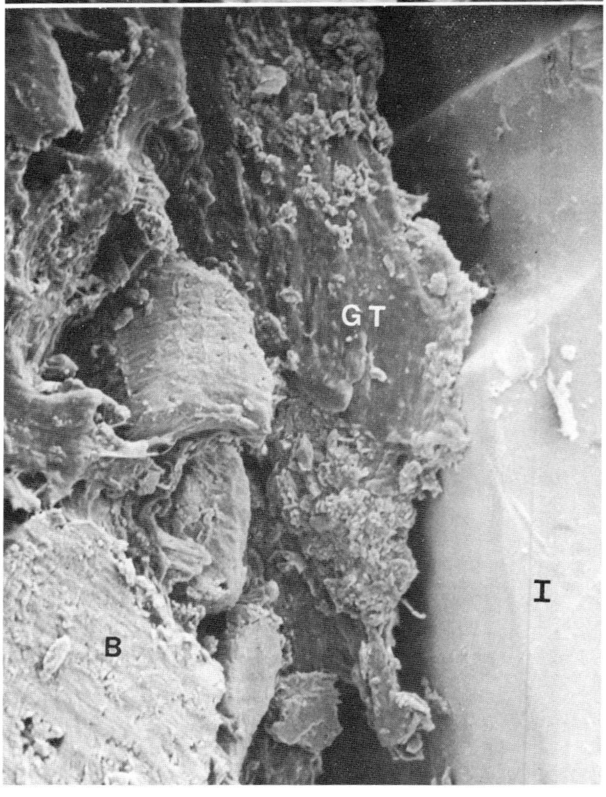

Fig. 8-22. Block section (*top left*) and scanning electron micrographs (*top right,* × 20; *bottom right,* × 1,000) of the clinically failing endosteal blade-vent implant in the dog mandible 12 months after insertion. The implant (I) was surrounded by a dark space next to which was an irregular, poorly organized zone of tissue that resembled granulation tissue (GT). This granulation tissue was surrounded by a well-organized calcified tissue (B) that appeared to be bone.

be immobile. The traumatized specimen demonstrated a radiolucent zone of tissue surrounding the implant. The periodontal probe could be extended to the apical portion of the implant body; a plus 2 mobility was demonstrated. For these reasons, this implant was deemed to be a clinical failure.

The block sections were placed in 80 per cent alcohol for drying. The specimens were then cemented to an aluminum disc and placed in a vacuum evaporator. The entire surface was uniformly coated with a layer of gold-palladium alloy (Fig. 8-17). The specimens were then examined with a scanning electron microscope.

In addition, a human mandibular third molar and a randomly selected blade-vent implant were mounted and coated as controls. The mandibular third molar was examined for normal surface detail (Figs. 8-18, 8-19). Normally, the surface texture of the enamel is smooth, and that of the cementum is pitted. The cementum covers the surface of the root of the tooth, and the periodontal ligament attaches the cementum to the alveolar bone.

Scanning electron micrographs of the control endosteal blade-vent implant are shown in Figure 8-20. The junction of the neck of the implant with the abutment head (post) resembled the cemento-enamel junction of the natural molar tooth. The smoothness of the implant head resembled the enamel of the natural crown, and the pitted surface of the neck was similar to that of the cementum on the surface of the root.

The scanning electron micrographs of the cross section of the successful implant revealed a tissue that was closely adapted to the implant (Fig. 8-21, *top left*). At a higher magnification, three distinct areas were noted: (a) the implant; (b) a well-organized type of soft tissue surrounding the implant, which may represent the "periodontal implant membrane;" and (c) the peripheral area, which appeared to be more highly calcified and probably represented the surrounding bone (Fig. 8-21, *top right*).

At still higher magnification, a well-organized, highly adaptive soft tissue was seen at the surface of the implant—the "periodontal implant membrane" (Fig. 8-21, *bottom*).

The scanning electron micrographs of the clinically failing implant revealed a clear zone around the implant, a thin area of irregular tissue that probably was granulation tissue, and a calcified tissue that was adjacent to the granulation tissue and that appeared to be the surrounding bone (Fig. 8-22).

BIBLIOGRAPHY

Armitage, J., Natiella, J., Greene, G. Jr., and Meenaghan, M.: An evaluation of early bone changes after the insertion of metal endosseous implants into the jaws of rhesus monkeys. Oral Surg., *32:*558-568, 1971.

Babbush, C. A.: Endosseous blade-vent implants: a research review. J. Oral Surg., *30:*168-175, 1972.

Bernier, J. L., and Canby, C. P.: Histologic studies on the reaction of alveolar bone to Vitallium implants. J. A. D. A., *30:*188-197, 1963.

Bhaskar, S. N.: Synopsis of Oral Histology. St. Louis, C. V. Mosby, 1962.

Chiarenza, A.: The implant sulcus. Oral Implantol., *4:*330-339, 1974.

Chung, S.: The periodontal ligament. Periodont. Abst., *21:*108-118, 1973.

Council on Dental Materials and Devices, Council on Dental Research: Current Evaluation of Dental Endosseous Implants. J. A. D. A., *88:*394-395, 1974.

Ferguson, A. B. Jr.: Metal and Engineering in Bone and Joint Surgery. Baltimore, Williams & Wilkins, 1959.

Homsy, C. A., Kent, J. N., and Hinds, E. C.: Materials for oral implantation—biological and functional criteria. J. A. D. A., *86:*817-832, 1973.

James, R. A.: A histological study of the nature of epithelium surrounding implant posts. Oral Implantol. *3:*105-122, 1972 (Part I); 137-159, 1973 (Part II).

Julius, R. B.: The reliability of metallic implant and anatomic cephalometric superimposition techniques for the maxilla and mandible. Am. J. Orthodontics, *65:*318-319, 1974.

Ludwigson, D. C.: Requirements for metallic surgical implants and prosthetic devices. Metal Engineering Quart., *5:*1-6, 1965.

Molinari, J. A.: The immunology of implants. Oral Implantol., *3:*160-174, 1973.

Newman, C., and Van Huysen, G.: Tissue reaction to Vitallium implantation. J. Pros. Dent., *4:*850-854, 1964.

Piliero, S. J., *et al.:* Histopathology or oral endosteal metallic implants in dogs. J. D. Res., *52:*1117-1127, 1973.

Venable, C. S., and Stuck, W. G.: General considerations of metals and buried appliances in surgery. Internat. Abst. Surg., *76:*297, 1943.

9 Prosthodontic Considerations of Dental Implants

THE RELATIONSHIP BETWEEN IMPLANT DENTISTRY AND PROSTHODONTIC TECHNIQUES (THE SYMBIOTIC RELATIONSHIP)

The prosthodontist should regard the surgically successful dental implant with the same importance that he would the successful endodontically treated tooth. In either case, the proper prosthodontic techniques are essential for the successful retention and use of the natural or man-made abutment tooth (Fig. 9-1).

The transition from the temporary (provisional) prosthesis to the permanent removable or fixed superstructure should be atraumatic. The temporary prosthesis (see Chaps. 5 and 10) should include as many of the characteristics required in the permanent prosthesis as is at all feasible (Fig. 9-2); occlusion, contours, pontics, margins, and esthetics should be considered as carefully in the fabrication of the temporary acrylic-resin prosthesis as in the fabrication of the final superstructure. (Naturally, the differences of the relative strengths of materials used must be taken into consideration.) Through such considered designs of both the temporary and the final prostheses, the following goals should be achieved:

1. The transition from temporary prosthesis to final prosthesis should be easily tolerated and accepted by the patient.
2. The functional capability of the final prosthesis should be predictable by the operator at the time of its insertion, because modifications and improvements on the temporary acrylic-resin splint would have been incorporated in the design of the final prosthesis.
3. The well-fabricated acrylic-resin splint can serve as a good functional and esthetic appliance, providing comfort for the patient during the lengthy amount of time that is required for the impressions, try-ins, indices, mountings, and laboratory steps of each prosthetic phase. Thus, the operator can give, without haste, due

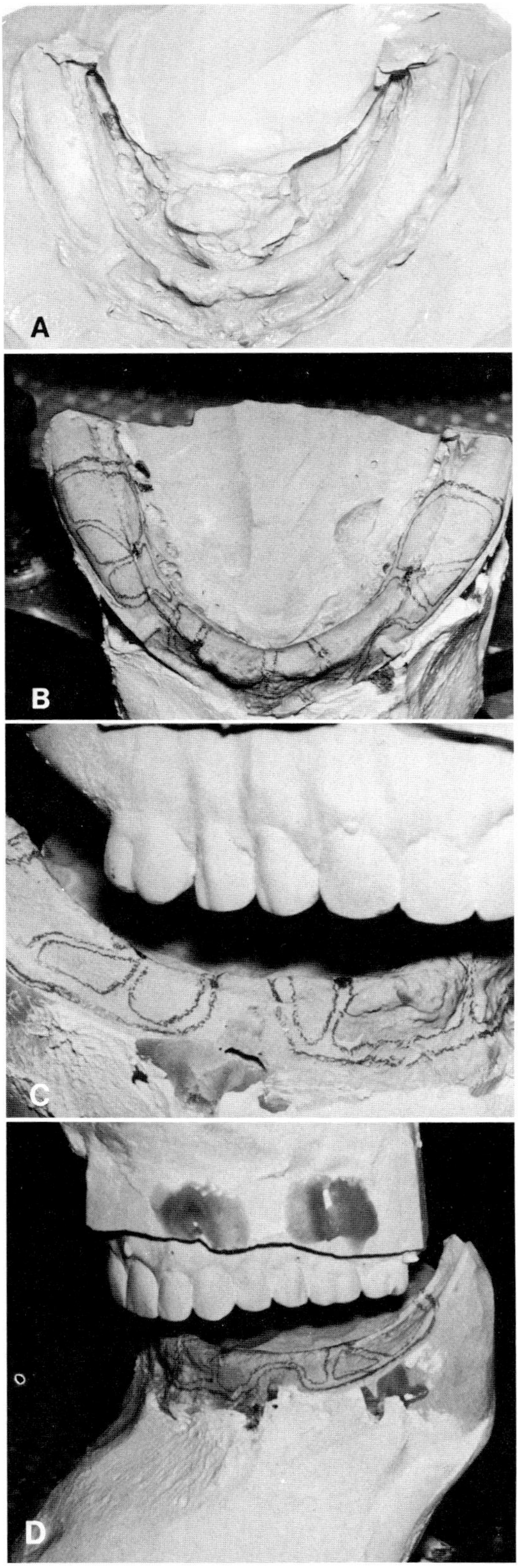

Fig. 9-1. Prosthodontic techniques that are basic to subperiosteal implant fabrication. (*A*) shows a die-stone model that has been poured for a complete mandibular subperiosteal implant. (*B*) shows this same model that has subsequently been trimmed and mounted on an articulator. The design of the implant frame and the locations of the posts have been outlined by the implantologist for the wax-up of the implant, prior to any other prosthetic considerations (*B* to *D*). This mounting will also be used for the fabrication of a temporary removable complete lower denture (see Chap. 5, on Temporization).

consideration to proper prosthodontic techniques that precede the insertion of the final prosthesis.

When fabricating any superstructure, it is important to bear in mind that the superstructure must not impede the functional longevity and cleansability of the implant components and their surrounding tissues. Plaque control, for example, is as important around the implant neck as it is around any natural abutment tooth. Also, the need to minimize lateral stresses should be considered when modifying any superstructure design. Therefore, not only must the implant be properly inserted surgically in order to support a functional prosthesis, but the prosthesis must be designed to enhance the environment for the survival of the implant.

THE CHOICE BETWEEN THE REMOVABLE AND THE FIXED PROSTHESIS

The choice between the use of a fixed superstructure or a removable appliance is dependent on the following factors:

1. Severe bone loss, leaving a highly resorbed residual ridge, may preclude the use of a fixed superstructure. The fixed appliance in such a situation may be esthetically unacceptable because of its excessively bulky and elongated teeth that would be created because of the lack of a denture base. Such elongated and bulky teeth could also be detrimental to the soft-tissue environment. The use of an acrylic-resin

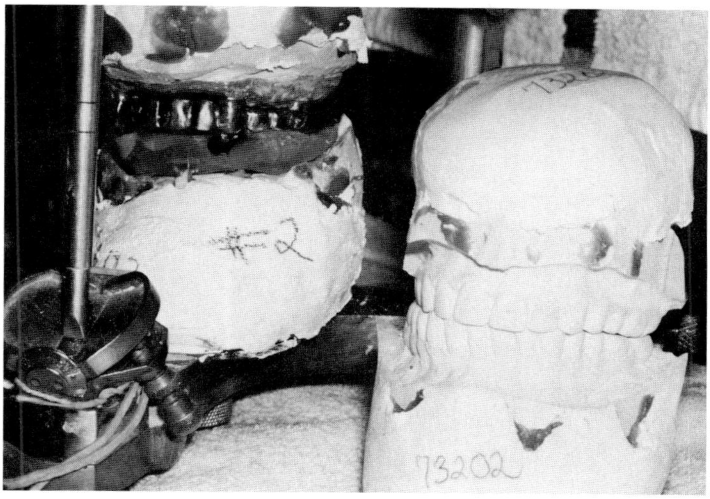

Fig. 9-2. A semi-adjustable articulator mounting (*left*) for the fabrication of the final prostheses, and a simple hinge mounting (*right*) of models of the temporary prostheses. The simple articulation of the temporary fixed splints or removable appliances serves as a guideline that should be followed in the construction of the permanent prosthesis.

denture base, which is possible in the removable superstructure, can aid in the supportive, and thus the esthetic, role of the superstructure.

The operator must also bear in mind the relatively excessive weight of a fixed appliance—compared with a removable appliance—that would be placed on an arch with severe ridge resorption. This factor is especially important in the upper arch. A constant gravitational pull on a heavy, fixed, upper-arch appliance could be damaging to the supportive structures of any implant in the long term.

In many implant cases, the amount of ridge resorption indicates the use of either a removable or a fixed appliance simply because of the capability of the particular appliance to support the surrounding soft tissues of the cheeks and lips.

2. In those cases where physical considerations are not overriding, psychological acceptability may influence the choice of the fixed or removable appliance. If the amount of ridge resorption is not great, either a removable or a fixed appliance may be used. The patient may then be given the choice. If he would feel more comfortable and stable with a fixed prosthesis, then, all things being equal, a fixed superstructure may be used. In cases that involve both natural and implant abutments, the same principles apply. The only proviso in such cases—i.e., of natural-tooth abutments with a removable prosthesis—is that the natural teeth be protected with cast copings that act as intermediaries between the natural teeth and the removable retainer.

THE REMOVABLE PROSTHESIS

The removable prosthesis for the complete implant consists of three components: (a) the implant superstructure frame, (b) the acrylic-resin base, and (c) the replacement teeth.

The basic difference between the complete removable implant denture and the standard complete denture is that the complete removable implant denture is not supported by any soft-tissue base. The complete removable implant denture is supported solely by the four posts of the implant frame or the four posts of individual implants (Fig. 9-3). In this manner, there is no impingement of the soft tissue lying between the base of the superstructure and the frame of the implant. This also ensures (a) stability of the denture, and (b) lack of interplay between the denture superstructure and the implant, which may transfer or create destructive forces to the implant, as projected through pliable soft

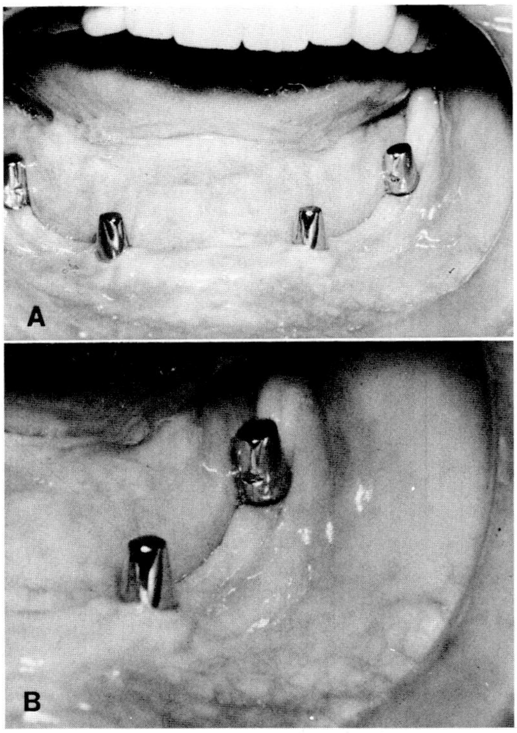

Fig. 9-3. The four posts of a complete mandibular subperiosteal implant extrude through attached gingival tissue (*A*). The patient has diligently kept the posts clean. These shiny posts, with proximal indentations (*B*), serve as abutments for the support of a complete removable denture. The small indentations in the posts secure the superstructure cast-frame clasps.

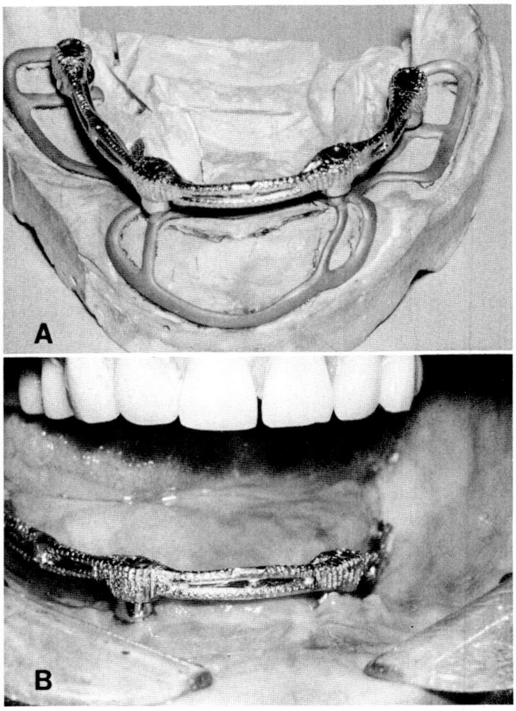

Fig. 9-4. The cast superstructure frame seated on the subperiosteal implant posts on the working model (*A*), and in the mouth (*B*). This frame is later embedded in the acrylic-resin base of the complete removable lower denture. The casting is fabricated at the same time as the subperiosteal implant frame. The try-in in the mouth precedes the fabrication of a wax bite-block.

tissue and rigid implant abutments. The main function of the implant posts for the removable prosthesis is to inhibit lateral displacement of the denture. The secondary role of the implant posts for the removable prosthesis is the retention to vertical displacement, which is especially applicable to the maxillary complete-arch denture.

The implant posts that are to support removable prostheses should be highly polished and should have a slight indentation that can receive the metallic interlocking clasp arm of the superstructure frame. The superstructure frame acts as a stabilizer for the denture base (Fig. 9-4). Not only is this frame rigid, but its clasp placement at each of the implant posts enables the complete denture to actually snap into place. This frame not only adds rigidity to the acrylic-resin base during processing procedures, but the nature of its clasp design allows the operator to manipulate the slightly flexible clasp arms in order to ensure stability of the denture at subsequent recall appointments (Fig. 9-5).

Once the superstructure has been tried in the mouth, the wax bite-block can be fabricated over the superstructure frame. Then the standard procedures of bite-block contouring and bite registration can be performed (Fig. 9-6). This will in turn lead to the wax try-in that is advised for all complete-denture prosthesis procedures. It is preferable that every complete-arch im-

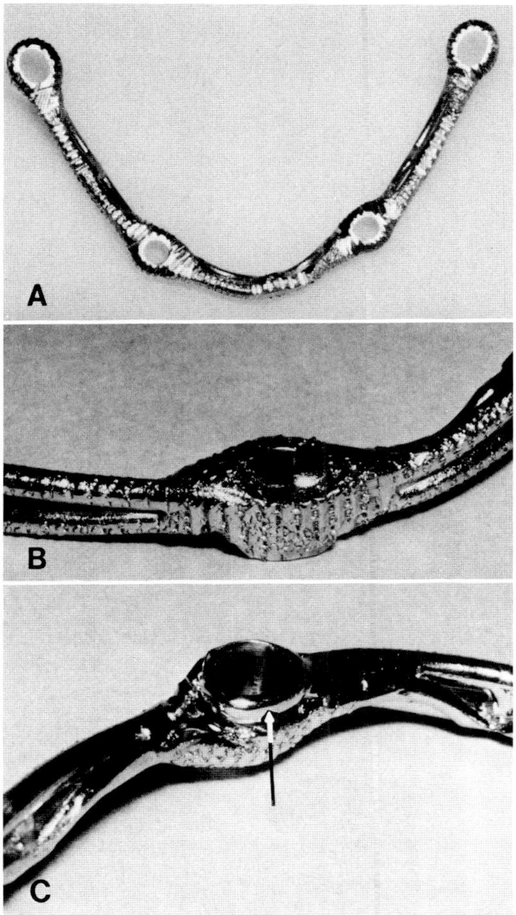

Fig. 9-5. Different views of the cast superstructure frame.* Occlusal view (*A*) of the complete frame on which the denture teeth will be superimposed. A closer occlusolabial view (*B*) of a portion of the frame that will seat on the abutment post, showing the positive occlusal stop that prevents overseating of the denture. A gingivolingual view (*C*) of the same portion of the frame, showing the adjustable clasp arm (*arrow*) that will engage the indentation of the implant post.

plant case receive a group-function occlusion, to distribute the forces over as great an area of the arch as possible. In the same manner as the snowshoe effect of the subperiosteal implant frame dissipates the forces transmitted through the implant, so

*Howmedica, Inc., New York, New York.

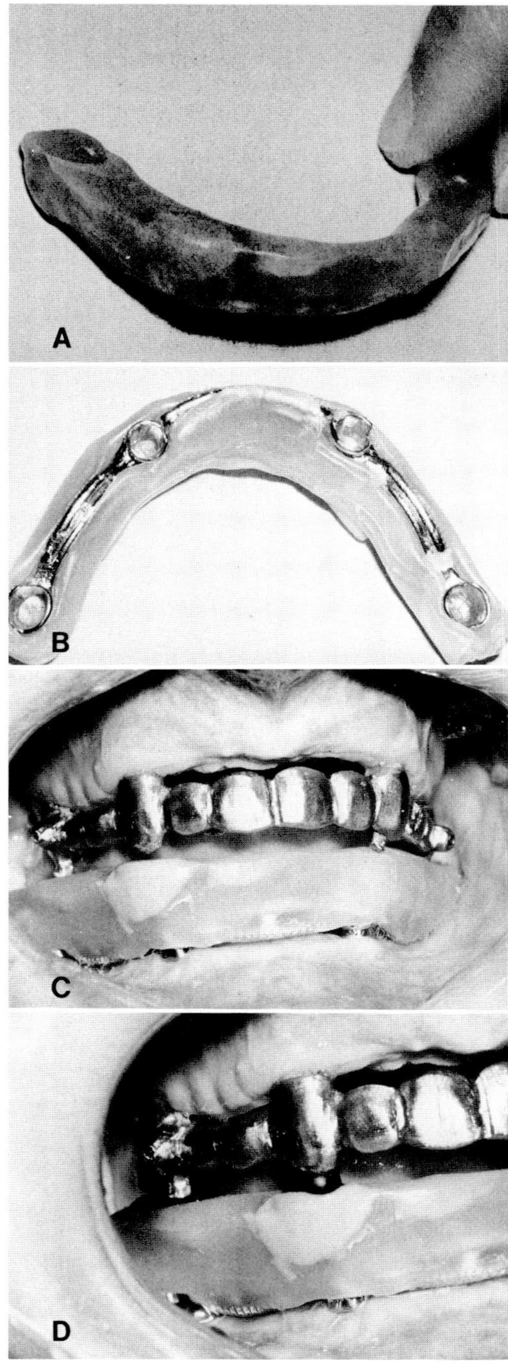

Fig. 9-6. A wax bite-block (*A*), and its use on the stable superstructure cast frame (*B*). The wax bite-rim engages, and is luted to, the cast frame. It does not, however, impinge upon the underlying soft tissues (*C, D*). Occlusal vertical dimension at centric relation has been recorded and registered.

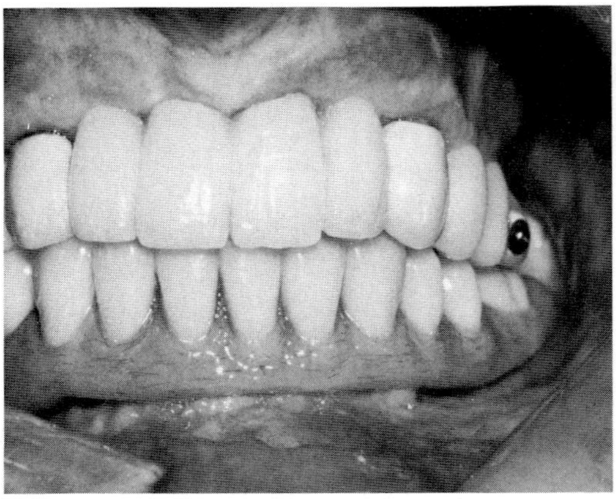

Fig. 9-7. A complete lower subperiosteal implant supporting a complete lower denture. The denture is supported by the implant posts only, and the flanges do not impinge upon the underlying soft tissues. The flanges support the lips and cheeks and are underextended, as compared with the standard complete denture.

should the implant superstructure be designed to dissipate the forces of occlusion over as great an area as possible (see Chap. 3). Such a design minimizes both lateral stresses and the concentration of forces in any given area.

The base of the removable prosthesis may be broad in a buccal or labial dimension, to support the labia. The base does not need any bulk in any other dimension. Its only other function is to support the replacement teeth. There is no need for flange extension in any direction, nor should there be any soft-tissue contact on the ridge aspect of the base (Fig. 9-7).

THE FIXED PROSTHESIS

The fabrication of a fixed appliance in any implant case does not preclude the step-by-step phases that are necessary for any good fixed prosthetic or crown and bridge technique. The principles for the design of the fixed superstructure are the same as those for any periodontal prosthesis. The only modifications are those that are specifically designed to enhance the long-term function of the implant and its accessibility to sound oral physiotherapy.

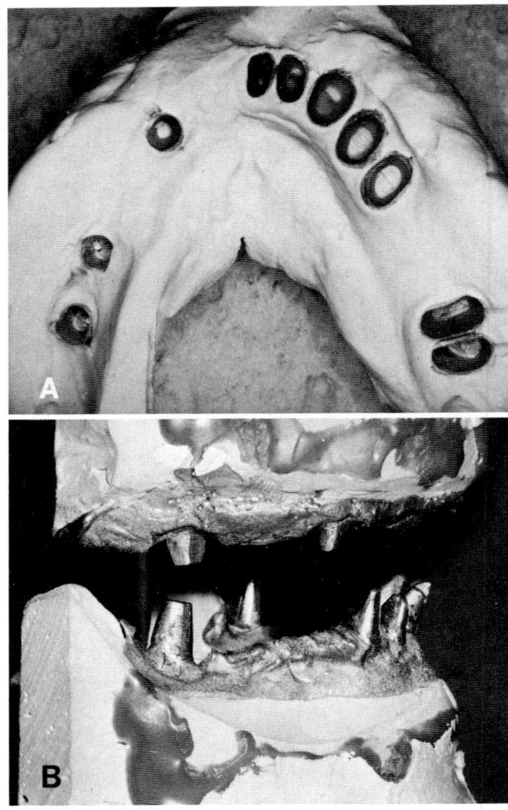

Fig. 9-8. At every stage of the assemblage of the fixed prosthetic superstructure, the path of insertion and the passiveness of seating are checked. The complete-arch Truplastic* index includes implant retainers and natural tooth retainers (*A*). Later, a soldering model (*B*) is poured, and the assemblage thus created is tried in the mouth prior to any veneering.

Tooth Alignment—Factors of Occlusion and Path of Insertion

The alignment of the implant abutment post with natural teeth in the same arch and with the opposing dentition is a contributing factor to the ease of manipulation of the fixed superstructure. In any case, the superstructure must seat *passively* over the implant abutments or the combination of implant abutments and natural-tooth abutments (Fig. 9-8).

*William Getz Corp., Chicago, Illinois.

The ability of the operator to control many variables is definitely augmented by the use of the subperiosteal implant. Because the subperiosteal implant is not preformed, but is designed specifically for the case at hand, the placement of the abutment post relative to both the opposing dentition and the path of insertion with natural abutment teeth can be completely oriented in the wax-up laboratory phase.

Also, the height (length) of the subperiosteal implant post may be extended or shortened at will as a laboratory procedure. The implant abutment of the subperiosteal frame can be maneuvered to create a satisfactory occlusal relationship with the opposing dentition, while simultaneously establishing a path of insertion with the natural abutment teeth.

When using the preformed abutments of the blade implants, however, we are limited by only being able to mechanically bend the abutments into position by distorting the implant neck. Not only is this practice limited in its scope, but its validity may be questionable with regard to weakening and placing new stresses on the implant neck and frame (see Chap. 12).

With regard to tooth alignment, it is important to note that priority is always given to the extrusion of the implant post through gingiva-type tissue rather than mucosal tissue. This would at times limit the operator because some posterior occlusal relationships would have to be constructed to form a crossbite relationship. Although such articulation may not be considered to be ideal, it is clinically valid in implant cases where soft-tissue factors take precedence over occlusion, *providing* that the occlusion can still serve to dissipate overall stresses.

Telescope Cast Copings as Implant Modifiers

The realignment of either a subperiosteal or a blade-vent implant abutment post can best be achieved by using a cast coping as an intermediary between the implant post and the superstructure retainer (Fig. 9-9). (Such telescope cast copings can also be used to realign the posts of blade implants without having to distort the implant neck.) The cast copings can be used for alignment for a path of insertion as well as alignment to accommodate an opposing dentition.

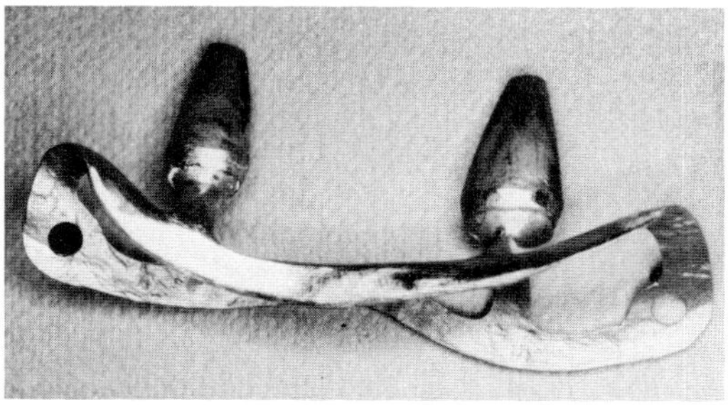

Fig. 9-9. Cast-gold telescope copings superimposed on the posts of a subperiosteal implant. *In this case,* the post lengths that were thus created did not fall within the circumference of a circle that is normally suggested for implant designs (see Chap. 3, subperiosteal implant design). As long as the superimposition of a telescope coping does not infringe on the basic rules of sound implant design, the coping may be used as an implant modifier.

Also, in instances where a large discrepancy would exist between the occlusal surface of the implant abutment and the projected occlusal table of the prosthesis, a decrease of the torque could be facilitated by using the intermediary cast coping. This truly exemplifies the telescopic characteristics of the cast coping, which diminish the chances of breakage of the cement bond that would be caused by excessive space between the occlusal table of the retainer and the occlusal surface of the implant post.

The Margins of the Fixed Superstructure Retainer

The margins of any full crown retainer that is seated on an implant abutment are all supragingival (Fig. 9-10). The very nature of a well-placed implant dictates this supragingival placement of the fixed superstructure. The margins of the crown retainer as related to the implant abutment

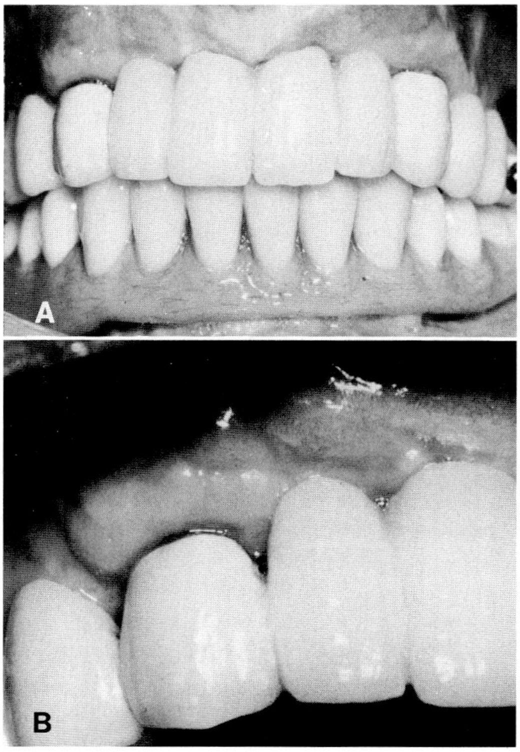

Fig. 9-10. An upper fixed prosthesis supported by a complete subperiosteal implant (*A*). The retainers in the cuspid areas have gingival margins that are short of the base of the implant posts (*B*). Often, the soft tissues that surround such an implant post have a darkish hue. This should not be misconstrued as a sign of unhealthy tissue. It may be the result of the metallic implant material being seen through a portion of the superimposed soft tissues.

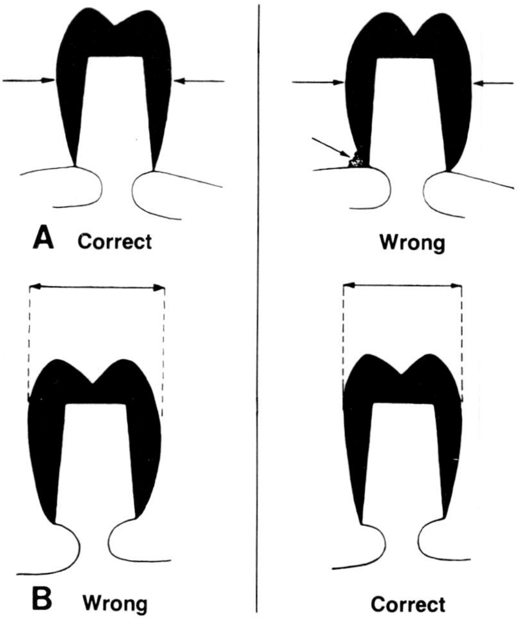

Fig. 9-11. The overcontouring of buccal or lingual axial crown surfaces can lead to the gingival accumulation of plaque (*A, right*). It is wise to modify the convex forms of these surfaces so as to have only slightly convex to flat planes (*A, left*). Within this convention, it is suggested to narrow the buccolingual width (*B*) of the occlusal food tables. This, in turn, will establish a more vertical placement of force upon the implant post.

are either feather- or knife-edged in design. The gingival aspect of these margins should be underextended and must never be overextended. Any overextension will not only be a direct irritant to the gingival soft-tissue collar, but would harbor putrefying material in this critical soft-tissue area. The confluence of superstructure to substructure should be as smooth as the intersection of the margins of a cast retainer to the finish line of any prepared natural-abutment tooth. This smooth confluence would not only eliminate the possibility of plaque accumulation, but would also enable the contours of the superstructure retainer to accommodate the surrounding gingival cuff. The aims of marginal placement are:

1. A smoothness of the surface of both the cast superstructure retainer and the implant post.
2. The confluence of adjoining cast surfaces.
3. The accessibility of all such areas to oral-hygiene procedures.

The Axial Crown Contours of the Fixed Superstructure Retainer

The accumulation of plaque can also be caused by overcontoured axial surfaces of the superimposed crowns (Fig. 9-11). Overcontoured crowns do *not* provide gingival protection. To the contrary, all axial

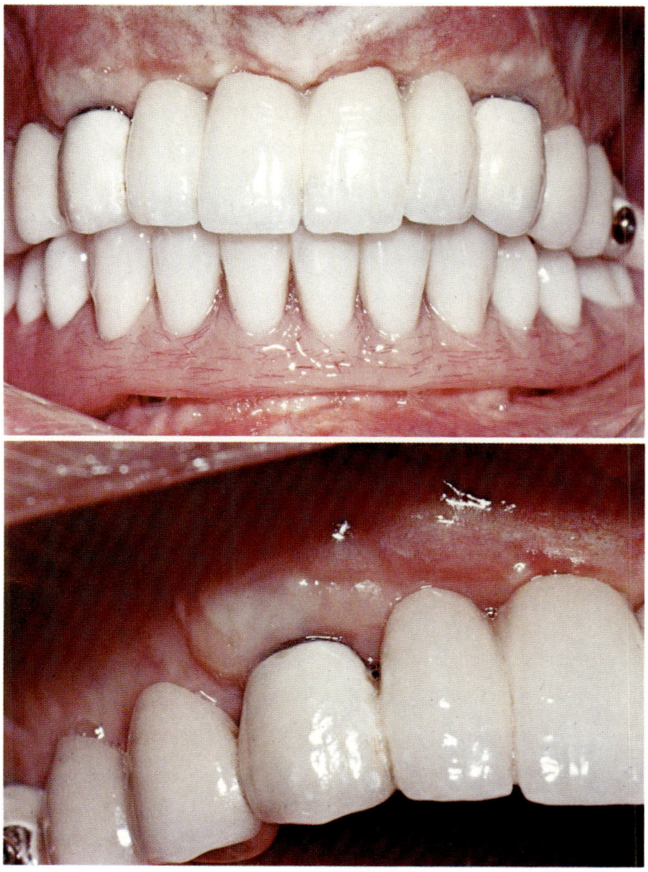

Plate 9–1. See Figure 9–10.

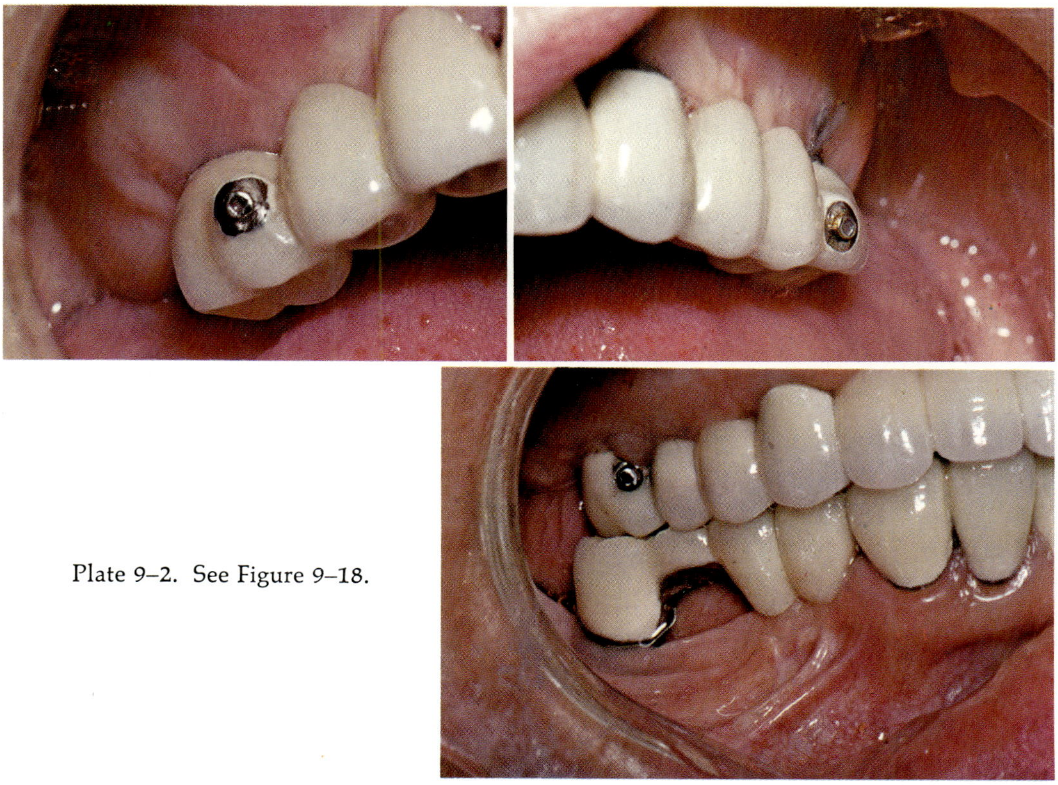

Plate 9–2. See Figure 9–18.

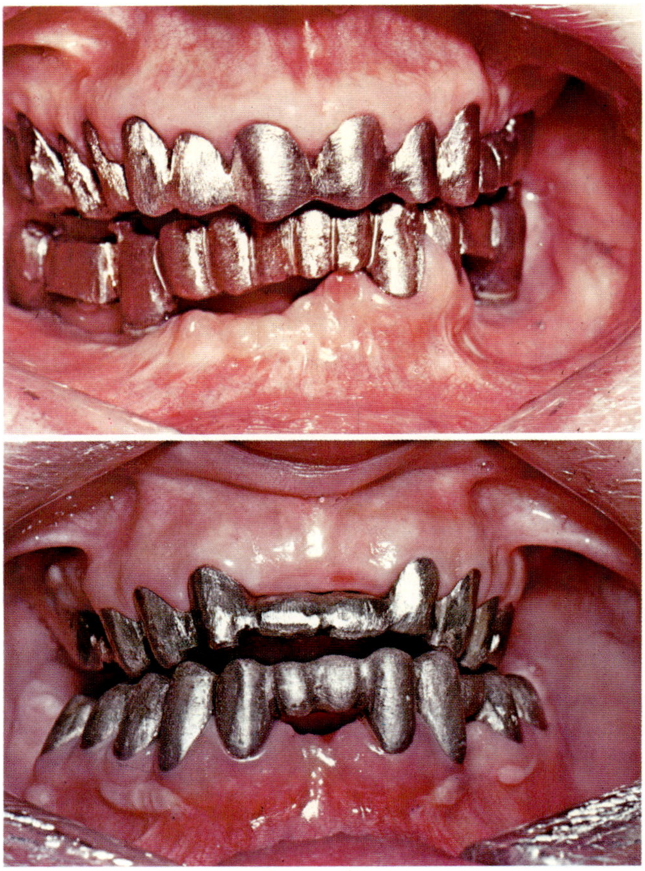

Plate 9–3. See Figure 9–21.

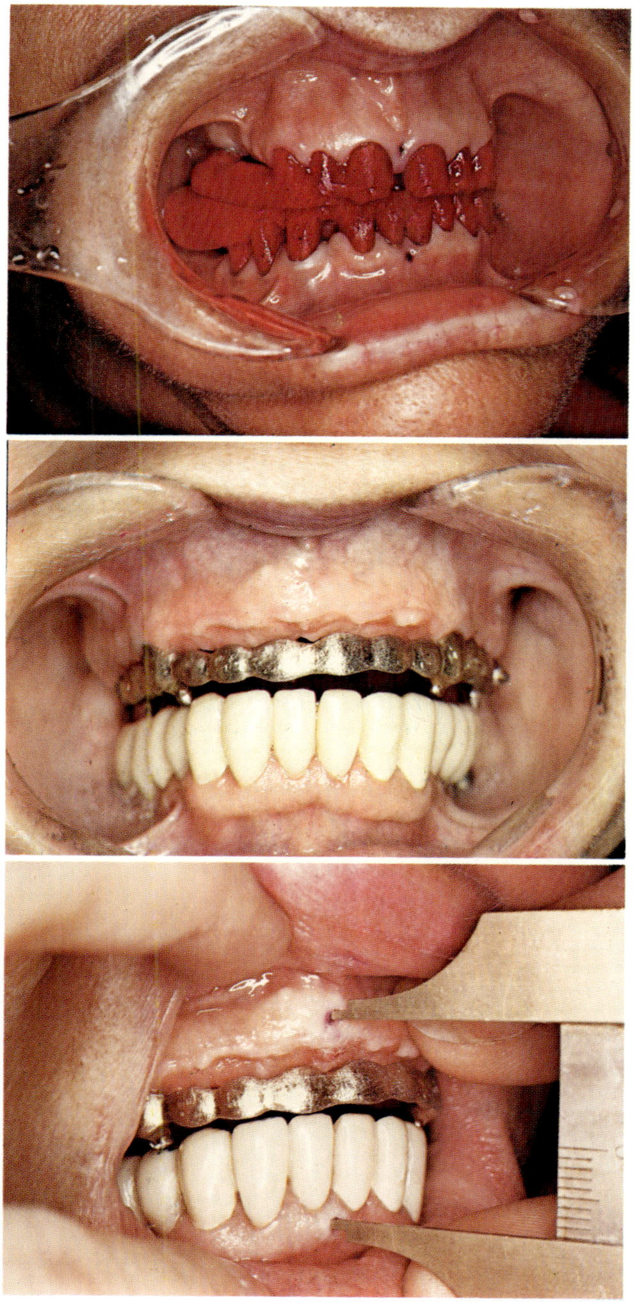

Plate 9–4. See Figure 9–22.

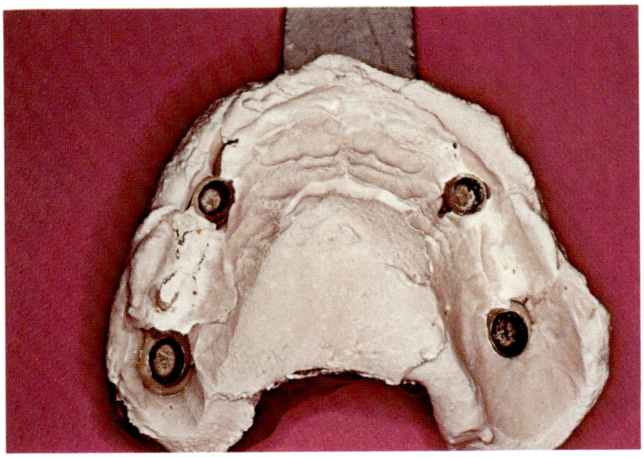

Plate 9–5. See Figure 9–23.

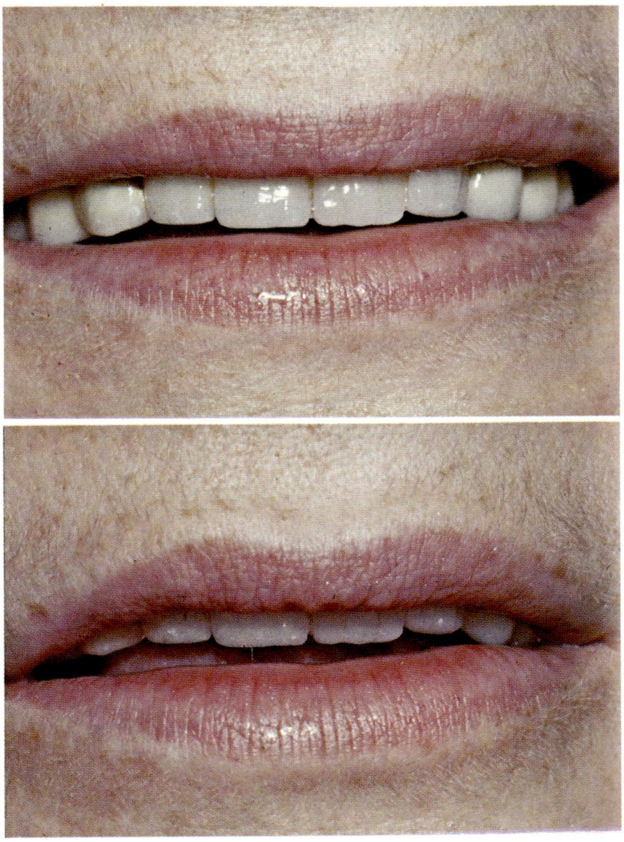

Plate 9–6. See Figure 9–24.

crown surfaces should be undercontoured. Undercontouring (a) enables the tongue, lips, and cheek to come in contact with and stimulate the soft tissues around the implant necks; (b) eliminates an area that would foster the accumulation of plaque; and (c) provides access for the patient to clean these areas with toothbrush, dental tape, and pipe cleaners (see Chap. 12, Home Care).

Related to these contours—but applicable only to the buccal and lingual surfaces—is the necessity to narrow the normal buccolingual width of the occlusal food tables. Still in harmony with sound occlusal concepts, the rationale for narrowing this portion of the crown retainers and their adjoining pontics within the same arch is related to stress distribution. In order to minimize lateral stresses and detrimental effects on the underlying bone due to torque at the occlusal level, it is best to maintain all occlusal forces in as much of a vertical plane as possible. To this end, it is advisable to eliminate many of the tangential forces that would be imparted through the implant retainer during mastication; this is achieved by narrowing the area of initiation of such adverse forces. In all cases, the occlusal surfaces should conform to the basic precepts of good occlusal anatomy and proper occlusal harmony. All interproximal contours should be similar to the design of wide major embrasures that exist in any natural dentition to accommodate and to passively house the surrounding soft tissues.

Pontic Design

There are generally two types of pontic design that should be used in conjunction with implant fixed-superstructure prostheses. These are: (a) the modified sanitary pontic, and (b) the modified ridge-lap pontic.

The modified sanitary pontic is routinely used in the mandibular posterior areas adjacent to terminal implant abutments (Fig. 9-12). Actually, it would be preferable to use this pontic design in all areas if it were not for the dominant esthetic factors in the anterior regions, and the unsanitary nature of food accumulation that would occur in the maxillary posterior regions. The modified sanitary pontic is designed in a Gothic-arch form so that it is confluent with the proximal surfaces of the adjoining abutment retainers and does not come in contact with the subjacent soft tissues. This design is beneficial because: (a) it prevents impingement of the soft tissues between the implant frame and the superstructure; (b) the Gothic-arch form provides strength at the solder joint areas; (c) it provides the patient with access to pontic areas for oral-hygiene procedures; (d) the Gothic-arch form in a mesiodistal direction establishes a smooth-flowing parabolic area, without indentations where plaque and food debris may accumulate (Fig. 9-13).

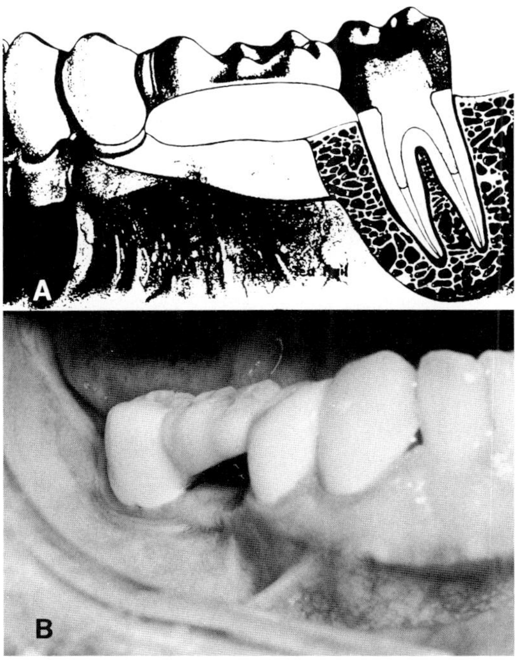

Fig. 9-12. The modified sanitary pontic in the mandibular posterior areas of both conventional *(A)* and implant *(B)* fixed prostheses. This design establishes a confluence of the proximal retainer surfaces with the undersurface of the pontics, without impinging on the subjacent soft tissues.

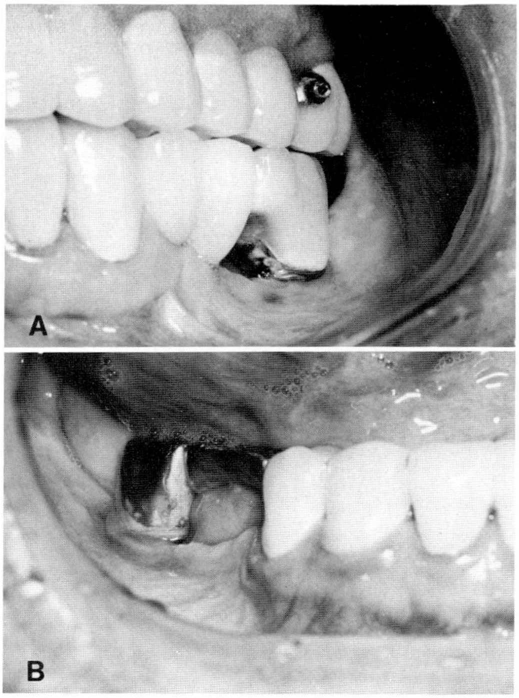

Fig. 9-13. Two different cases with mandibular terminal implants that support, in part, fixed prosthetic appliances. The modified sanitary pontics provide accessibility to the patient for home-care attention. The patient in (*A*) was not diligent in the removal of plaque on the mesial aspect of the distal retainer. This area, which may not have been accessible with other pontic designs, is accessible for the removal of such debris.

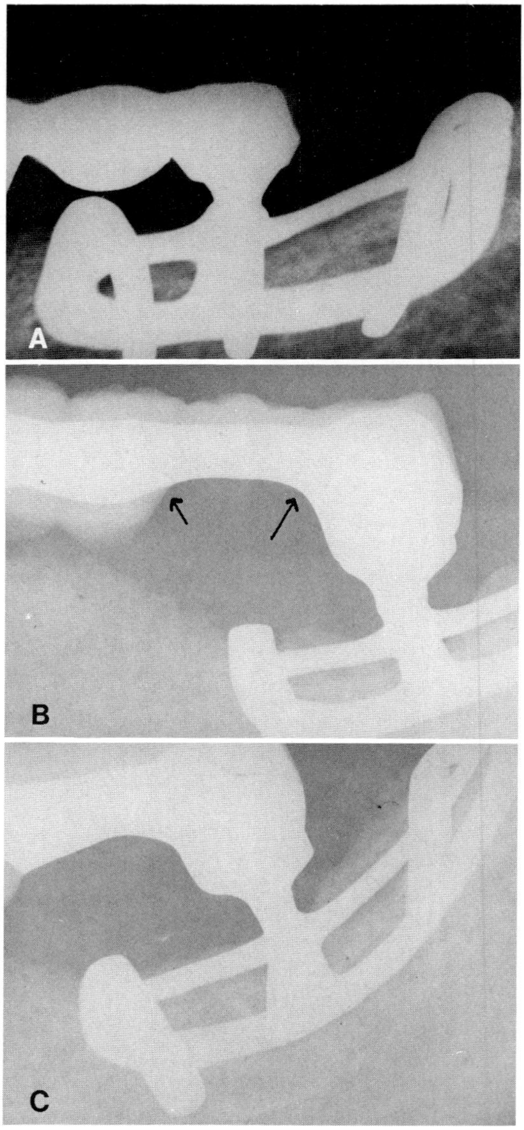

Fig. 9-14. Radiographs showing the relationship of pontics to underlying subperiosteal implant frames. The gingival aspect of a conventional ridge-lap pontic is shown in proximity to the peripheral border of the implant frame (*A*). This is a dangerous position because impingement by the pontic and any inflammatory process of the soft tissues may expose a portion of the implant frame unnecessarily. In two other cases (*B, C*), the distance that is left between the base of the modified sanitary pontic (*arrows*) and the frame of the subperiosteal implants is shown. The margins of each of the crown retainers are short of the bases of the implant posts.

The use of the modified sanitary pontic is more important with the subperiosteal implant than with the blade-vent implant. Any ridge-lap pontic would excessively approximate the soft tissues overlying the subperiosteal implant (Fig. 9-14). This may be hazardous because of the potential for compression of these soft tissues between the implant frame and the base of the pontic. Also, such pontic areas are amenable to the accumulation of soft debris. The direct irritation and inflammatory response, caused by excessive approximation and compression of the soft tissues by the ridge-lap pontic, may lead to the exposure of adjacent implant struts.

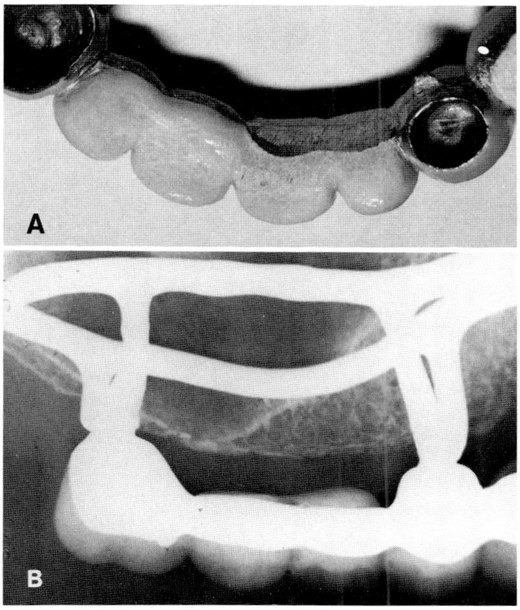

Fig. 9-15. The nature of the modified ridge-lap pontic design can be seen in a photograph (*A*), but cannot be ascertained radiographically (*B*). The photograph shows the modification of the standard ridge-lap pontics (*A, left*) for a central and lateral incisor to the modified ridge-lap pontics (*A, right*). At this biscuit-bake stage, the gingival portion of the pontic porcelain is removed, so that there is contact with only labial or buccal tissue. It is obvious that radiographs do not suffice in portraying the nuances of ridge-lap pontic contours and the design of the superimposed fixed prosthesis.

All other pontics used in areas where esthetics is of overriding importance—precluding the use of a modified sanitary pontic—should be of the modified ridge-lap design (Fig. 9-15). This pontic has contact on the labial aspect of the gingival base, for esthetic appearances. There is no contact on the lingual aspect, so that the base of the pontic is S-shaped from the labial contact, through the gingival surface, to the axial crown contour of the lingual surface (Fig. 9-16). This design eliminates soft-tissue impingement and provides ready access for dental floss. Such labial contact may be broadened in the maxillary anterior region to avoid both excessive sali-

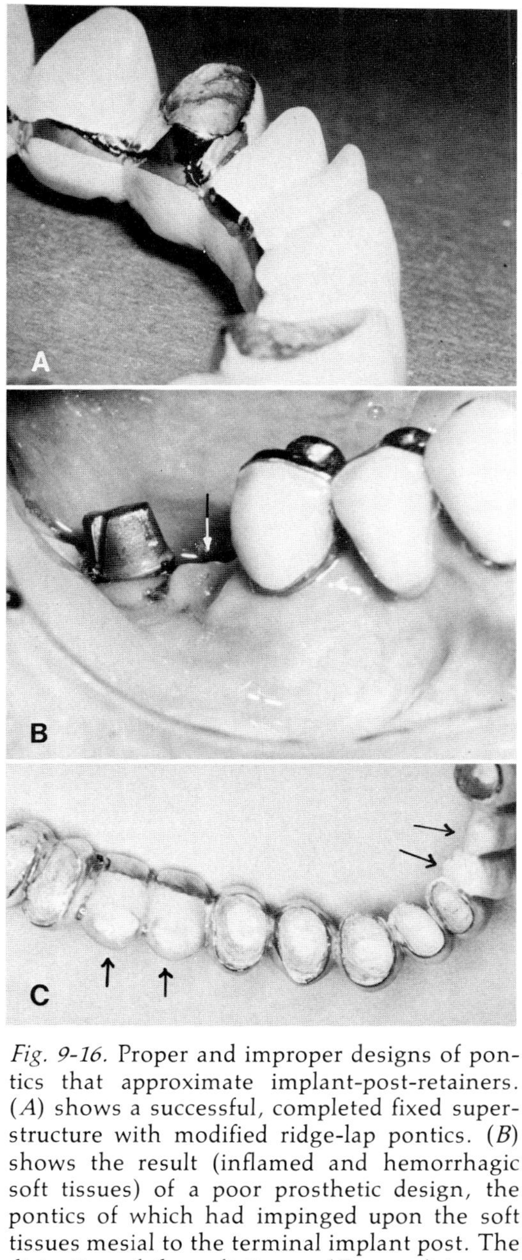

Fig. 9-16. Proper and improper designs of pontics that approximate implant-post-retainers. (*A*) shows a successful, completed fixed superstructure with modified ridge-lap pontics. (*B*) shows the result (inflamed and hemorrhagic soft tissues) of a poor prosthetic design, the pontics of which had impinged upon the soft tissues mesial to the terminal implant post. The distortion of the soft tissues (*B, arrow*) is seen after removal of the distal portion of this fixed bridge. (*C*) shows the undersurface of a fixed prosthesis with a standard ridge-lap design that had been temporarily cemented in the mouth for 2 weeks. The cement has not yet been removed. Each of the pontic areas (*arrows*) exhibits an accumulation of plaque; it is for this reason that the modified sanitary pontic or the modified ridge-lap pontic is prescribed, rather than this standard ridge-lap design.

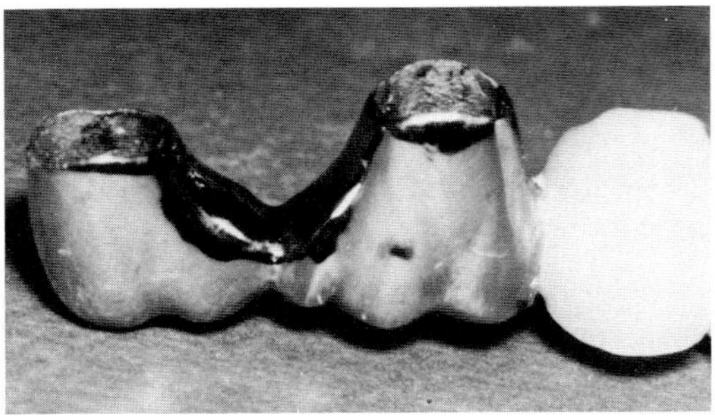

Fig. 9-17. Two cast retainers for a double-post blade implant are joined to form a type of modified sanitary pontic. These are to serve as distal retainers on a terminal blade implant. The buccal and lingual axial crown surfaces are only slightly convex, and the buccolingual dimension of the food tables is narrow.

vation during speech and unsightly dark areas between pontics. Otherwise, the standard use of the modified sanitary pontic and the modified ridge-lap pontic can be instituted in all cases that involve implants. With pontics, as with retainers, the goals are: to reduce the bulk of material; to avoid impingement on the surrounding soft tissues; and to provide the patient as much facility as is possible for oral home-care procedures (Fig. 9-17).

The Re Seté Pins

A safeguard for the retention of an upper-arch fixed prosthesis is the use of the Re Seté pin* (Fig. 9-18). There is no need to use such additional retention on the lower arch. Nevertheless, in view of the effects of gravitational pull and of possible overbite situations, it is advisable to use Re Seté pins within the retainers of the superstructure on the terminal implant abutment posts. There is never any need to use more than two of these pins in any given arch.

In conjunction with these pins, it is best to use a nonpermanent cement for the insertion of the permanent fixed prosthesis. There is no need to use a permanent ce-

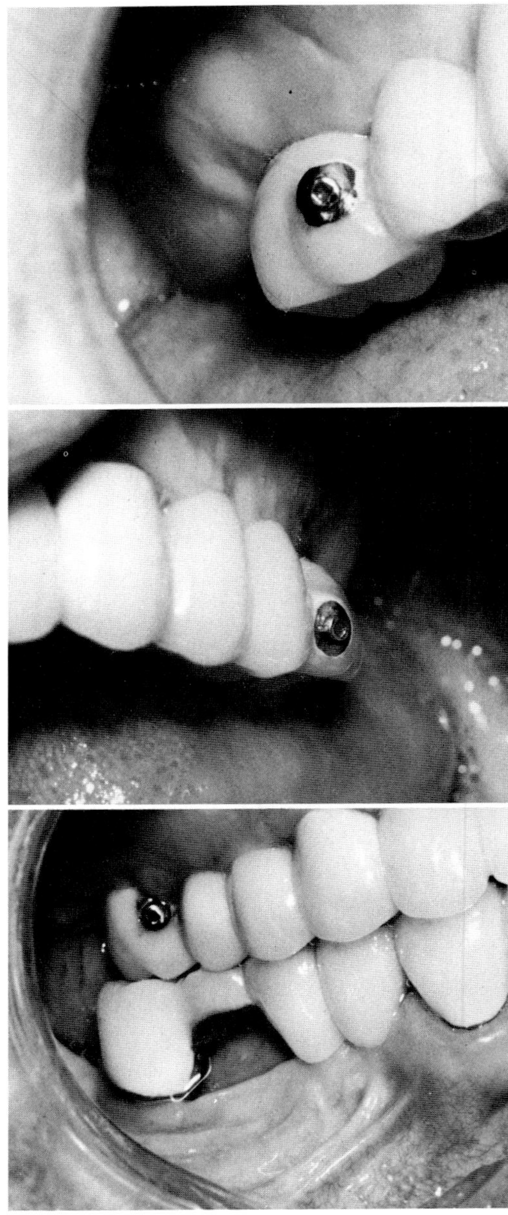

Fig. 9-18. Re Seté pins in accessible areas within the terminal retainers of implant abutment posts. These fine screws not only aid in the retention of metal to metal; but they make possible the removal of the superstructure if and when it is necessary. The soft tissue in each of these cases is sound. It is not surprising to find struts nearly exposed in areas that have a taut and thin, yet healthy, superimposed soft tissue. In each of these cases, the embrasures are shaped to accommodate the interproximal soft tissues as well as to make possible proximal home care.

*Whaledent, Inc., Brooklyn, New York.

ment, in conjunction with Re Seté pin retention, if (a) the implant posts are not tapered more than 5 degrees; (b) the implant posts have a sandblasted finish; (c) the crown retainers are well-adapted inner castings; and (d) the entire frame of the superstructure as a single unit fits passively yet securely over the combined implant posts. It is advisable that the dentist be able to remove the superstructure. Such removal is readily achieved by loosening the Re Seté screws and the subsequent reverse tapping of the superstructure. It is important that the dentist be able to remove the superstructure in case accessibility is later required for observation or intervention of the implant frame or neck. The removal of the fixed prosthesis may be necessary in order to check any specific area or to afford access for any surgical intervention such as curettage or removal of a strut. These procedures may become necessary at any time on any implant.

It is important to manipulate these screws properly at the time of cementation. *Before* the nonpermanent cement sets, each pin is tightened with the hand wrench that accompanies it. This sequence of procedures prevents the cement bond in any area from being broken. If the threaded screws are tightened after the cement has been set, the cement bond may break. Therefore, not only do the Re Seté thin screws provide additional retention; they also afford accessibility for the correction of any possible implant problem.

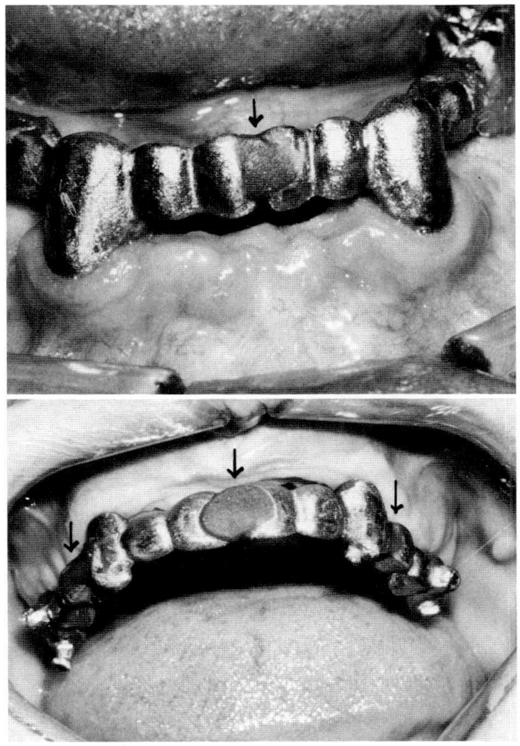

Fig. 9-19. Two different cases exemplifing the necessary intermediary steps in the construction of a fixed prosthesis. The individual units are being tried in the mouth, to verify adaptation, margins, contours, and overall acceptability. After these factors have been found to be satisfactory, the units are luted in place with Dura Lay* (*arrows*). This is a preparatory step to the plaster index impression. As in any other prosthetic phase, the soft tissues must be sound; this is achieved by proper temporization.

GENERAL CROWN AND BRIDGE PROCEDURES

All the principles that are inherent in sound fixed prosthetic and periodontal prosthesis procedures are basic to the follow-through of any implant insertion. The kinds of superstructure impression techniques and articulation methods to use are strictly within the judicious domain and conscientiousness of the individual practitioner. Any impression technique, however, must produce an accurate, acceptable die and excellent working models that can be mounted, regardless of the techniques employed. Therefore, certain sequential procedures must be followed in order to ensure as predictable an end result as is possible.

There must be at least one try-in of the individual units (Fig. 9-19). The use of a complete-arch single casting for a fixed

*Reliance Dental Manufacturing Co., Worth, Illinois.

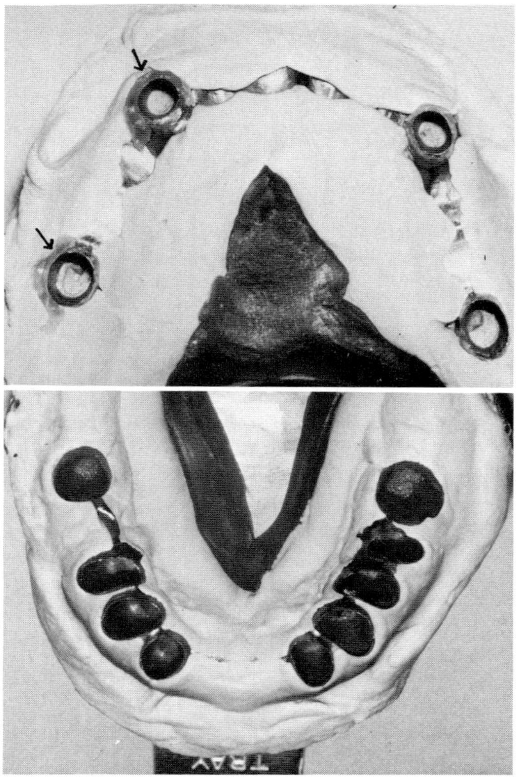

Fig. 9-20. Two complete-arch Truplastic* indices showing the positive seating of the retainers within the material. In cases that are to receive modified ridge-lap pontics, it is only necessary to capture the labial or buccal aspects of the residual ridges. It is suggested that each of the implant posts be rimmed (*arrows*) with soft Surgident Wax† prior to taking this index; this precautionary step will preclude the setting of stone within the undercuts of the implant posts.

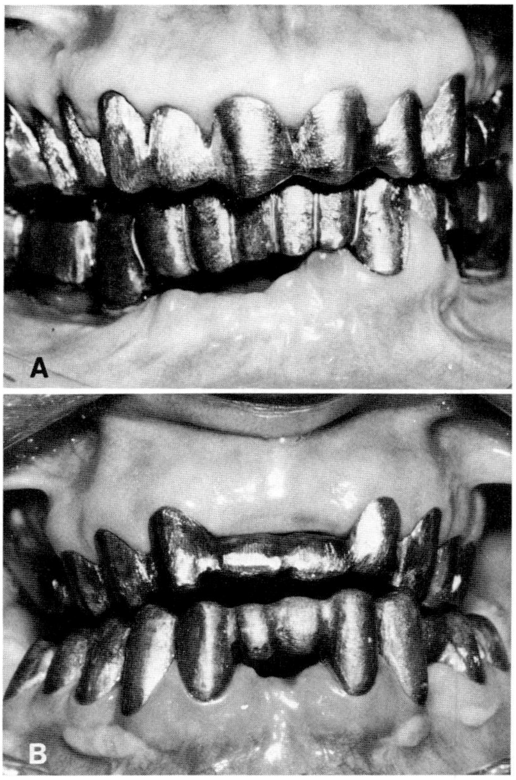

Fig. 9-21. The try-in stage of the united frame castings is shown in cases with (*A*) and without (*B*) implant abutments. The criteria of soft-tissue accommodation are the same in both cases: not only must the frames seat properly, but modifications may have to be made at this stage to accommodate the soft tissues, especially in the major embrasures.

prosthetic superstructure is unacceptable. The try-in of individual units ensures: (a) proper internal adaptation of the castings; (b) proper marginal placement and adaptation; and (c) proper pontic relationships that can be modified chair-side by the operator even if it necessitates the retake of any single abutment impression. Only after the operator is satisfied with each *individual unit* can they be luted in place and an overall index taken for soldering procedures (Fig. 9-20). Then, the cast frame try-in should precede any veneering of either acrylic resin or porcelain (Fig. 9-21). In this manner, any warpage or distortion can be detected. Such detection and the correction of same would avoid improper seating. The subsequent torque on any implant may be avoided by severing one or more solder joints in order to retake the index for another try-in.

Through each of these steps, the occlusion should be checked and rechecked, particularly to ensure proper centric positioning at an acceptable occlusal vertical di-

*William Getz Corp., Dental Products, Chicago, Illinois.

†Lactona Corp., Los Angeles, California; Philadelphia, Pennsylvania.

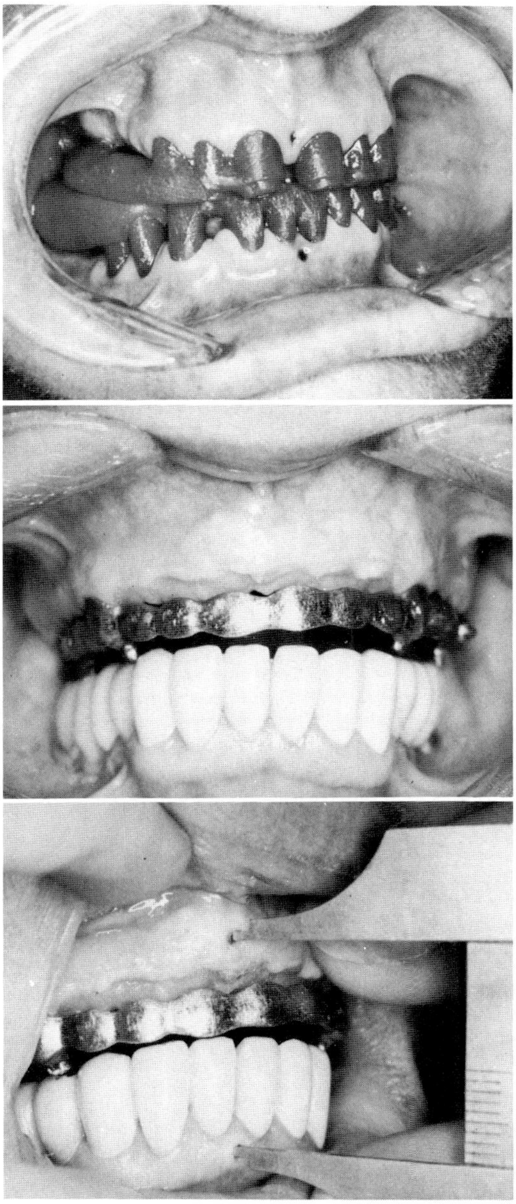

Fig. 9-22. At each of the stages of prosthesis construction, the occlusal vertical dimension is verified in centric. Thus, the prosthodontist must attend to: (a) mechanical design and adaptation; (b) soft-tissue adaptations to and accommodation of retainers and pontics; and (c) verification of centric and occlusal vertical dimension for the establishment of occlusion.

mension (Fig. 9-22). Before proceeding to the laboratory veneering phase, the dentist must make sure that the single-unit cast

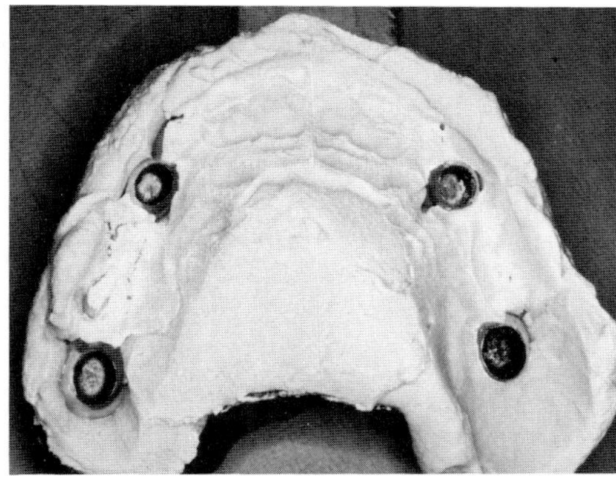

Fig. 9-23. A Truplastic* impression taken over a fixed prosthesis that was at the biscuit-bake try-in stage. The importance of the various try-ins at each stage of prosthetic construction cannot be overemphasized. In this case, the pontic areas had to be recaptured in order to add porcelain to some of the labial segments of the ridge-lap pontics. Another try-in will precede the final glaze.

frame can be securely inserted and passively seated, and that a proper occlusal relationship is established. If a porcelain occlusion is to be used, at least one biscuit-bake try-in should be made, prior to the final glaze (Fig. 9-23). The crux of the prosthodontic procedures is that no shortcuts are to be taken; this applies to any sound crown and bridge procedures and is especially applicable to implant procedures where the success of the implant is so dependent on the fabrication and design of the superstructure that it is intended to support.

The advent of the clinically acceptable dental implant has been a milestone in fixed prosthodontics. The addition of implant fixed prostheses to the treatment-planning armamentarium of the prosthodontist does not imply that removable prostheses are obsolete. Rather, another dimension has been added to the science of fixed-removable prosthodontics (Fig. 9-24).

The predictability of success in implan-

*William Getz Corp., Dental Products, Chicago, Illinois.

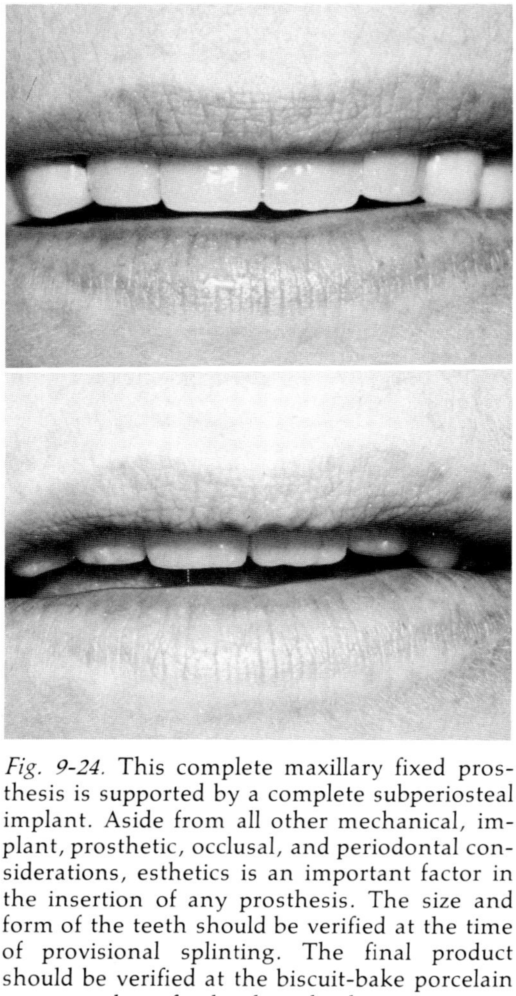

Fig. 9-24. This complete maxillary fixed prosthesis is supported by a complete subperiosteal implant. Aside from all other mechanical, implant, prosthetic, occlusal, and periodontal considerations, esthetics is an important factor in the insertion of any prosthesis. The size and form of the teeth should be verified at the time of provisional splinting. The final product should be verified at the biscuit-bake porcelain stage, and is finalized with the appropriate staining. Esthetics is one of the many important phases that require months of work between implant case selection and implant prosthesis insertion.

tology, based on case selection and site selection, makes possible the use of more fixed prostheses, thus fulfilling the literal meaning of fixed prosthodontics. All things being equal, the treatment of choice *usually* tends toward the fixed rather than the removable prosthesis. The most obvious reason for such a preference is the enhancement of the functional stability and the comfort of the stomatognathic system. It is to be hoped that the longevity of this system is increased by the insertion of a fixed appliance. The use of dental implant fixed prostheses may eliminate the physical and psychological stresses that are placed on the patient by removable appliances.

BIBLIOGRAPHY

Amsterdam, M., and Abrams, L.: Periodontal prosthesis. *In* Goldman, H. M., and Cohen, D. W. (eds.): Periodontal Therapy. ed. 5. St. Louis, C. V. Mosby, 1973.

Eissmann, H. F., Radke, R. A., and Noble, W. H.: Physiologic design criteria for fixed dental restorations. D. Clin. North America, *15:*543-568, 1971.

Jones, R.: The Physiological Role of Dental Occlusion in the Masticatory System. Montreal, University of Montreal Dental Press, 1967.

Lovdal, A., Arno, A., and Waerhaug, J.: Incidence of clinical manifestations of periodontal disease in light of oral hygiene and calculus formation. J. A. D. A., *56:*21-33, 1958.

Lucia, V. O.: Modern Gnathological Concepts. St. Louis, C. V. Mosby, 1961.

Perel, M. L.: Axial crown contours. J. Pros. Dent., *25:*642-649, 1971.

———: Periodontal considerations of crown contours. J. Pros. Dent., *26:*627-630, 1971.

———: A modified sanitary pontic. J. Pros. Dent., *28:*589-592, 1972.

Posselt, U.: Physiology of Occlusion and Rehabilitation. ed. 2. Oxford, Blackwell Scientific Publications, 1968.

Pugh, C. E., and Smerke, J. W.: Rationale for fixed prostheses in the management of advanced periodontal disease. D. Clin. North America, *13:*243-262, 1969.

Ramfjord, S., and Ash, M. Jr.: Occlusion. ed. 2. Philadelphia, W. B. Saunders, 1971.

Ross, I. F.: Problems connected with combined periodontal therapy and fixed restorative care. D. Clin. North America, *16:*47-57, 1972.

Stein, R. S.: Pontic–residual ridge relationship: a research report. J. Pros. Dent., *16:*251-285, 1966.

Tylman, S. D.: Theory and Practice of Crown and Fixed Partial Prosthodontics. ed. 6. St. Louis, C. V. Mosby, 1970.

Weinberg, L. A.: Atlas of Crown and Bridge Prosthodontics. St. Louis, C. V. Mosby, 1965.

10 Periodontal Perspectives of Dental Implants

Myron Nevins, D.D.S.

THE ROLE OF IMPLANTOLOGY AND PERIODONTAL TREATMENT PLANNING

Even today, the practicality of the terminal-extension free-end saddle denture remains an enigma in periodontal treatment planning. There are proponents of various precision and semi-precision attachments. The different opinions relative to impressions temper one's attitude about the ability of the soft tissues to offer continuous support for a removable prosthesis. There are proponents of bicuspid occlusions; and there are those who believe that it might be rational to keep teeth that are severely damaged periodontally, rather than utilizing any of the above approaches.

The past decade has introduced the terminal metal implant substitute for the natural distal abutment as another member of our treatment-planning armamentarium. Great enthusiasm has been engendered by the proponents of this type of implant, and although many have sought to temper it, the success rate of the terminal implant must be given serious consideration. Any new form of treatment is difficult to integrate into the dental practitioners' armamentarium; however, it may be advantageous to try a new form of treatment *for a particular circumstance.* It is certainly necessary to alert the patient to the success rate of the implant so that the patient can be prepared for the possibility of failure (see Chap. 2).

The Implant Candidate—Four Categories

The first category of implant candidates consists of individuals who present with partial dentures. Some patients are satisfied with this prosthetic solution, and if the periodontium is capable of supporting a removable or a combination fixed and removable prosthesis, it is logical for these

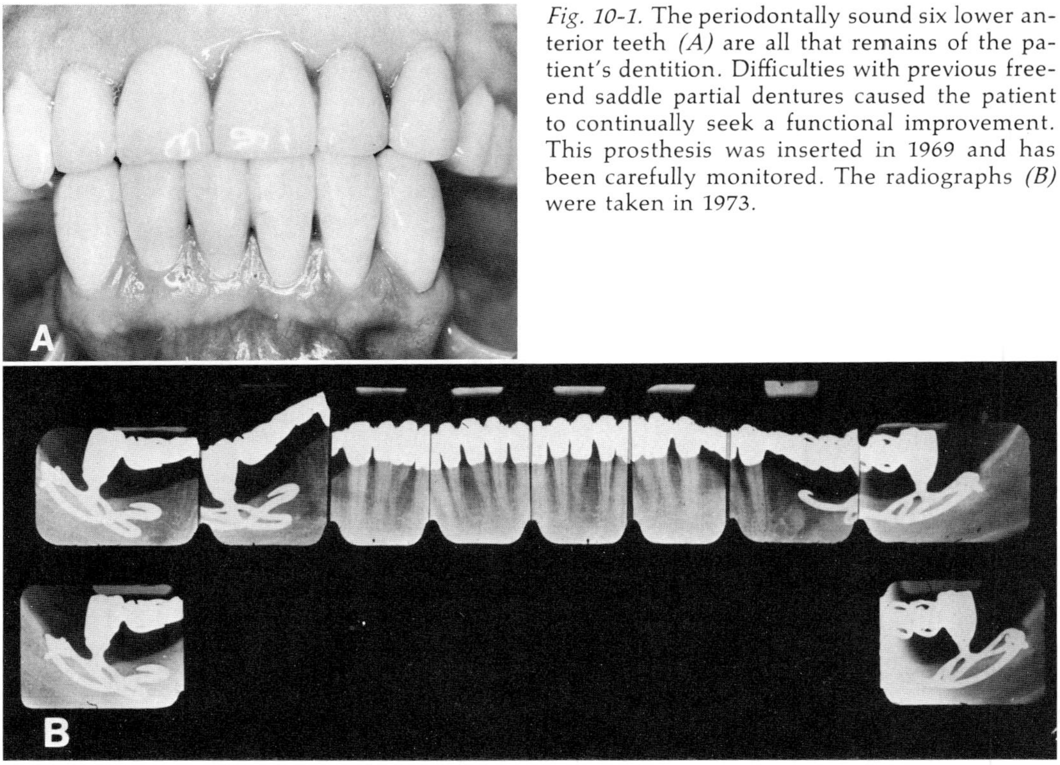

Fig. 10-1. The periodontally sound six lower anterior teeth *(A)* are all that remains of the patient's dentition. Difficulties with previous free-end saddle partial dentures caused the patient to continually seek a functional improvement. This prosthesis was inserted in 1969 and has been carefully monitored. The radiographs *(B)* were taken in 1973.

patients to retain such prostheses. Some patients, however, are dissatisfied with their partial dentures and appeal to members of the dental profession for a better solution. It could be that their appliances were inadequately constructed, and similar appliances could therefore prove satisfactory. Some individuals with properly constructed appliances, however, simply are not comfortable with their partial dentures (Figs. 10-1, 10-2). In cases of properly constructed appliances, we have to contend with the free-end saddle type of removable appliance and any type of removable partial denture that is tooth-supported, where the posterior abutments may become so periodontally involved that they are beyond periodontal management and must be removed. The dental implant can be considered as a method of providing a firm prosthesis that may enhance the function and comfort of the individual in both examples.

The age and systemic health of the patient must be considered. Although it would appear rational to limit implantology to young healthy individuals, it is often the geriatric patient who benefits most from implants (see Chap. 2). It is frequently difficult for an individual who has had the use of his natural teeth for a long period of time to adapt to an artificial removable dentition later in life.

It would be irrational to consider the soft tissue and hard tissue acceptance of a foreign substance if the patient suffers from any pathology or requires any medication that would have a direct bearing on the quality of the tissues involved. Some gastrointestinal disorders—colitis, for example—require a supervised diet; dental implants may help patients with such disorders counter their abnormalities more successfully.

The second category of patients presenting for implant therapy consists of individ-

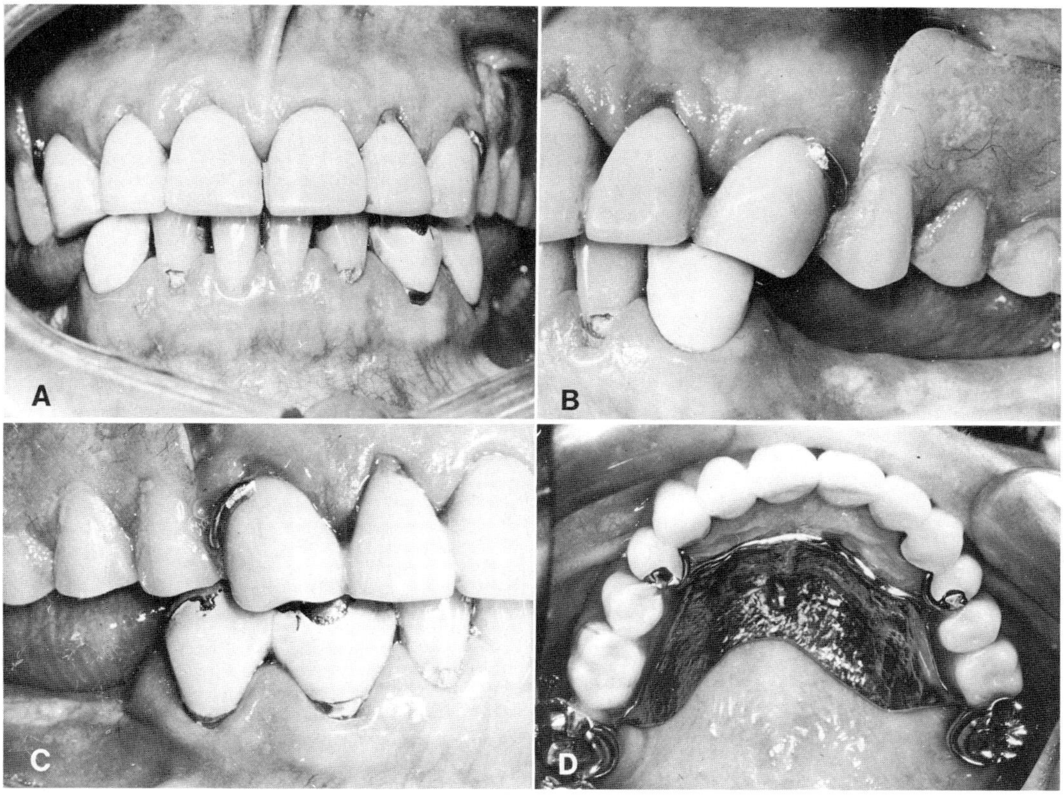

Fig. 10-2. This patient presented with difficulties related to mastication and esthetics. The remaining teeth were stable, with significant amounts of periodontal supporting structures. Subperiosteal terminal implants were used in the maxilla, due to the proximity of the maxillary sinus *F, (arrows)* Intra-osseous implants were utilized in the mandible, due to the large quantities of alveolar bone that were present. *(A to C)* As the patient presented to the office. *(D)* The finished maxillary prosthesis with removable cross-arch support for further stabilization. *(Please see next page.)*

uals who have several missing teeth that are not presently replaced. These patients are unable to masticate properly and are dissatisfied with their appearance. It is imperative to consider the degree of periodontal involvement and the stability of the remaining natural dentition. If posterior teeth are missing in one arch or in both arches bilaterally, it may be possible to build posterior segments on one side and an abbreviated or bicuspid form of occlusion on the other side. In many instances of abbreviated occlusion, it is necessary to examine the remaining natural dentition during the initial presentation of the patient, and to consider to what degree it has withstood the damaging factors of stress.

It is obligatory to develop a trial situation (provisionalization) for a realistic period of time before finally deciding on a bicuspid form of occlusion. Individuals with a long facial form may find it difficult to masticate properly with unusually long edentulous posterior ridges, and there are patients with esthetically unacceptable extensive smile lines caused by edentulous ridges that are portrayed as dark shadows. It frequently is necessary to allow the patient to evaluate this type of situation before contemplating any final form of restorative

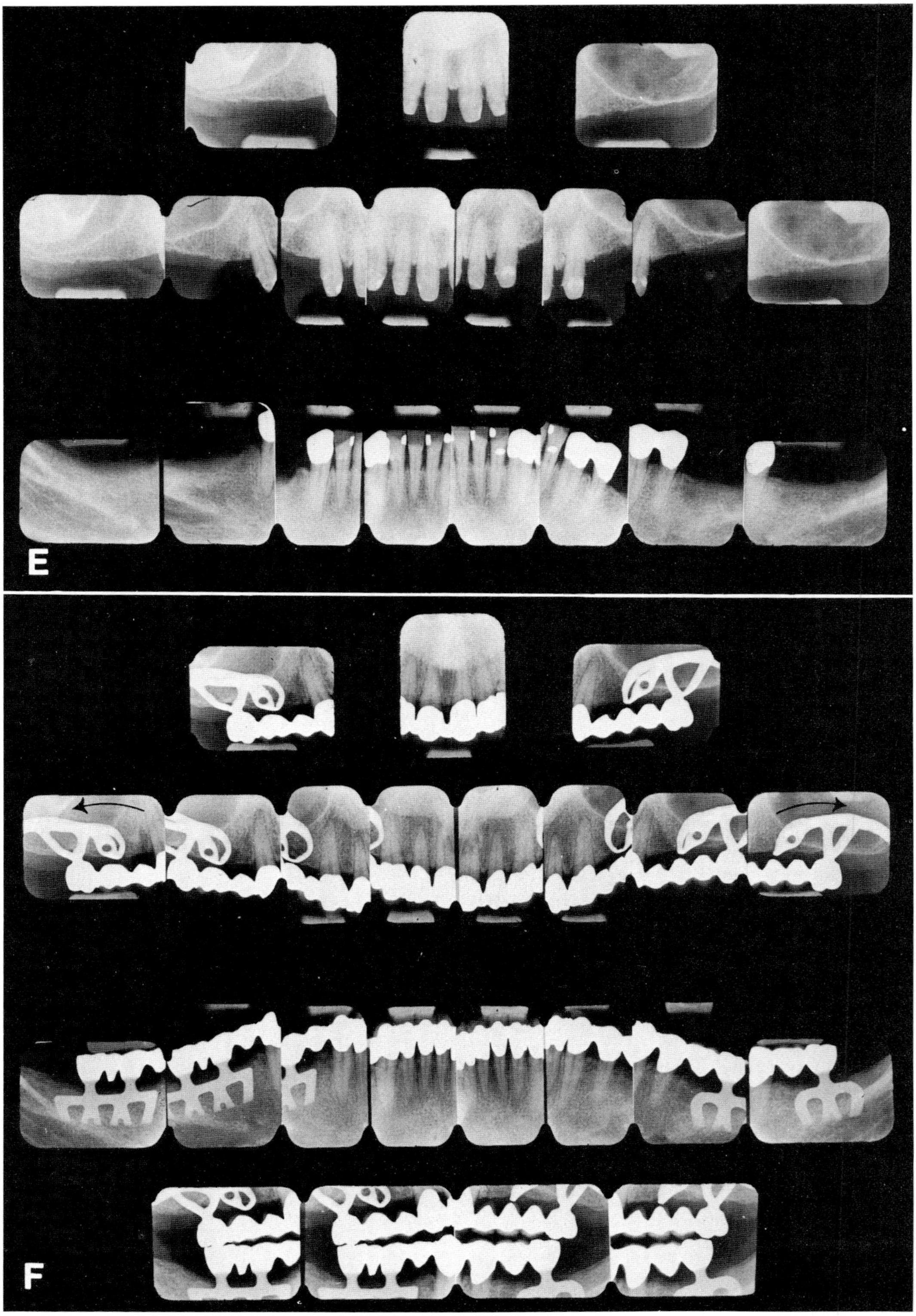

Fig. 10-2 (Continued.) (E) Pre-treatment radiographic survey. *(F)* Post-treatment radiographic survey.

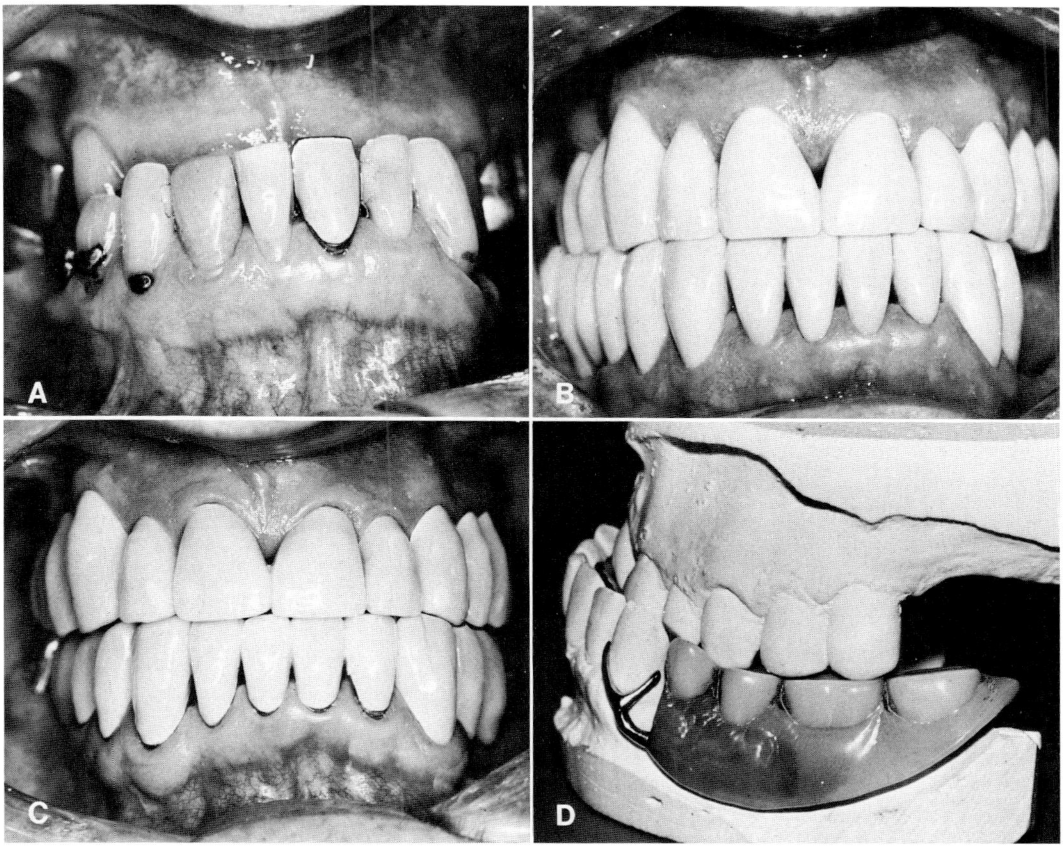

Fig. 10-3. (A) Overclosed pseudo-Class III dentition. *(B)* One week after the provisional bridges have been placed. *(C)* Two years later, upon completion of the prosthesis (note the difference in quality of the periodontal tissues). *(D)* Study models with previous partial denture in place, supplying teeth for the lower left quadrant. *(Please see next page.)*

dentistry. If the candidate has not previously had a removable prosthesis, the dentist should first test the removable prosthesis provisionally before reaching a final conclusion. The implant, however, should be considered as a possible solution to this problem.

The third implant candidate is the individual with no removable prosthesis and few or no missing teeth, who has suffered severe periodontal destruction. This individual, because of extenuating factors, may be maintained as is without definitive periodontal and/or prosthetic correction. The dentist may consider therapy that would include extraction of selected posterior teeth and the construction of partial dentures. This form of therapy might be unwise if the remaining periodontally involved teeth do not seem stable enough to serve as abutments for a removable prosthesis. There is an inherent danger in considering implantology for this type of patient without giving due consideration to techniques that might salvage a reasonable portion of the natural dentition for the construction of a fixed prosthesis, thus precluding the need for implants or a removable prosthesis.

Sectioning techniques for molar teeth have exhibited respectable long-term results, and they must be contemplated *be-*

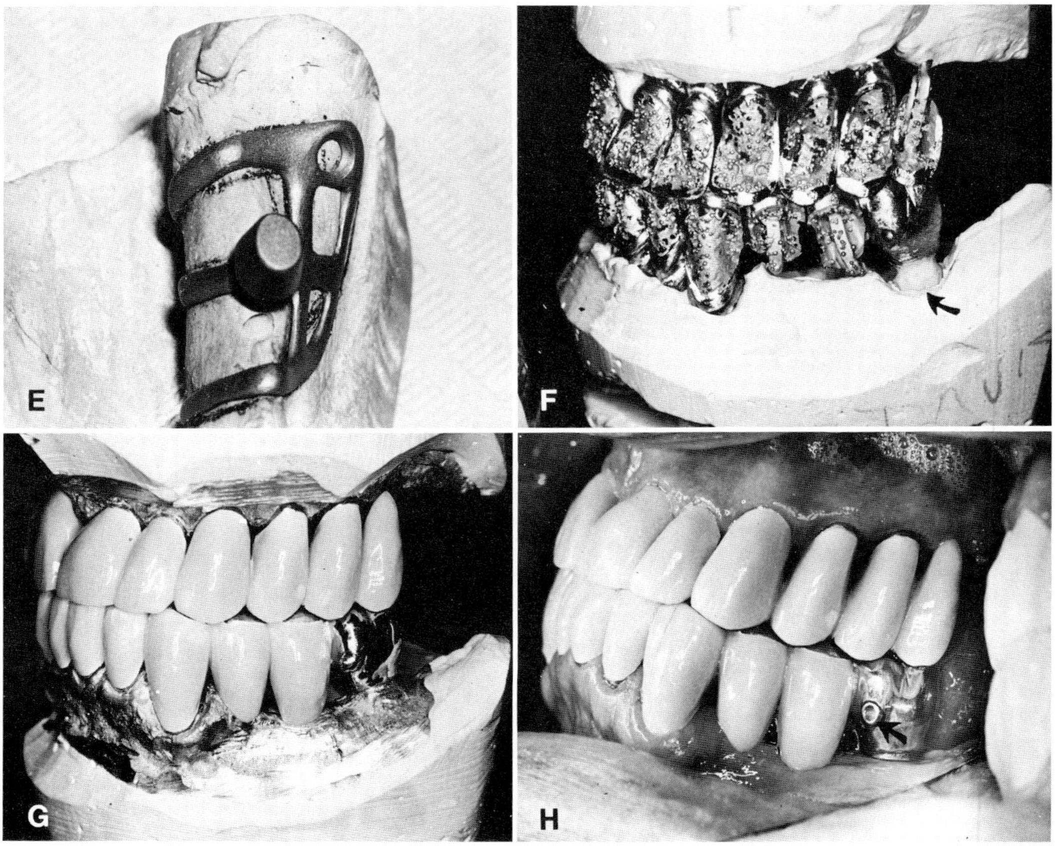

Fig. 10-3 (Continued.) (E) Subperiosteal implant for the lower left quadrant. *(F)* Mounting of prosthesis at the casting stage *(arrow to die of implant)*. *(G)* Mounting of the finished prosthesis. *(H)* Prothesis delivered to patient as a fixed restoration. Note the Re Seté threaded screw *(arrow)* on the retainer for the implant. This is to compensate for the difficulty of cementing metal surface to metal surface. *(Please see next page.)*

fore the extraction of stable posterior periodontally involved teeth. If such teeth have undue mobility, it would seem that the preservation of parts of these teeth would be less likely. It would be mandatory to first test a fixed prosthesis for a reliable period of time before inserting an implant. If the preliminary fixed prosthesis were to be unstable, clinical experience indicates that the implant would not stabilize any mobile segment of the natural dentition for a significant period of time. Any movement in the natural section seems to detract from the stability of the implant as the forces of mastication, and those forces from tooth contact when not masticating, are exerted. It would seem that the implant as a substitute for missing teeth would be most successful in those individuals for whom an artificial dentition or fixed bridgework could be built with success without the implant, but for whom the implants would offer an esthetic and/or functional improvement; this is a clinical impression and must be substantiated over longer periods of time (Fig. 10-3).

The fourth category of implant candidates consists of those patients whose crown and bridge abutments have failed. This would most appropriately be described as an example of *conversion,* because we would be converting fixed

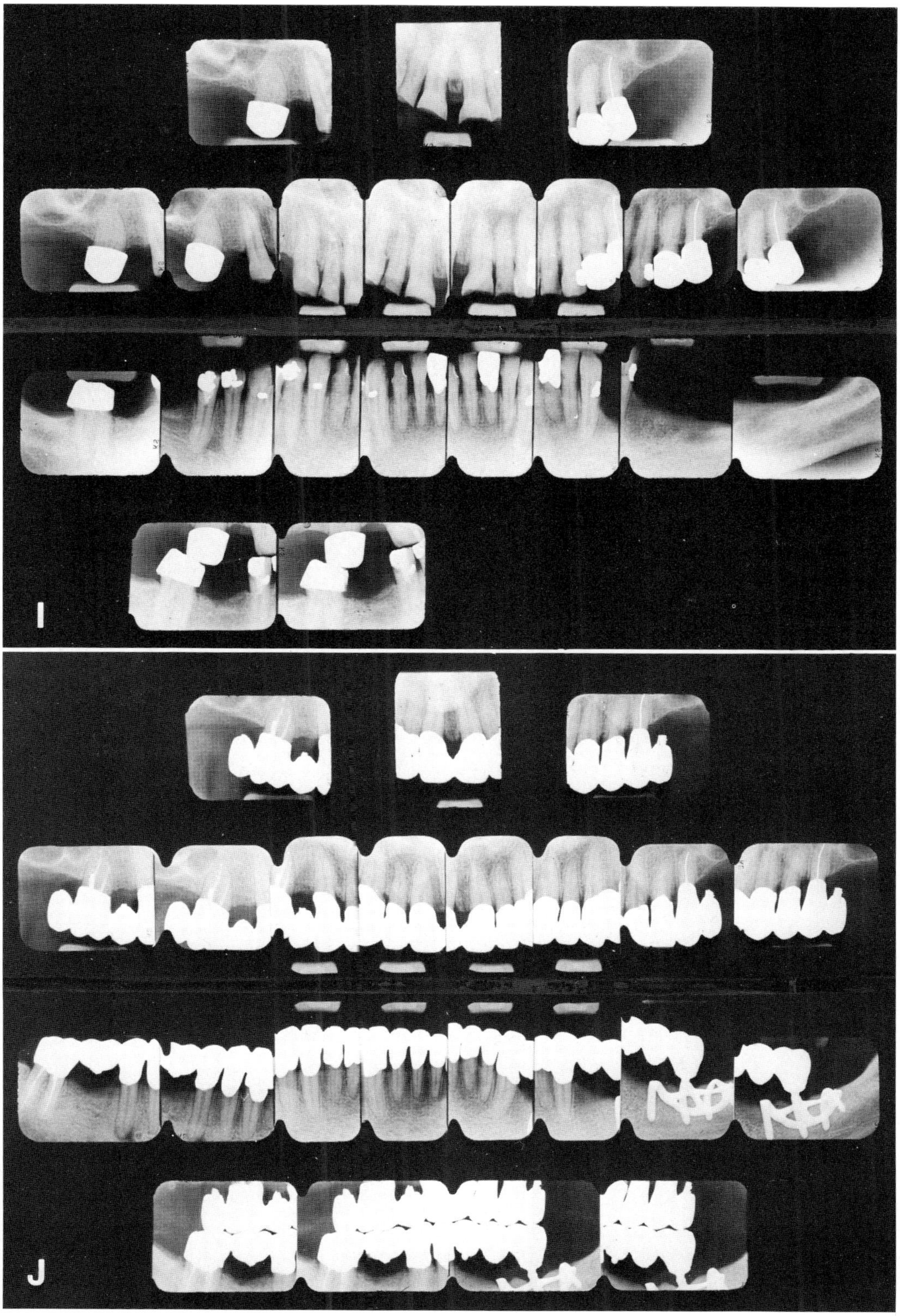

Fig. 10-3 (Continued). (I) Pre-treatment radiographic survey. *(J)* Post-treatment radiographic survey (note the mental foramen at the apex of the lower right bicuspid).

bridgework from the natural abutment to an artificial abutment (Fig. 10-4). There is a long-range complication associated with the construction of a final prosthesis for an individual with this problem. It is first necessary to remove the damaged posterior natural abutment and to allow significant healing of the hard and soft tissues. Depending on the quantity of the remaining structures and the rate of healing of the individual, there is a probable wait of about 3 to 9 months. The implant should only be inserted after the tissues have completely healed; and for reasons that will be developed later in this chapter, it is advisable to wait at least 6 months after implant insertion before providing a new fixed permanent prosthesis. This will require some degree of patience on the part of the dentist and the patient.

EVALUATION OF THE PATIENT

It is imperative to evaluate carefully any candidate for dental implantology. Those patients who are familiar with implantology must be informed realistically as to the probability of success. It is proper to inform them of the other modalities available for the replacement of missing teeth. They must understand that there is a risk of failure in implantology and that this failure might take place not only during the provisional phase, but also after the delivery of a final prosthesis. It is necessary to judge the patient's ability to accept failure before initiating dental implant procedures. Indeed, the patient's emotional stability and his ability to accept failure should be prerequisites for implant case selections. An individual who lacks the desire or ability to practice above-average dental hygiene during initial debridement procedures, for example, should not be considered.

The preceding paragraphs indicate the need to know more about the patient than his number of missing teeth. It is important to consider all aspects of therapy as carefully as one would consider the substitute for the missing tooth. In ensuing paragraphs, the reader will observe the progression of procedures from the consideration of the implant candidate, to the final decision to utilize implants and the care of the patient upon their insertion.

DEVELOPMENT AND DETERMINATION OF THE TYPE OF THERAPY

During the initial appointment, the implant candidate is asked to enter an introductory phase of therapy, during which careful records are accumulated. These records include the results of a full-mouth radiographic survey, possibly a panradiograph, carefully taken study models, and jaw-to-jaw and occlusal relationships. The necessity for ordering any battery of systemic tests to be done by a competent physician is determined by the dentist after a careful survey of the patient's past medical history. A lengthy debridement procedure is undertaken during several visits in order to determine the patient's motivation and ability to accept more complicated dental procedures.

The carefully selected candidate is then presented with a comprehensive treatment plan that includes alternatives that would provide him with a properly functioning dentition. (The use of the term *function* here includes esthetics.) It is possible to provide most patients with more than one alternative, depending on what conditions prevail in the existing dentition. Possible alternatives might be a bicuspid occlusion, continued use of partial dentures, or the utilization of an implant. In most cases it is unusual for the insertion of the implant to be the next step in patient management. The clinician should first consider the success rate of implants to that of definitively treated posterior natural abutments with severe periodontal implications.

The armamentarium of the periodontist today is varied, and he can provide successful management of many difficult prob-

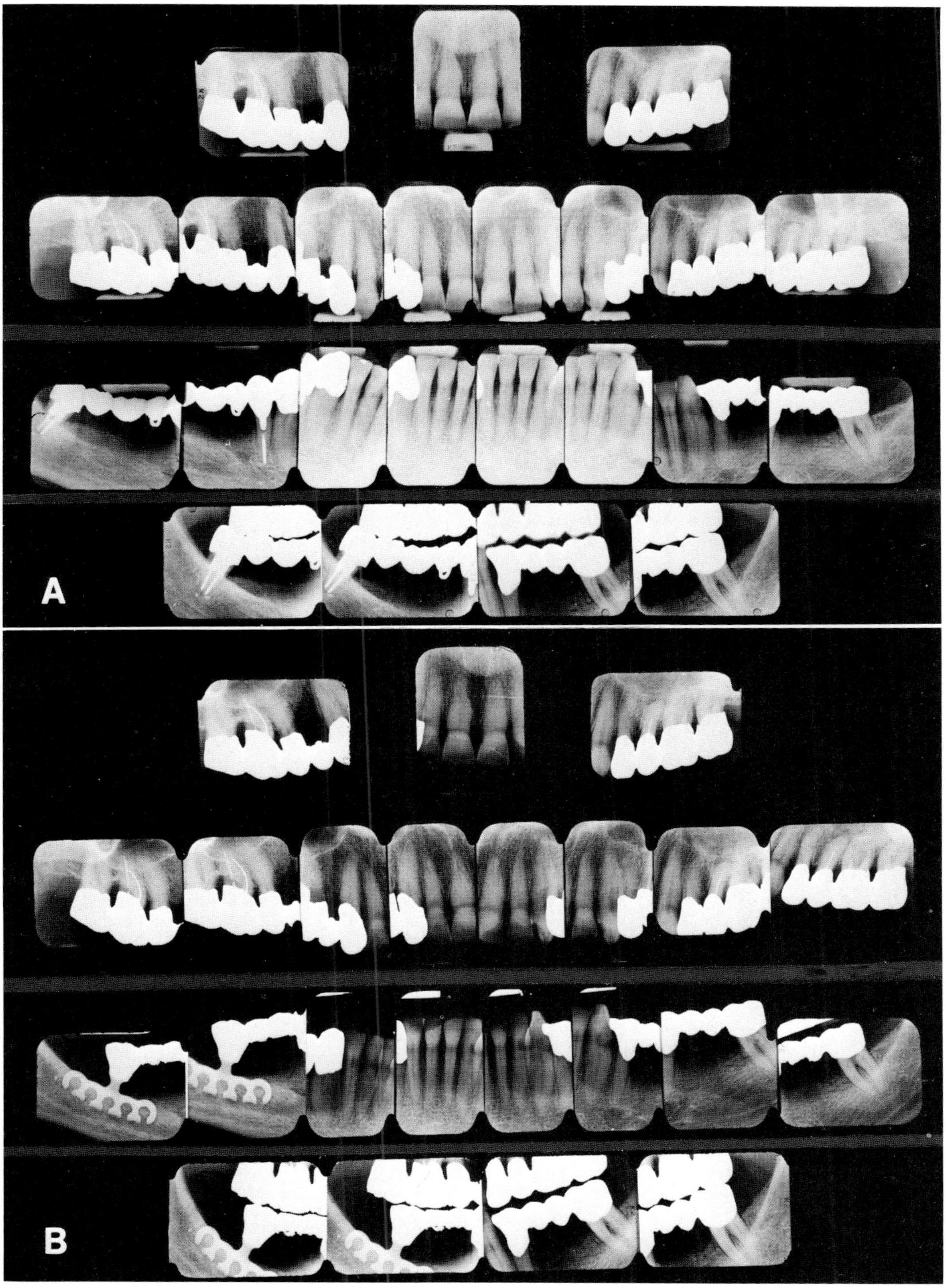

Fig. 10-4. (A) Full-mouth radiographic survey (1967) of prosthesis inserted in 1960. *(B)* Full-mouth radiographic survey (1973) after failure of lower right molar and its replacement with an intra-osseous implant. In 1960, the upper right first molar had been sectioned but the upper left first molar had not been. The sectioned molar has fared better.

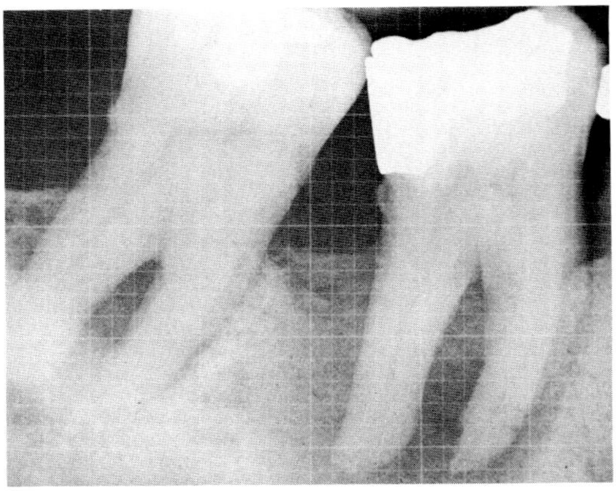

Fig. 10-5. Periodontally unsound molar teeth. An implant would seem to have a better prognosis for long-term success.

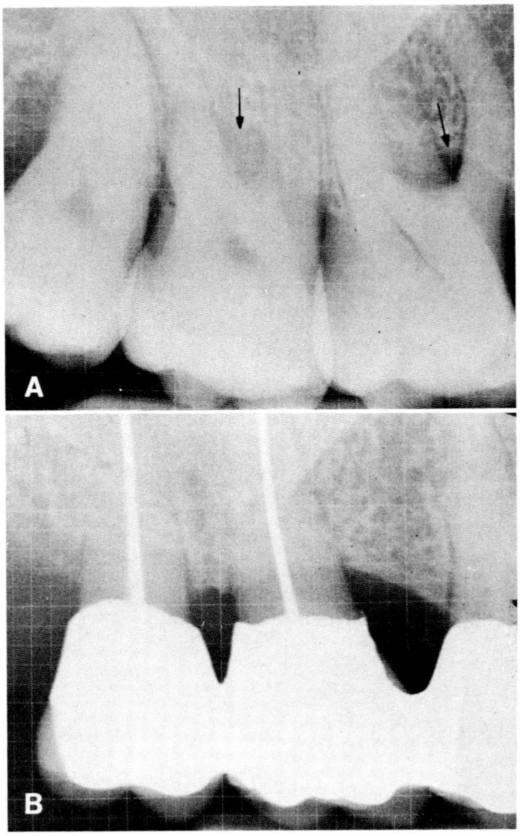

Fig. 10-6. (A) Pre-operative radiograph showing advanced alveolar bone loss in the intra-radicular areas *(arrows)* and interproximally. *(B)* Post-treatment radiograph showing retention of two palatal roots. The maxillary first and second molars were stable before being sectioned, and the individual palatal roots were virtually stable.

lems. A major issue with proposed posterior abutments for fixed prosthesis is the loss of intra-radicular bone in multirooted teeth (Fig. 10-5). If a tooth with a bifurcated root involvement is stable, it might be reasonable to contemplate the use of one or two remaining roots to support fixed bridges (Figs. 10-6, 10-7). It is unreasonable to think of a single root of a multirooted tooth as being stable if the tooth as a whole is severely mobile; we probably would not consider sectioning this tooth. It is also necessary to take into account the edentulous span that one is considering to restore prosthetically; it might very well be that a root of a stable tooth will not remain stable if it is overtaxed with the stresses of occlusion through its use as an abutment.

Many posterior teeth may be stable even though they have deeply involved periodontal infrabony pockets (Fig. 10-8). Bone-addition procedures should be considered, because this form of therapy is well documented and very likely could improve the condition of the teeth.

Many patients present with posterior teeth that have drifted and tilted because of early loss of adjacent teeth. These teeth frequently have accentuated pocket depths. It is best to treat such teeth by emphasizing two factors: (a) tooth position, and (b) a superimposed soft-tissue inflammation. The periodontal health of many of these teeth improves dramatically when the teeth are repositioned. An example of such a situation is a lower molar tooth that is tipped in a mesial direction and that would have to be uprighted before it could be considered for use as an abutment for fixed bridgework (Fig. 10-9).

Of major concern to all clinicians performing fixed prosthodontics have been the problems of caries in posterior natural

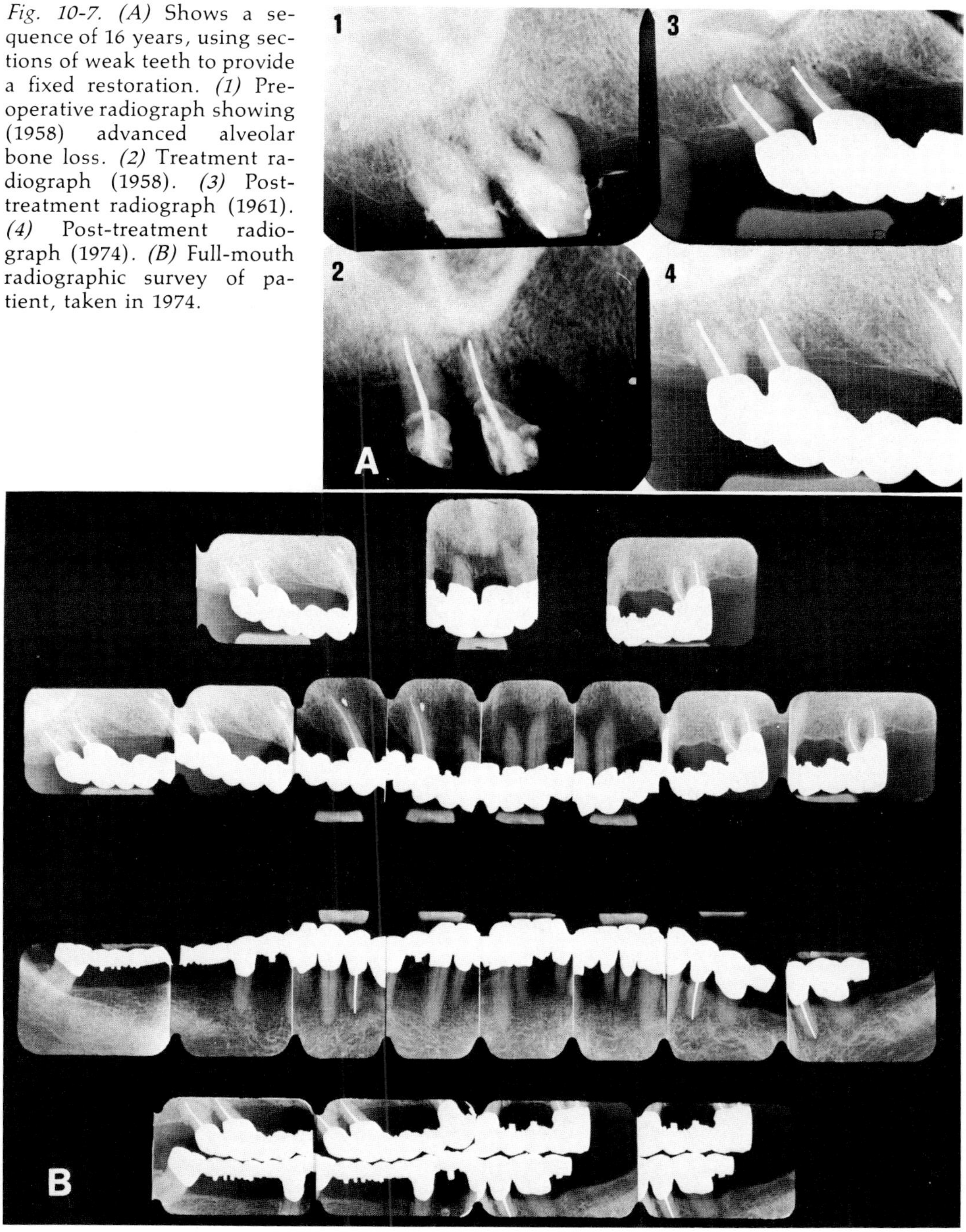

Fig. 10-7. (A) Shows a sequence of 16 years, using sections of weak teeth to provide a fixed restoration. *(1)* Preoperative radiograph showing (1958) advanced alveolar bone loss. *(2)* Treatment radiograph (1958). *(3)* Post-treatment radiograph (1961). *(4)* Post-treatment radiograph (1974). *(B)* Full-mouth radiographic survey of patient, taken in 1974.

abutments and of moderate to lengthy edentulous spans. A long clinical crown, which would provide more square millimeters of contact between the tooth preparation and the retainer, should be a clinical prerequisite because it would lessen the chance of a distal cement washout, which could easily lead to gross decay of

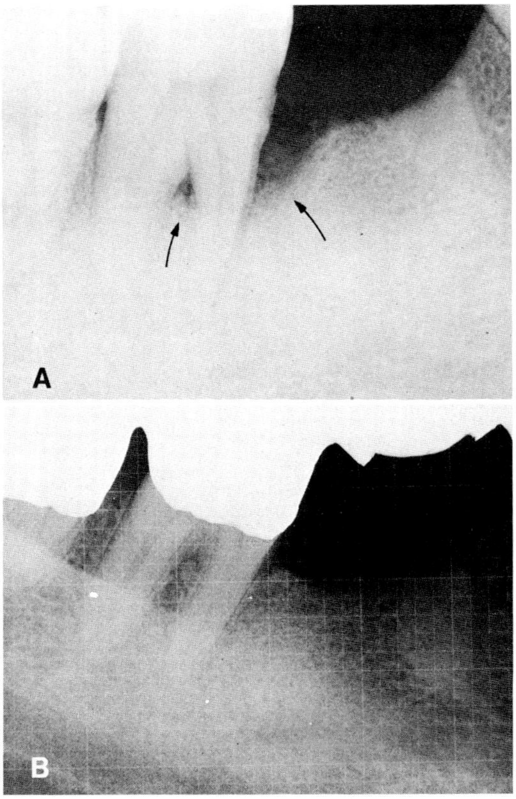

Fig. 10-8. (A) Pre-treatment radiograph (1965) showing mesial infrabony lesion and intra-radicular lesion *(arrows). (B)* Post-treatment radiograph (1974) showing osseous correction.

the natural-abutment tooth. If an existing posterior natural-abutment tooth has had such advanced carious destruction that a provisional bridge cannot possibly be afforded retention, and that any further periodontal surgery would not expose usable suprafurcation tooth structure, one should consider this abutment to be a liability and utilize an implant to replace it.

It is the responsibility of the clinician to carefully plan treatment by weighing all of the above factors in his decision. In some instances there could be a greater percentage of success with an implant than with a very weak natural-tooth abutment (Figs. 10-10 to 10-12). The various implants and the sites proposed for them would have to be carefully evaluated in order to make intelligent decisions.

PROVISIONAL PERIODONTAL PROSTHESES

Most terminal implants are considered for use with fixed prostheses. It would seem likely, therefore, to follow the initial education and evaluation of the patient with the development of a trial restoration to evaluate weakened posterior abutments. With a free-end saddle partial denture, the clinician also has an opportunity to test the patient's ability to manage a provisional removable prosthesis. If the provisional removable prosthesis is successful, the clinician may utilize it as the final prosthesis. If the provisional prosthesis is unsuccessful, a further discussion of the possibility of inserting an implant would be indicated.

The clinician may decide to test the patient's ability to manage an abbreviated dentition unilaterally or bilaterally in order to provide the patient with a prolonged opportunity to evaluate the decision as to whether such a dentition can provide comfort, function, and esthetics for that particular case (Fig. 10-3). This trial period would enable the clinician and the patient to test the use of fixed posterior single-cantilevered pontics, that are part of an anterior provisional fixed prosthesis, as a solution to esthetic and functional problems. It is not the purpose of this discussion to present the merits of cantilevered pontics; however, it is suggested that a single-unit cantilever used as a distal extension from an extensive fixed prosthesis may be as advantageous as the use of a combined fixed *and* removable prosthesis.

If the trial apparatus is to be of value in determining the merits of the final prosthesis, it must be constructed as carefully as any final prosthesis (Fig. 10-3). The patient must be able to clean *all* areas without causing any further deterioration of the remaining periodontium. The provisional prosthesis must be conceived occlusally in such a fashion that it will be of help in garnering information for the final occlusal scheme. If the patient is dissatisfied with

(Text continues on p.171.)

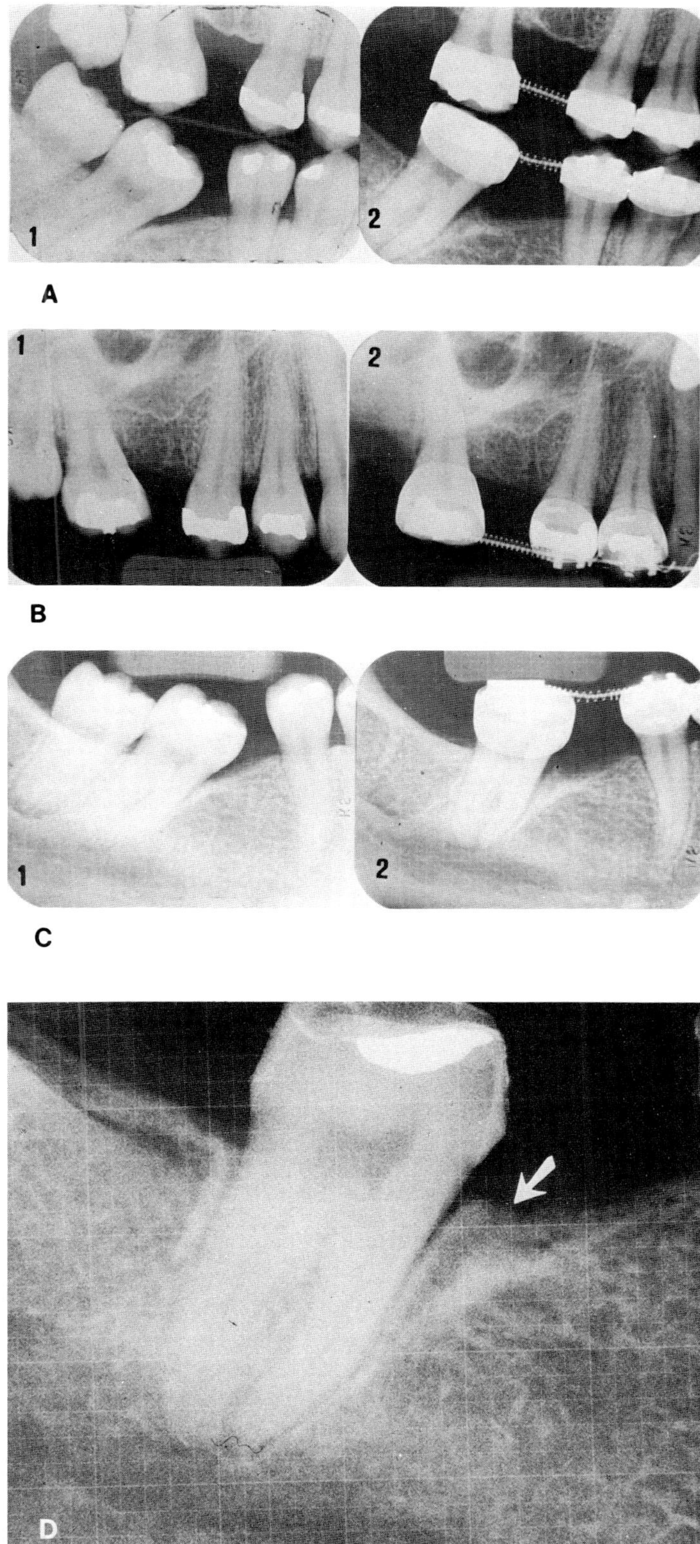

Fig. 10-9. (A) (1) Pre-treatment bite-wing radiograph showing upper and lower first molars missing and remaining molars tipped in a mesial direction. *(2)* Bite-wing radiograph after third molars have been extracted and second molars tipped distally. *(B) (1)* Pre-treatment radiograph of maxillary molars. *(2)* Post-orthodontic-treatment radiograph. *(C)* (1) Pre-treatment radiograph of mandibular molars. *(2)* Lower right second molar after orthodontic tooth movement. *(D)* Periapical radiograph of lower right molar, depicting the improved periodontal status of this tooth as a potential abutment for a fixed restoration. The arrow shows change in the mesial bone morphology. The new position of the tooth obviates the restorative problem of parallelism. (Orthodontics by Dr. Roger Wise, Swampscott, Massachusetts)

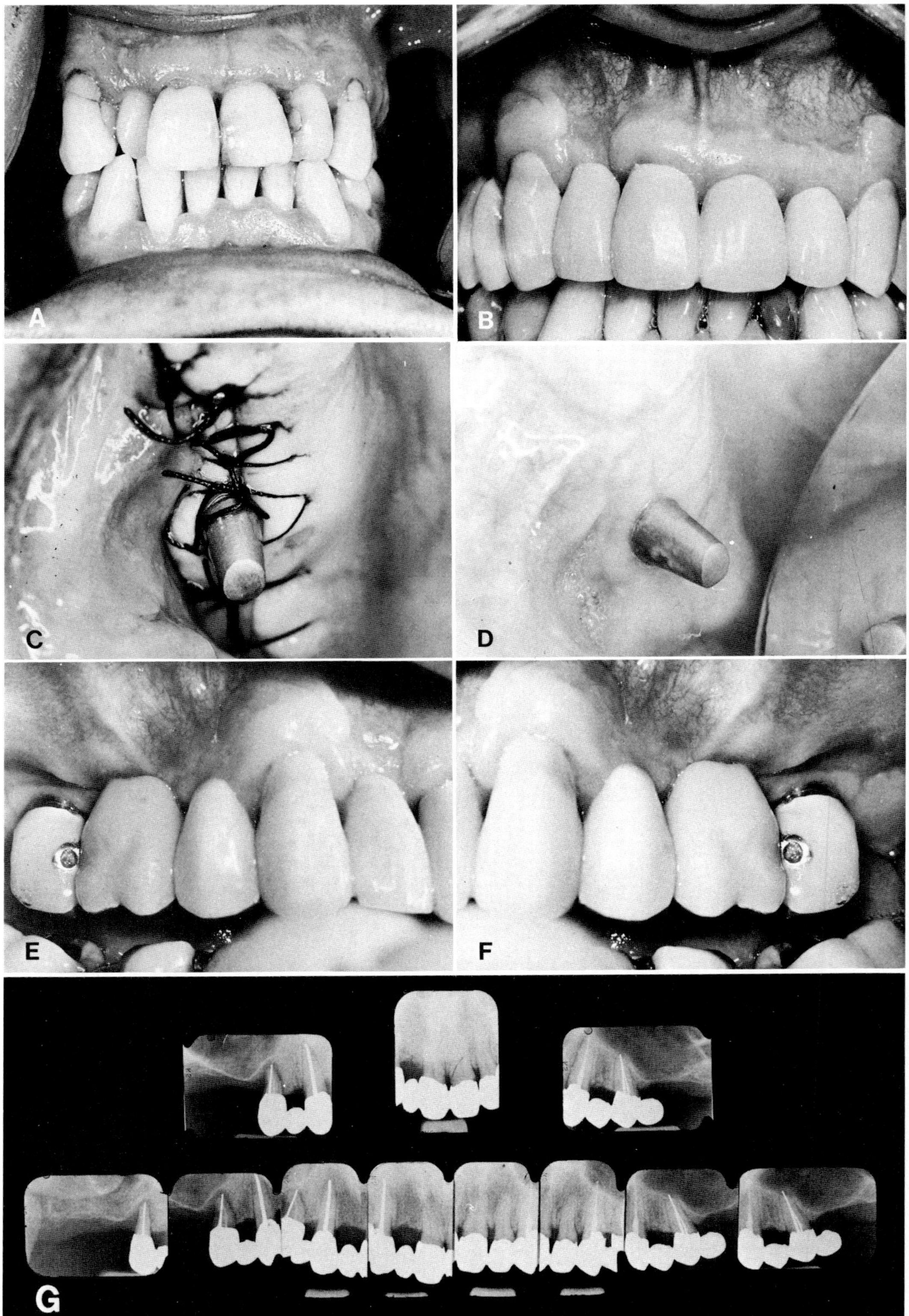

Fig. 10-10A to G. (See legend opposite.)

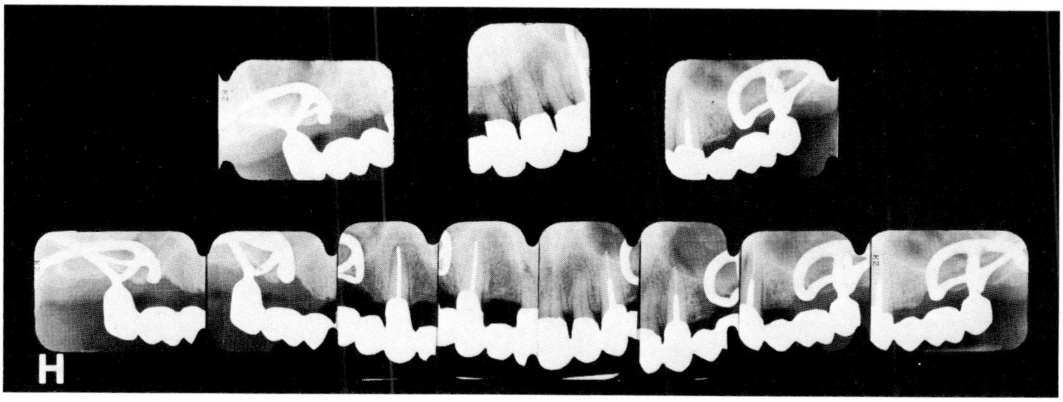

Fig. 10-10. *(A)* Pre-treatment clinical photograph (1954). *(B)* Clinical photograph, (1974) after insertion of maxillary subperiosteal terminal implants. *(C)* Day of insertion of upper right implant (1970). *(D)* Upper right implant 6 months after insertion. *(E)* Upper right implant after delivery of prosthesis. *(F)* Upper left implant after delivery of prosthesis. *(G)* Upper radiographs (1969) showing periodontal failure of the upper right second bicuspid. The upper left second bicuspid subsequently fractured during prosthetic therapy. *(H)* Post-treatment upper radiographic survey showing maxillary terminal subperiosteal implants and the prosthesis in place.

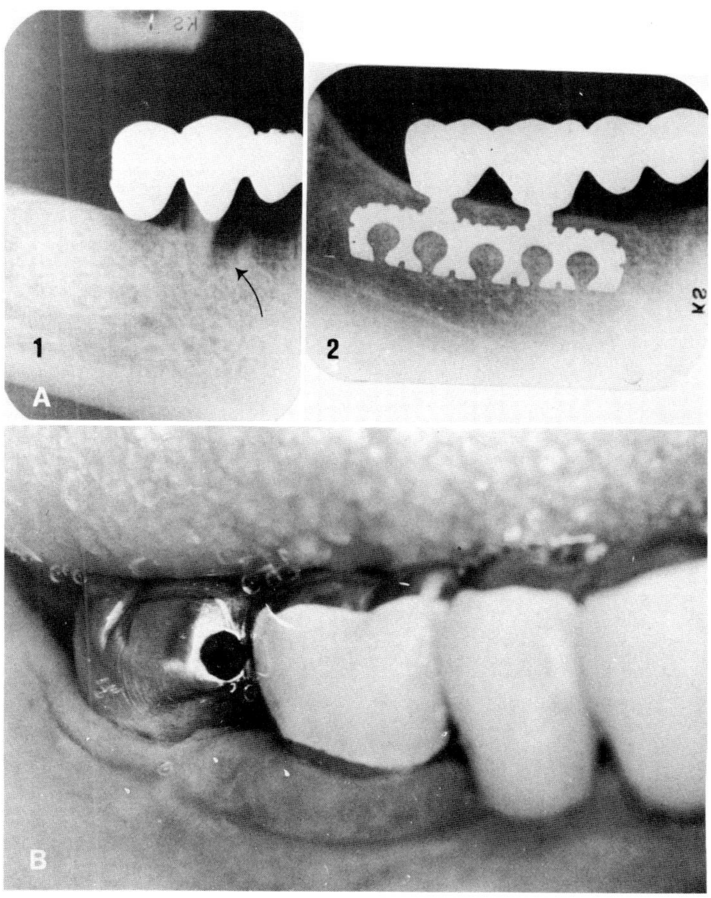

Fig. 10-11. *(A)* *(1)* The remaining natural abutment on the right side is severely damaged periodontally *(arrow)*. *(2)* A new prosthesis, with an intra-osseous implant taking the place of the periodontally damaged natural abutment. *(B)* The clinical photograph of this quadrant.

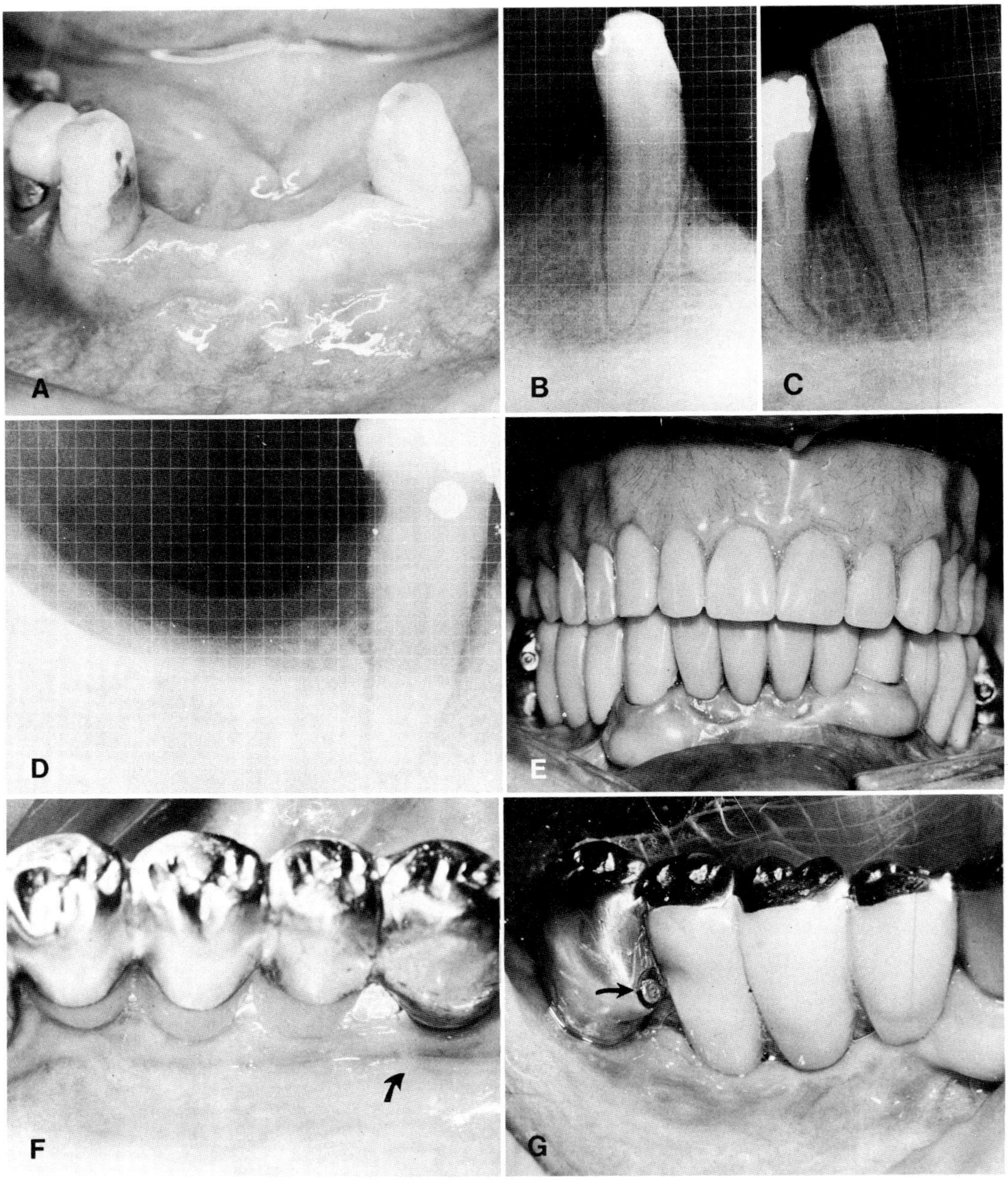

Fig. 10-12. (A) Clinical pre-treatment photograph of the four remaining teeth in this arch. *(B)* Radiograph of the stable left cuspid. *(C)* Radiograph of the periodontally stable lower right cuspid. The lower right first bicuspid required endodontic therapy, which proved to be unsuccessful; this tooth was extracted. *(D)* Radiograph of the lower right second bicuspid, which displayed a Class-III mobility. The decision was ultimately made to remove both bicuspids and to construct a provisional prosthesis that would utilize the two cuspids and two subperiosteal implants as abutments. *(E)* The finished lower prosthesis 4 years after delivery. *(F)* Lingual view of the right implant *(arrow)*. *(G)* Buccal view of the right implant *(arrow to Re Seté threaded screw)*. *(Please see next page.)*

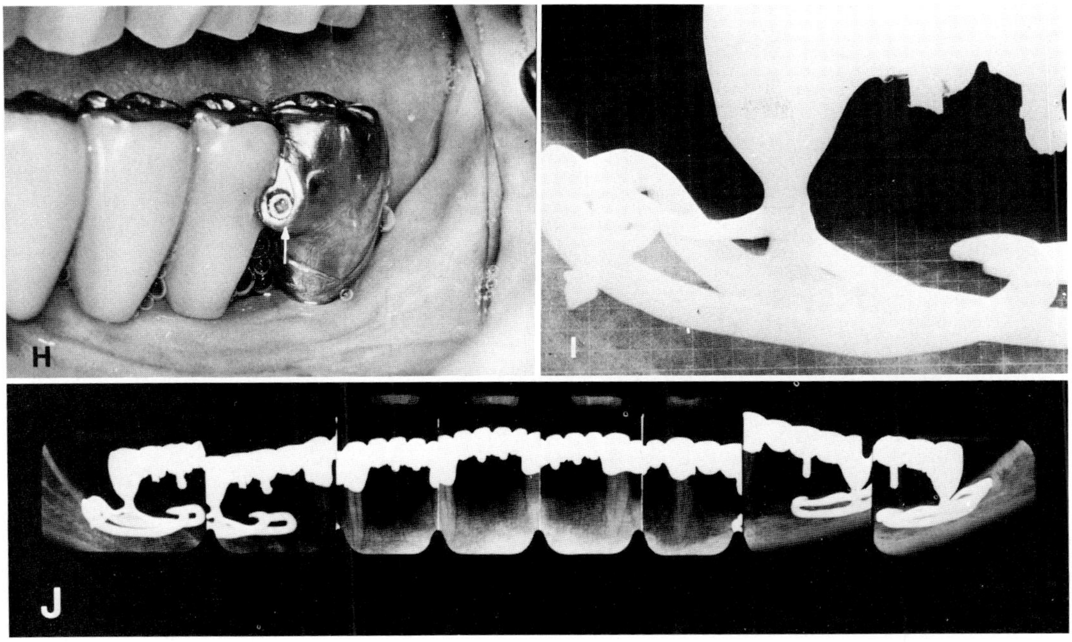

Fig. 10-12 (Continued). (H) Buccal view of lower left implant. *(I)* Radiograph of the lower right implant. Note the careful fit of the casting. *(J)* Lower radiographic survey 4 years after insertion.

the appearance or functioning of the provisional prosthesis the tendency is to convert from the provisional prosthesis to a fixed prosthesis too quickly, thereby limiting the opportunity to gain knowledge from this important phase of therapy.

THE LONG PERIOD OF PATIENT EVALUATION

The clinician has the opportunity to evaluate the patient during periodontal therapy, and during what is commonly referred to as "relining" the provisional fixed bridge. (It is wise to avoid the term *temporary bridge,* because this would indicate that there is no value other than to serve as a temporary retainer; it is this thought process that too frequently encourages the clinician to forge ahead without the proper data.)

Periodontal therapy is instituted after a period of time during which extraction sockets have healed and the patient has become accustomed to proper care of his provisional prosthesis. It is more difficult to care for this artificial prosthesis than for one's natural teeth, and it is frequently necessary to educate the patient further with regard to this care.

It is during this phase of therapy that attempts are made to treat posterior abutments. If minor tooth movement is to be instituted as a form of corrective treatment, it is usually done before provisionalization is completed. There are times, however, when minor tooth movement is not encountered until the provisionalization has been completed. In these latter instances, the retainers used to secure orthodontic appliances are provided in the provisional bridge. An example of such reversal of orthodontic-prosthodontic sequential treatment might be a lower molar tooth that is sectioned during periodontal surgical correction that has roots too close together to develop an embrasure (Fig. 10-13).

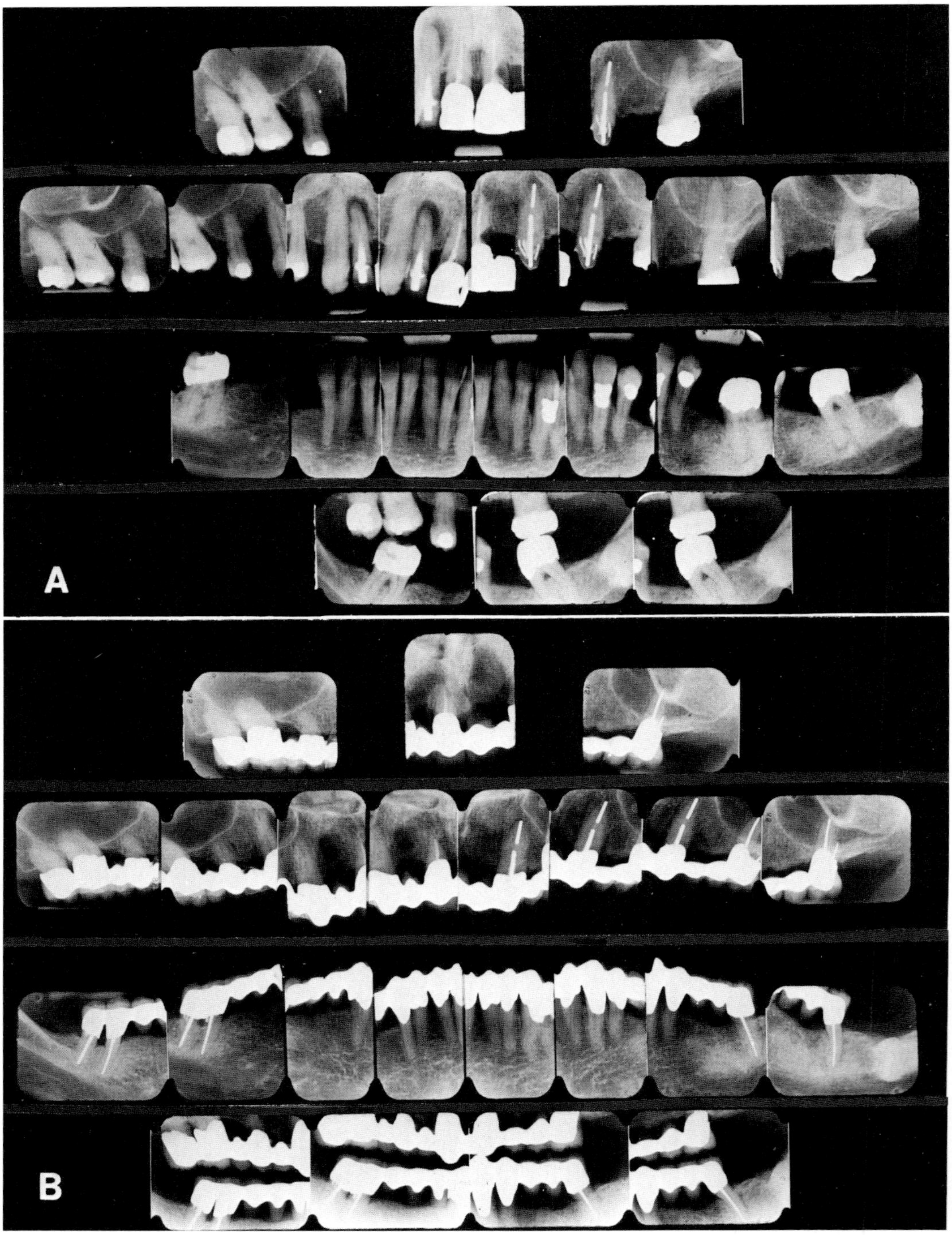

Fig. 10-13. *(A)* Pre-treatment full-mouth radiographic survey. Both remaining lower molar teeth have intra-radicular problems. The lower right cuspid and both bicuspids are missing, presenting a long edentulous span, with the lower incisors having to lend anterior support for the prosthesis. The right molar tooth was stable, and it was decided that maintenance of both roots would be preferable for reasons of periodontal support. The presence of the first bicuspid and cuspid on the left side precluded the necessity of a similar endeavor, and only the distal root was utilized. *(B)* Post-treatment radiographic survey. *(Please see next page.)*

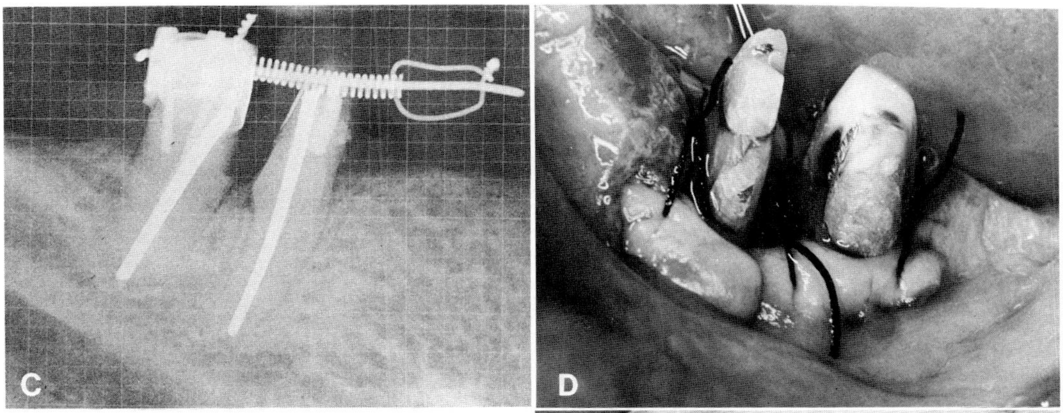

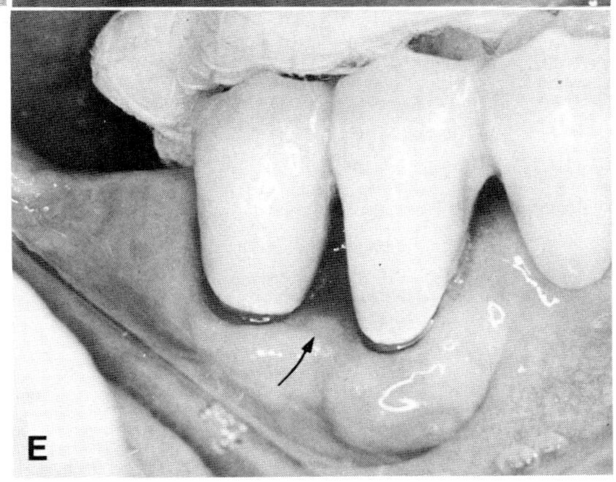

Fig. 10-13 (Continued). (C) Radiograph taken at time of insertion of the orthodontic appliance into the provisional bridge. *(D)* Photograph at time of subsequent periodontal surgery, after roots were separated and ledges on roots were removed. *(E)* Clinical photograph of final prosthesis, with embrasure *(arrow)* that is easily managed by the dentist prosthetically and by the patient.

The stability of the provisional prosthesis should be tested. If necessary, additional natural abutment teeth should be used, to eliminate mobility. If, however, all available natural abutments in the arch have been utilized and the prosthesis remains mobile, the practitioner must reconsider the course of treatment. It is this type of development that has led to many premature clinical failures. The clinician should continually impress upon the patient the possibility of failure and of the consequent necessity to resort to different forms of treatment.

If, after periodontal corrective therapy has been accomplished, the provisional prosthesis is found to be stable, the dentist should begin refurbishing the bridge. If a tooth has been sectioned to serve as an abutment, it should be reprepared and the acrylic retainer relined, so that this abutment can play an active role in the stabilization of the segment of teeth that are to be included within the confines of the fixed prosthesis. The acrylic resin should approximate the new margin of the gingiva, in order to enable the patient to function properly and to practice adequate plaque control.

Frequently, the path of insertion of a prosthesis is altered after periodontal surgery. The initial tooth preparation changes direction as more clinical crown is exposed (Figs. 10-14, 10-15). Thus, if an implant were to be inserted prior to periodontal surgery, it would be unlikely that the post of the implant would be parallel to the final tooth preparations of the natural abutments. In cases of minor periodontal involvement, this is less of a problem, and one might consider an earlier insertion of an implant. Nevertheless, because of the possibility of failure with the earlier insertion of an implant, care should be taken

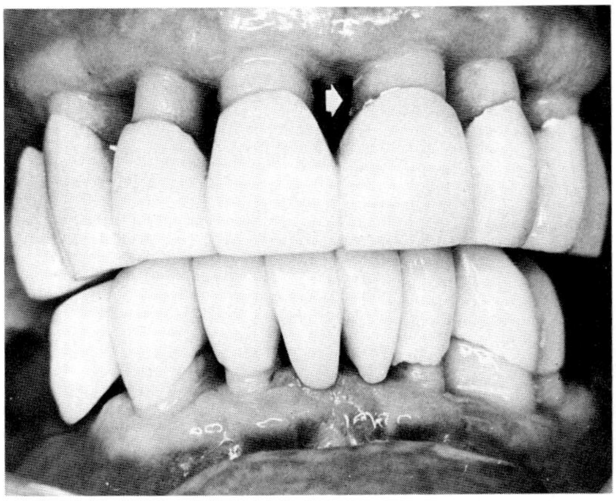

Fig. 10-14. Postoperative photograph showing the clinical discrepancy apparent after surgery of periodontally involved teeth. The arrow indicates the necessary extension of the tooth preparations to the gingiva.

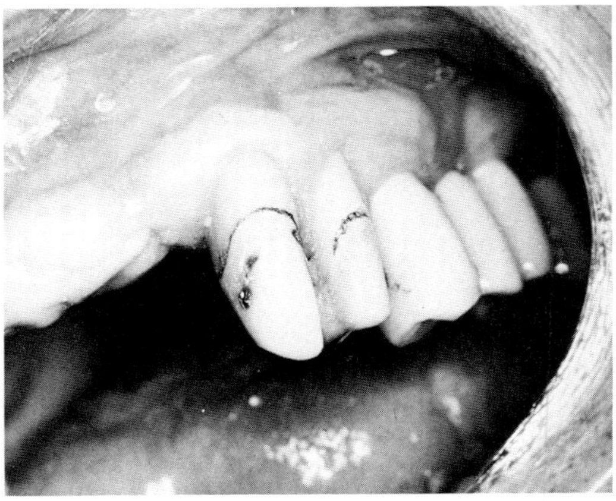

Fig. 10-15. The penciled lines on the tooth preparation indicate where the initial tooth preparation ended. Extension to the new gingival margins will alter the path of insertion of the provisional bridge.

not to introduce the implant into the definitive treatment plan until the preparatory and investigatory procedures have been accomplished.

REDISCUSSION OF THE TREATMENT PLAN WITH THE PATIENT

If at this time the patient still appears to be a responsible candidate for an implant, it seems feasible to discuss the situation further. It may be that although all therapies preparatory to inserting an implant have been very successful to date, the patient's tolerance is wearing thin, and therefore the dentist may opt for a different form of treatment. If, however, the patient continues to be responsive, it would be proper to proceed with implant procedures if: (a) a provisional removable treatment partial denture has been utilized and has been unsuccessful; or (b) an abbreviated occlusion has not given the patient the desired mastication or the desired esthetic effect.

It is necessary to clearly inform the patient that after the implant is inserted, it must be tested for a reliable period of time. Many of the failures encountered in implantology occur during the first few months after insertion. Again, it is integral to the success of this treatment that the provisional bridgework be of such a satisfactory quality that the patient will not be uncomfortable during this continued phase of observation.

SELECTION OF THE TYPE OF IMPLANT

The past decade has provided us with a variety of substitutes for natural teeth. Most have been composed of inert metal. During the past 2 years, however, attempts have been made to utilize materials that might be better accepted by the soft tissues. Most often, the selection of the type of implant is dependent on its site of insertion. It is necessary to consider different forms of implants for different anatomic locations.

The Upper Posterior Region

In most instances, a sinus is in some proximity to the site of extracted upper

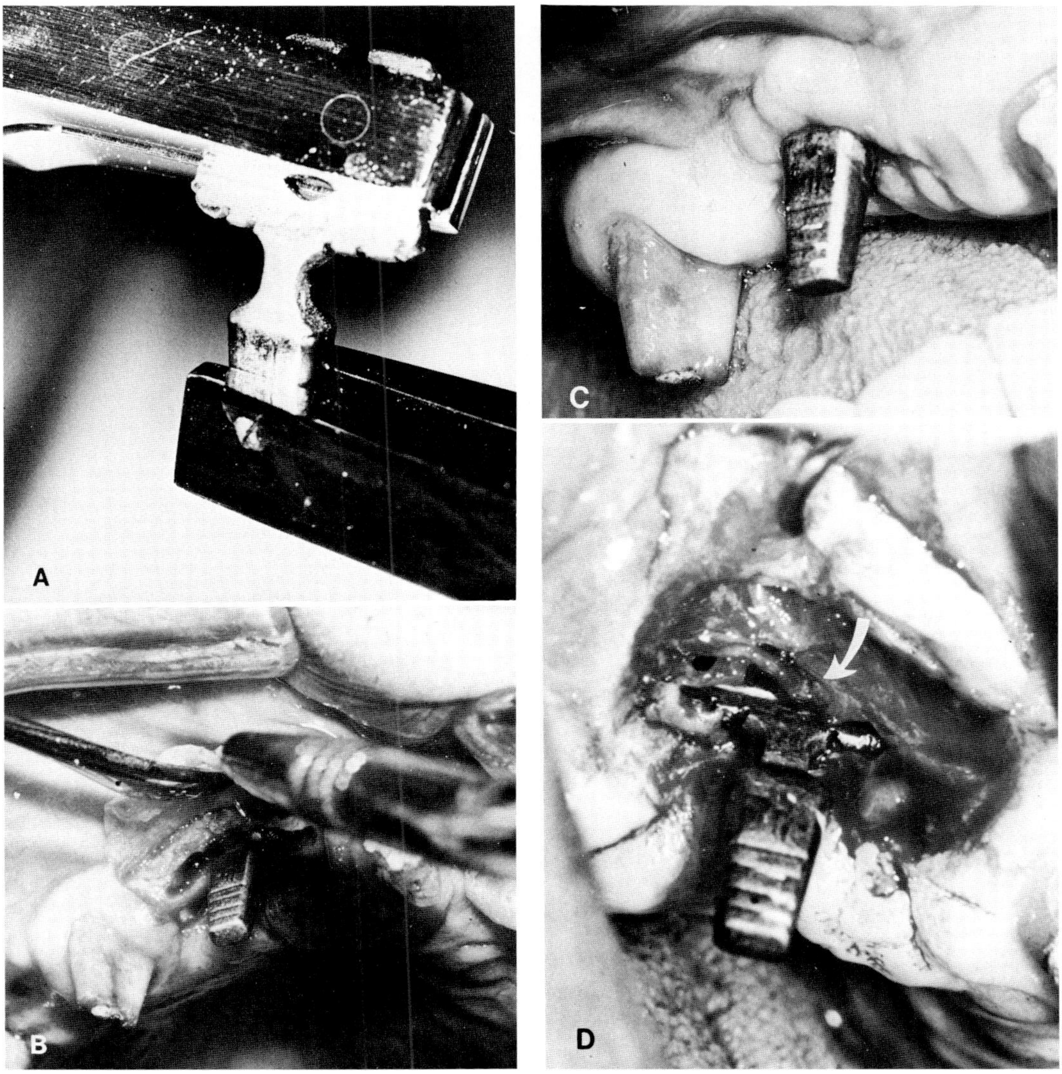

Fig. 10-16. (A) Bending an intra-osseous implant in order to place it parallel to the remaining natural abutment teeth. *(B)* Placing the implant in the position of the upper right cuspid. *(C)* The apparently successful implant 2 months after insertion. *(D)* The implant area reopened because of clinical mobility. Note the destruction of the labial plate *(arrow).*

molar teeth (Fig. 10-2F); this places some limits on the use of intraosseous implants. One rarely considers the use of an intraosseous implant that is designed to surround the sinus (rather than enter it), because there may not be enough supportive bone to provide adequate stability for this type of implant.

The success to date with terminal subperiosteal implants to replace upper posterior teeth indicates the validity of considering this form of therapy as a matter of course. It may be that the heavy palatal tissues offer better containment to the metal struts of the subperiosteal implant than do those tissues found in the mandibular posterior areas.

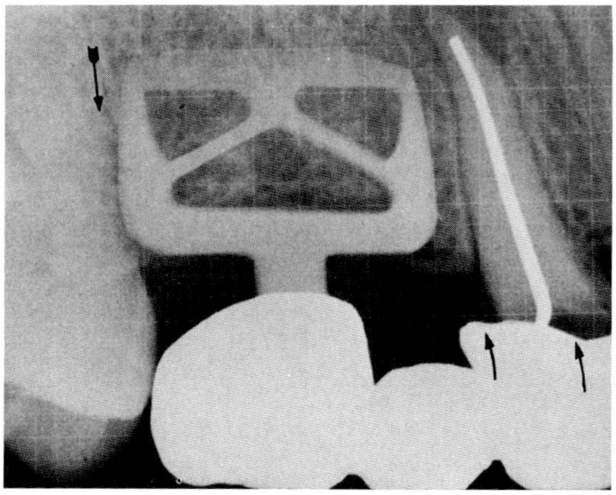

Fig. 10-17. Radiograph of an intra-osseous implant that replaces a single missing tooth. The periodontal support of the upper right second molar *(top arrow)* has been jeopardized. The poor fit of the retainer for the bicuspid *(bottom arrows)* represents a lack of expertise in more elementary dental treatments.

The Upper Anterior Region

This ridge is frequently knife-like, and the architecture of the premaxilla is such that a blade implant inserted into it would be in a labial position and would not even approximate parallelism with existing posterior abutments. It should be noted that this is an example of the reason that this form of implant should not be inserted without opening the soft tissues and observing the topography of the hard tissues. In instances where the ridge has been found to be flatter and wider, there has been some success with the intra-osseous implant.

The method of bending the blade implant at the neck has been less than totally successful (Fig. 10-16). This method, in effect, eliminates what predictability there is, relative to the distribution of forces from occlusion.

In the context of this discussion, one might have to consider the use of an implant to replace a single missing tooth (Fig. 10-17). The relative unpredictability of any implant, however, as compared with the relative predictability of fixed bridgework, contraindicates the use of an implant for the replacement of a single missing tooth. The possibility of damage to periodontal supportive structures of the adjacent natural dentition does not seem to validate the use of this form of therapy.

The Upper Bicuspid Region

This area appears to be the most appropriate candidate for maxillary intra-osseous implants. Both subperiosteal and intra-osseous implants have been utilized between natural anterior teeth and posterior abutments for unmanageable spans. The use of implants in this area seems to have few contraindications.

As one reaches the region of the cuspid, however, implantation becomes more difficult because of the lateral occlusal stresses that are routinely exerted in this region. In addition, placement of the implant in the cuspid region may be difficult because there is the distinct possibility of the loss of the thin plate of labial bone and the placement of the implant in a compromised position.

The Lower Posterior Region

In this area, both forms of implants have been used successfully. When possible, the use of the intra-osseous implant offers much less chance of complication than does the subperiosteal implant. The intra-osseous implant requires only one surgical intervention and does not require the degree of disengagement of muscular fiber connection that the subperiosteal implant does, thus carrying few postoperative sequelae. The blade implant has limitations in this area because of the anatomy of the mandible (Fig. 10-18). The lingual surface of the edentulous mandible curves towards the center of the mandible as it extends apically. In a badly resorbed mandible, therefore, the placement of the blade implant may cause perforation of the lingual plate. Another difficulty in placing intra-

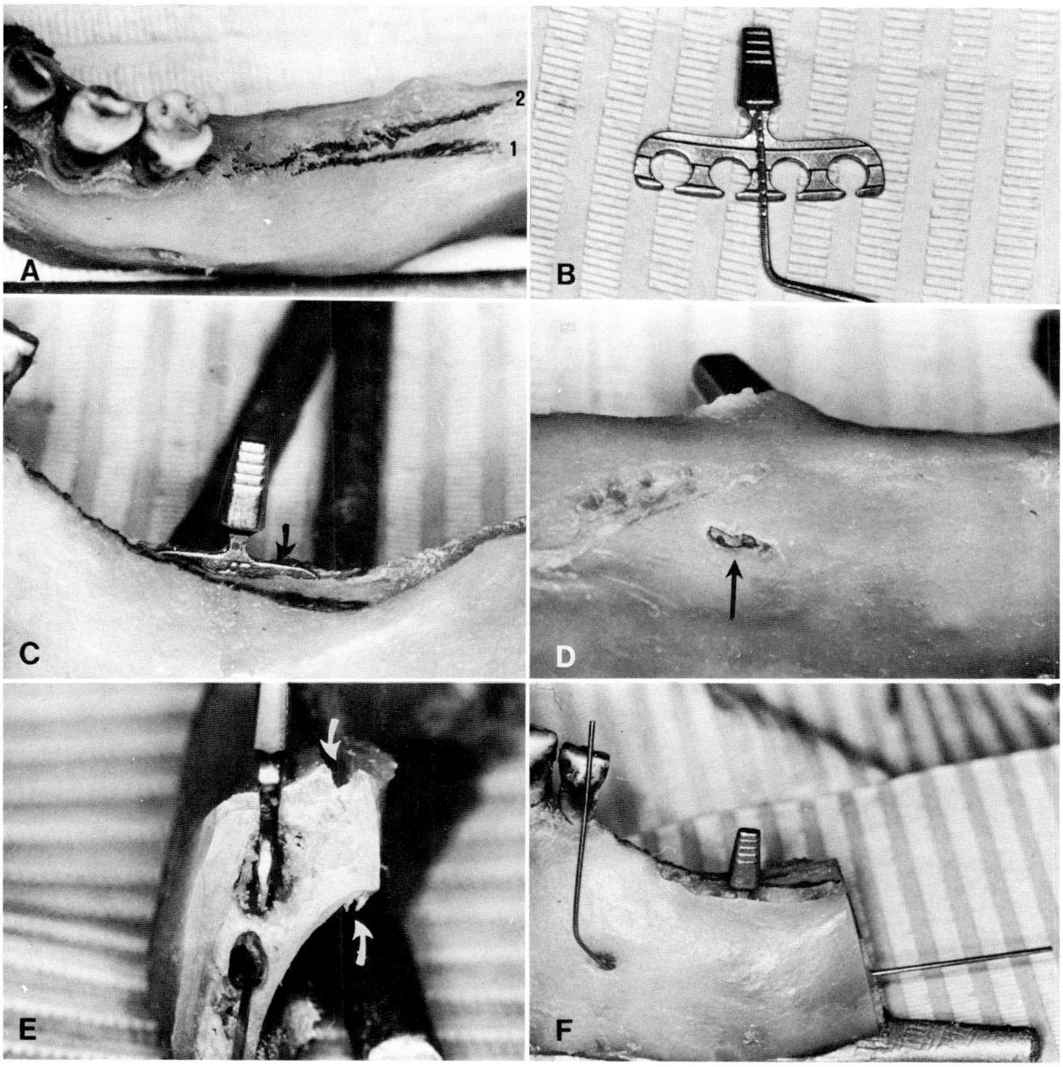

Fig. 10-18. *(A)* Mandible of cadaver, showing discrepancy between *(1)* where implant would be optimally placed for occlusal purposes and *(2)* where intra-osseous implant would be optimally placed for purposes of support. *(B)* Periodontal probe measuring the implant to be used for purposes of demonstration. *(C)* Implant being placed in position *(2)*. Note that the implant is not fully seated, as the upper ridge *(arrow)* is still visible. *(D)* Perforation of the lingual plate *(arrow)* with an intra-osseous implant. *(E)* The proximity of the intra-osseous implant to the mental foramen. It is necessary to recognize that the depth of the implant is only average, as shown in *(B)*, and that there is a substantial quantity of alveolar bone occlusal to the mental foramen. Note the possibility of perforation of the lingual plate *(arrows)*. *(F)* The intra-osseous implant fully seated in position *(1)*, with a wire tracing the mandibular canal to the mental foramen.

osseous implants in badly resorbed mandibular posterior areas is that the site of insertion may not align with the upper posterior occlusal scheme, and may even be in linguoversion. This, therefore, would place undue stress on the mandibular implant and diminish the probability of its success.

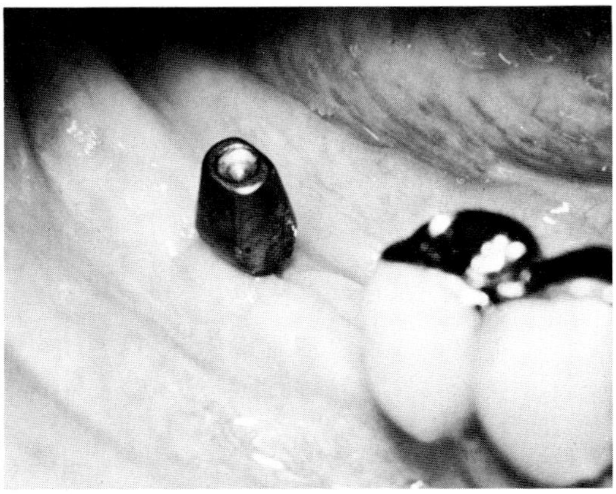

Fig. 10-19. Successful intra-osseous implant 3 months after insertion.

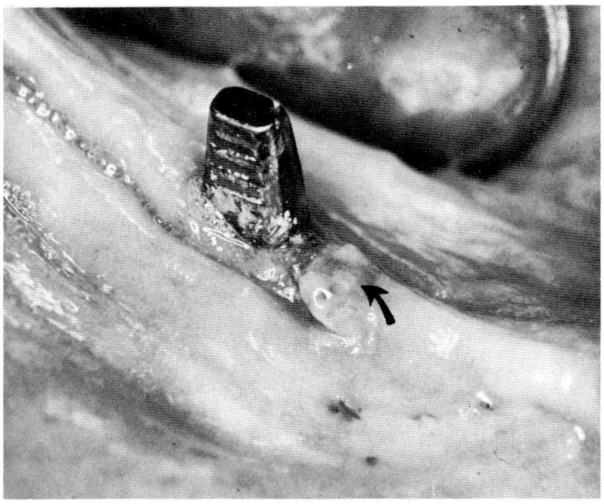

Fig. 10-20. Unsuccessful intra-osseous implant 3 months after insertion. There is a fistula *(arrow)* at the mesial aspect of the implant.

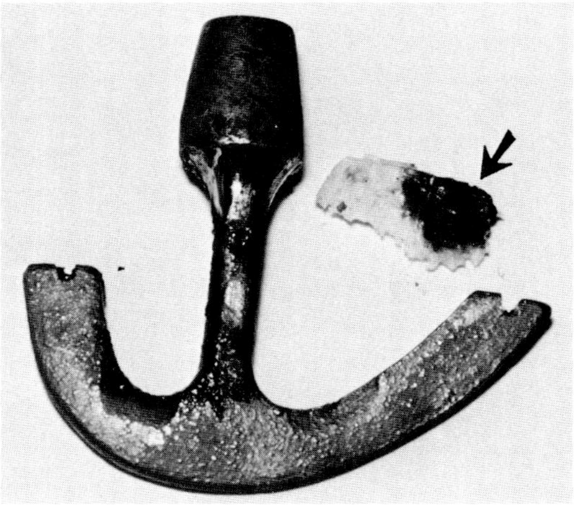

Fig. 10-21. Intra-osseous implant that has been removed. There apparently was a corrosive change in the metallic structure that caused the degeneration and staining of the bone *(arrow to portion of bone sequestrum).* This change in the metallic structure is an unusual finding.

One also must keep in mind that when many molar teeth are lost, the buccal portion of bone is also lost. The ridge then slants from a higher peak lingually to a more apical dimension buccally as one enters the area of the external oblique ridge. Again, the clinician should be discouraged from inserting an intra-osseous implant in an area in which the hard structures have not been exposed for visual observation. There is no way to determine the topography of the bone merely by observing the topography of the soft tissues (Figs. 10-19 to 10-21).

Terminal subperiosteal implants have been somewhat less successful in lower posterior areas than in upper posterior areas. It is difficult to ascertain the specific reasons for failure, but a likely explanation might be found by assessing the comparative strengths of the soft tissues of both arches.

The Lower Biscuspid Region

In a discussion of this region, it is necessary to be concerned with the mental foramen (Fig. 10-18F). There would never be a situation in which it would be so necessary to insert an intra-osseous implant in this region that one would risk jeopardizing the vascular or nerve supply to this area. The insertion of a subperiosteal implant slightly posterior to this area might be more readily tolerated.

The Lower Cuspid Region

Again, there is the possibility of a knifelike ridge caused by previous bone loss and the healing of the extraction wounds of lower cuspids. In the construction of almost any occlusion, the lower cuspid area has to be functional. It may be difficult to insert an intra-osseous implant in the lower cuspid area in such a position that it can function properly for a prolonged period of time. It is unusual to have to consider the insertion of an implant in the region of the lower incisor teeth and the lower cuspids, because the natural dentition in this area most frequently remains for the longest period of time.

INSERTION OF THE IMPLANT AND EXTENSION OF THE PROVISIONAL PROSTHESIS TO THE IMPLANT

It is possible to extend the provisional prosthesis so as to include the implant as a retainer either on the day of insertion or at a specified later time. It is wise, however, to allow for a period of initial healing after inserting the implant before including the implant in the trial prosthesis. The rationale for this is that:

1. The patient usually exerts pressure on the clinician to insert the implant. If the clinician is not at his optimum level of performance, errors may be made that may prove to be critical to the success of the implant.
2. The patient is deeply anesthetized during implant insertion procedures and may not be able to provide a proper occlusal response, thus making it difficult to achieve an optimal occlusal relationship. Also, as the implant wound is healing, it is best to exert as few harmful stresses on the area as possible; therefore, it is wise not to try to establish occlusal relationships during the healing period.
3. It seems correct to keep all provisional restorative materials away from the wound. Certainly, the introduction of acrylic-resin monomers does not enhance wound healing.

It may be preferable to allow about 3 weeks to pass after implant insertion before extending the provisional prosthesis to the implant. Once the provisional prosthesis is extended, it is necessary to cement it very carefully so that it does not loosen. If the provisional prosthesis does loosen, a "pumping action" is exerted on this artificial tooth substitute. Again, the relative uncertainty of the success of this procedure is such that unnecessary detrimental factors should not be introduced.

PERIOD OF OBSERVATION

Following the insertion of the implant, there are symptoms that may readily provide clues as to possible failure. Some are obvious, such as pain, swelling or unusual tastes. Pain may be relative to initial surgical procedures or, if encountered at a later time, could be indicative of more serious problems. Swelling is to be expected more with the insertion of the subperiosteal implant, because of the necessity of more extensive reflection of muscular insertions than with the blade implant. Beyond the short-term postoperative period, swelling most frequently is indicative of an infection. Unpleasant taste usually relates to infection or is an indication that the provisional bridge has become loose.

Other symptoms are vaguer and much more difficult to interpret. The patient may complain of a dull ache in the area of the implant. This may occur during the first attempts at mastication with the implant and could reflect the patient's inability to withstand the masticatory pressure in this area. Because of this direction of symptomatology, the experienced clinician should tell the patient prior to therapy that he cannot expect the same satisfaction with the implant that he once had with a full complement of natural teeth.

In many instances, the patient may be totally comfortable, and infections and other problems are only observed during periodic examination visits; this is often the case with a fistula or exposure of struts (Figs. 10-22 to 10-27). The patient frequently is unaware of mobility of the implant. It is unlikely that the symptoms mentioned in this paragraph are synonymous with success of the implant, and it

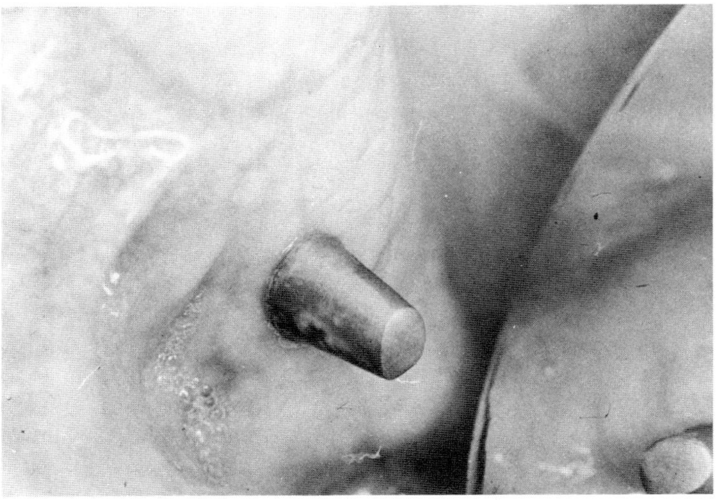

Fig. 10-22. Successful subperiosteal terminal implant, 6 months after insertion.

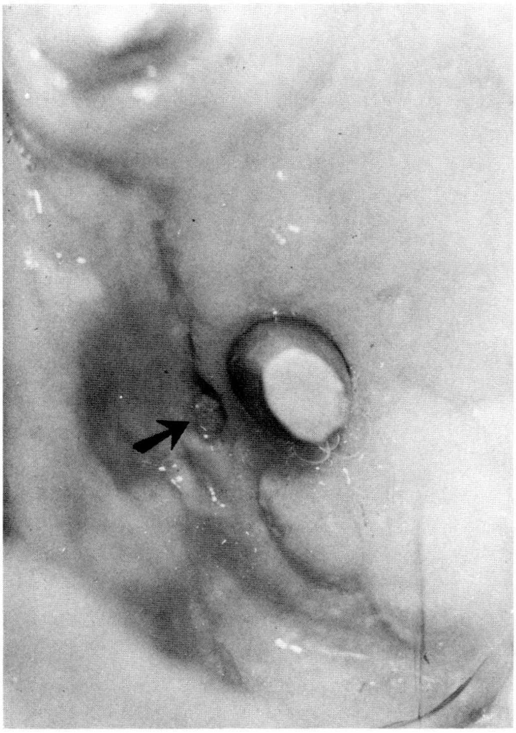

Fig. 10-23. Subperiosteal implant 4 months after insertion. Fistulation has resulted in the exposure of a strut *(arrow).*

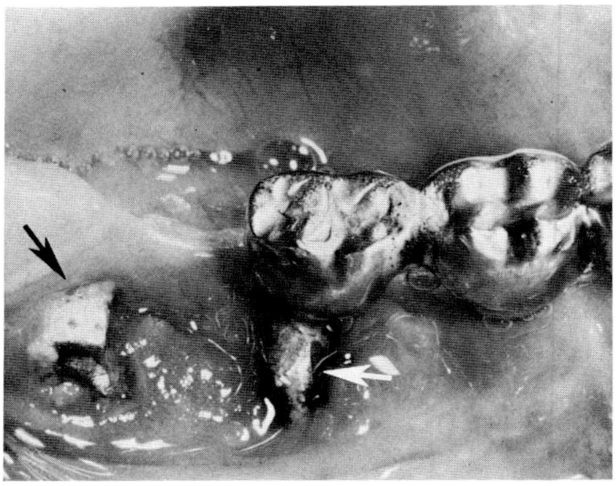

Fig. 10-24. An implant failure, with struts *(arrows)* obviously exposed.

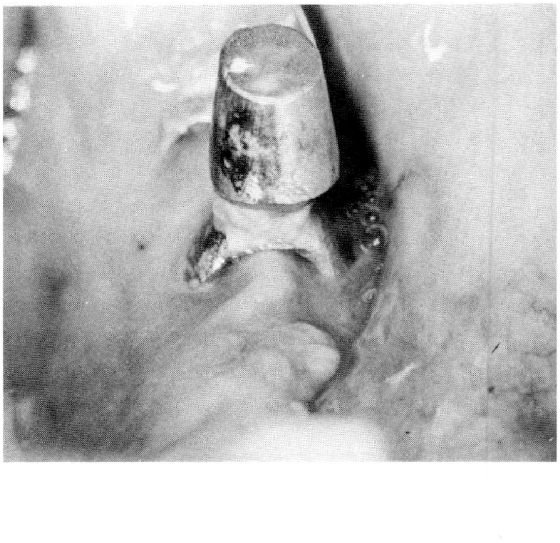

Fig. 10-25. An unsuccessful subperiosteal implant on the day of removal.

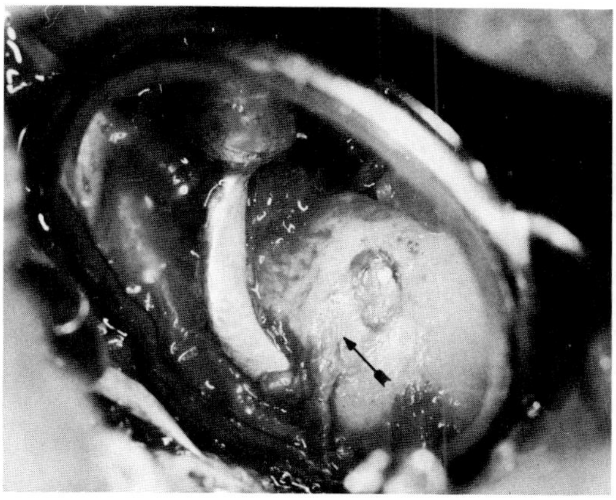

Fig. 10-26. Day of removal of a subperiosteal implant, where alveolar bone has grown over the strut arm *(arrow).*

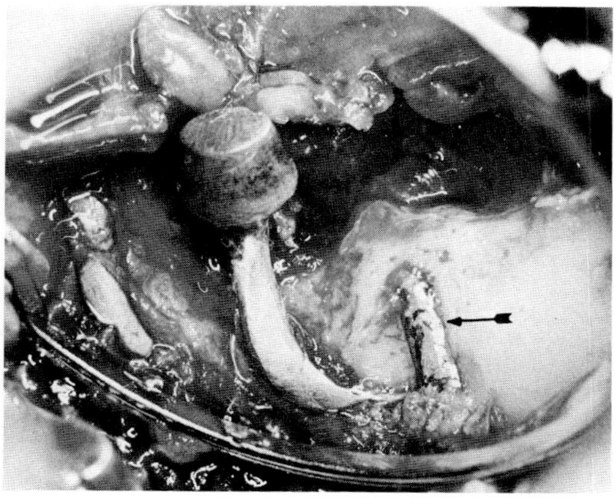

Fig. 10-27. The bone has been removed from the surface of the strut arm *(arrow)* (See Fig. 10-26.)

is always better to be aware of these problems before delivering a permanent prosthesis.

Radiographic changes are very difficult to interpret. With many intra-osseous implants, the radiographic changes only detect ultimate failure (Figs. 10-28, 10-29). It is doubtful that a patient would be unsupervised long enough for dramatic radiographic changes to develop. In most instances, there appears to be some radiolucency where the intra-osseous implant leaves the alveolar bone. This is a very difficult area to interpret, because radiolucency occurs in both health and disease. Also, in some instances, upon examination by surgical reentry, there appears to be no problem in the area of contact between bone and the neck of the intra-osseous implant. The radiograph may serve as a positive indication of a break in the metal of an implant (Fig. 10-30). A break in the metal of an implant has been observed infrequently.

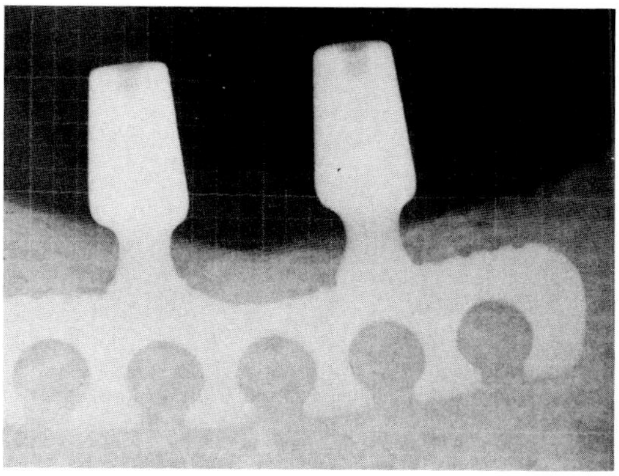

Fig. 10-28. Radiograph of a successful intra-osseous implant.

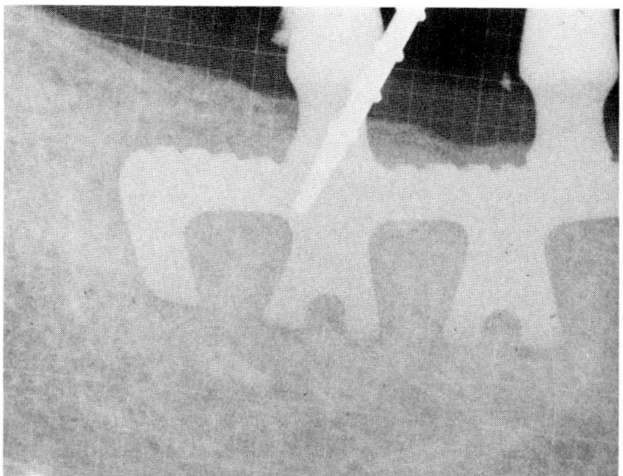

Fig. 10-29. Radiograph of an unsuccessful intra-osseous implant. Note the Hirschfeld point communicating from the oral cavity to a problem area.

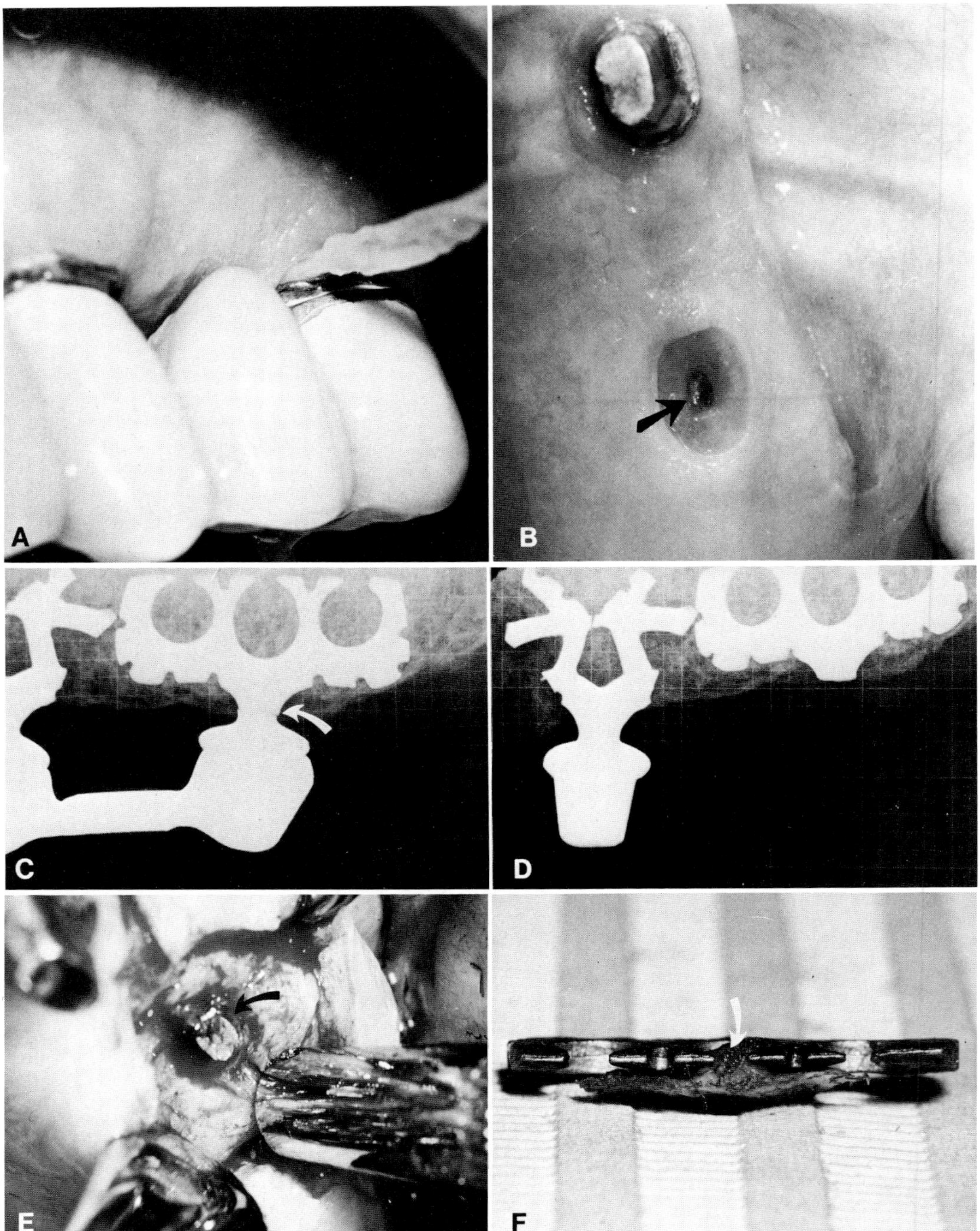

Fig. 10-30. An intra-osseous implant that has fractured at the neck. *(A)* Dental floss passing between the pieces. *(B)* The bridge is removed, and the neck of the implant is visible *(arrow)*. *(C)* Radiograph of the otherwise successful implant. Arrow denotes fracture line. Note the inadequate fit of the castings to the implant, compared with Figure 10-12 I. *(D)* Radiograph without bridge in place. It was fortunate that two separate implants were used, rather than one with two abutments. *(E)* Surgical exposure of the neck of the implant. This offers the opportunity to compare the radiographic appearance *(C)* to the surgically exposed osseous structures at the neck of the implant. *(F)* Implant with spicule of bone growing between the struts *(arrow)*.

Radiographs are of limited value in diagnosing early changes in the subperiosteal implant. Although radiographs have been frequently utilized to display success, it is common to be unable to relate the health of the implant with the status of the radiograph. *It may be that clinical observations are far more valuable than radiographs in evaluating early changes in subperiosteal implants.*

Clinical findings indicate that if the patient is asymptomatic 6 months after implant insertion, it is rational to proceed with the production of the finished prosthesis.

MAINTENANCE OF THE IMPLANT

It is necessary to teach the patient to care for the area of the implant in a fashion similar to that required for natural abutments. Most manual forms of plaque removal are advisable. One must seriously consider whether irrigating devices have an adverse effect, such as forcing debris into the gingival sulcus of the implant.

The office procedures for implant patients are very similar to those for patients with natural-abutment teeth. If the patient is observed for 6 to 12 weeks after insertion, there is usually no problem caring for implants. Changes are apparent at early stages, and one will not encounter catastrophic results except in the most unusual circumstances. The implant area is cleansed by an oral hygienist with a water-spray cleansing device. The implant sulcus is then gently cleaned with a fine, sharp curette. Only on rare occasions do we find so firm a connection of soft tissue to the metal that we cannot probe this area.

It is difficult to accept the philosophy that all implants have a questionable prognosis and that clinical therapeutics involving implants are irresponsible. This theory seems to come from those who have not had the opportunity to perform implantology and to continue a regimented post-therapeutic documentation with the patient. The problem of implant failures may not be so much with the philosophy and mechanics of implantology as with the application of implant therapy in a framework of less than an optimum dental and surgical educational background. If one has the opportunity to perform implant therapy and to observe his patients on a disciplined post-therapeutic regimen, one tends to take a more sanguine view of the field.

BIBLIOGRAPHY

Abelson, M. N.: Molar uprighting. D. Clin. North America, *16:*539-548, 1972.

Amen, C. R.: Hemisection and root amputation. Periodontics, *4:*197-204, 1966.

Amsterdam, M., and Rossman, S.: Technique of hemisection of multirooted teeth. Alpha Omegan, *53:*4-15, 1960.

Basaraba, N.: Root amputation and tooth hemisection. D. Clin. North America, *13:*121-132, 1969.

Brown, I. S.: The effect of orthodontic therapy on certain types of periodontal defects. J. Periodont., *44:*742-756, 1973.

Farrar, J. N.: Radical and heroic treatment of alveolar abscess by amputation of roots of teeth. D. Cosmos, *26:*79-81, 1884.

Hiatt, W. H., and Amen, C. R.: Periodontal pocket elimination by combined therapy. D. Clin. North America, pp. 133-144, March, 1964.

Kramer, G. M., and Reiser, G. M.: The tipped lower molar—therapeutic considerations. Alpha Omegan, *66:*33-39, 1973.

Messinger, T. F., and Orban, B. J.: Elimination of periodontal pockets by root amputation. J. Periodont., *25:*213-215, 1954.

Rosen, H., and Gitnick, P. J.: Separation and splinting of the roots of multirooted teeth. J. Pros. Dent., *21:*34-38, 1969.

Salman, L.: Root amputation. New York State J. Dent., *24:*79-86, 1958.

Sternlicht, H. C.: A new approach to the management of multirooted teeth with advanced periodontal disease. J. Periodont., *34:*150-158, 1963.

11 Endodontic Implants—Case Selection and Techniques

Edwin S. Mehlman, D.D.S.

THE NECESSITY OF INTERDISCIPLINARY, COMPREHENSIVE TREATMENT

Endodontic implants are a small but important segment of the implant armamentarium. These implants often serve as the key to salvaging an abutment tooth that may otherwise have a poor or a hopeless prognosis. Teeth that have an inadequate amount of natural attachment apparatus may receive intra-osseous root extensions in the form of endodontic implants. Thus, the endodontic implant serves not only as a stabilizer of mobile teeth, but as a man-made extension of the attachment apparatus. These characteristics of the endodontic implant are not unlike the supra-osseous coverage required for the subperiosteal implant or the intra-osseous expanse of an acceptable blade-vent implant (Fig. 11-1).

Because endodontic implants are often maligned, it should be noted that many of the failures seen are due to the lack of a total dental concept or philosophy on the part of the operator. Attention must be paid to periodontal therapy and comprehensive treatment planning in conjunction with the implant. Endodontic implantology must be performed in areas that have been made periodontally sound. A potential abutment tooth may require provisional splinting *and* periodontal procedures *prior* to the initiation of the implant procedure. After initial preparation, a sound endodontic routine remains an integral part of this implant procedure; i.e., the canal must be completely cleaned and shaped, sanitized, and sealed at the apical foramen (Figs. 11-2 to 11-4).

Too often, endodontic implants are not inserted according to these basic criteria and according to the interdisciplinary techniques that are required for a successful endodontically implanted abutment tooth. The implantologist may concentrate on the length and stability of the implant and may not consider sealing the apical foramen (Fig. 11-5); the endodontist may consider the apical seal but may not bear in mind the hopeless peridontal prognosis. Both the implantologist and the endodontist may

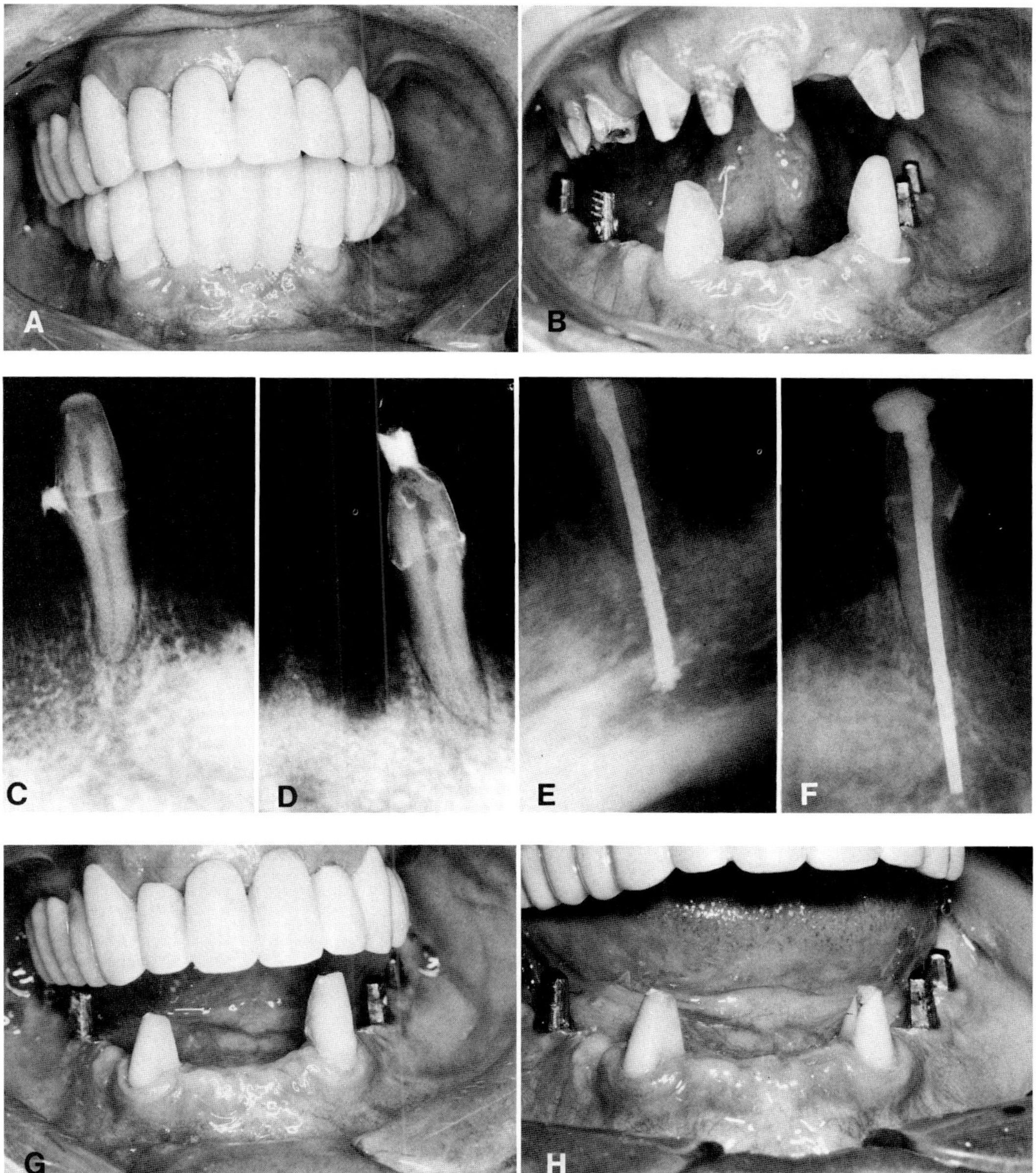

Fig. 11-1. *(A)* Temporary acrylic-resin splints prior to periodontal and endodontic treatments. *(B)* Splints removed after lower-arch periodontal treatment. Notice the extreme length of the clinical crowns of the lower right and lower left cuspids. Both teeth exhibited Class 2 mobility. *(C, D)* Radiographs of the lower right and lower left cuspids, showing the unfavorable crown-root ratio. *(E, F)* Endodontic implants inserted in order to stabilize mobile teeth and to extend the attachment apparatus to improve the crown-root ratio. *(G)* Lower right cuspid reprepared after periodontal and endodontic treatments have been completed. *(H)* Both lower cuspids reprepared after periodontal and endodontic treatments. Notice the improved length of the clinical crowns, which leads to a less stressful occlusal relationship, and, thus, to a more favorable prognosis for the implants and the natural teeth.

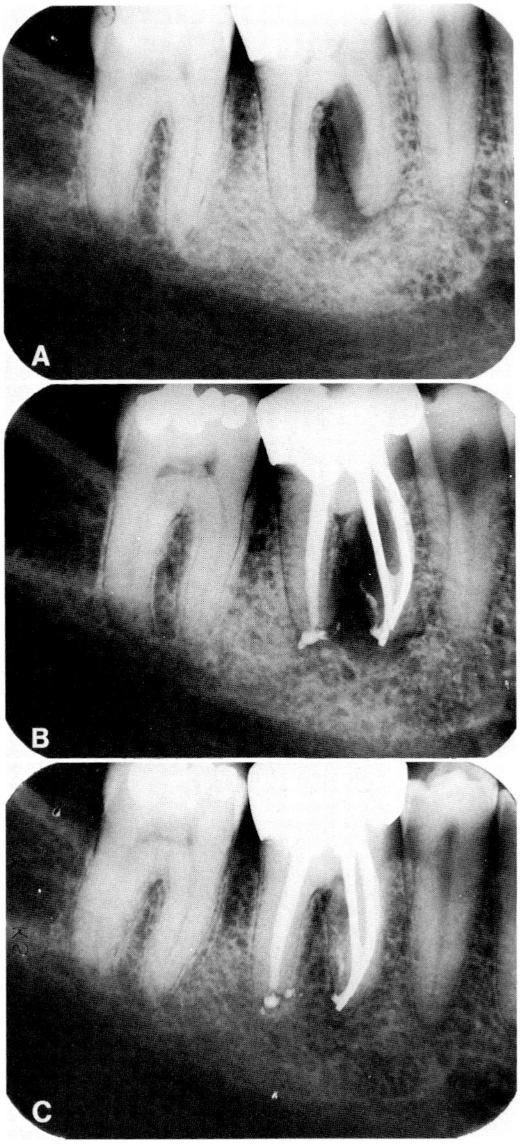

Fig. 11-2. (Figures 11-2 through 11-4 show examples of proper obturation of root canal systems.) *(A)* Radiograph for this patient, taken on 4/13/66, shows loss of bone in bifurcation of the lower right first molar. Periodontal probe in the sulcus reaches almost to the apex. The pulp of the tooth is necrotic. *(B)* Radiograph of same patient, taken on 5/3/66, shows proper obturation of the root canal system. *(C)* Radiograph of same patient, taken on 11/20/71, shows complete fill of bifurcation with new bone. No periodontal treatment was undertaken; this result was achieved by endodontic treatment only.

forget the occlusion of the restorative appliance that is to be placed on this important abutment. Lack of consideration of any of these aspects of treatment can lead to failure. Thus it can be seen how a technique such as this can be considered objectionable unless it is handled with a multidisciplinary approach, wherein a basic knowledge of implant techniques, periodontics, endodontics, and prosthodontics all contribute in some measure to the procedures.

The endodontic implant, by definition, is the only type of implant that has no contact with oral epithelium. This implant functions in a closed system (see Chap. 1). This gives the endodontic implant a distinct advantage for success over any other type of implant, provided that the indications and contraindications are thoroughly considered and that the proper technique is used. Orlay was among the pioneers in the field of endodontic implantology and contributed to the acceptance of endodontic implants. It was Frank, however, who established well-organized criteria for the selection of cases and who standardized the techniques for the use of the endodontic implant.

INDICATIONS FOR THE USE OF ENDODONTIC IMPLANTS

1. A horizontal fracture in the apical one-half to one-third of the root, which would necessitate the removal of the apical portion of the root. The resultant inadequate crown-root ratio would give the tooth a poor long-term prognosis (Figs. 11-6A, 11-7).

2. Internal resorption, in the apical one-half to one-third of the root, that perforates through to the outer aspect in an inaccessible area that cannot be repaired with amalgam. This would also necessitate the removal of the apical portion of the root (Fig. 11-6B).

(Text continues on p.189.)

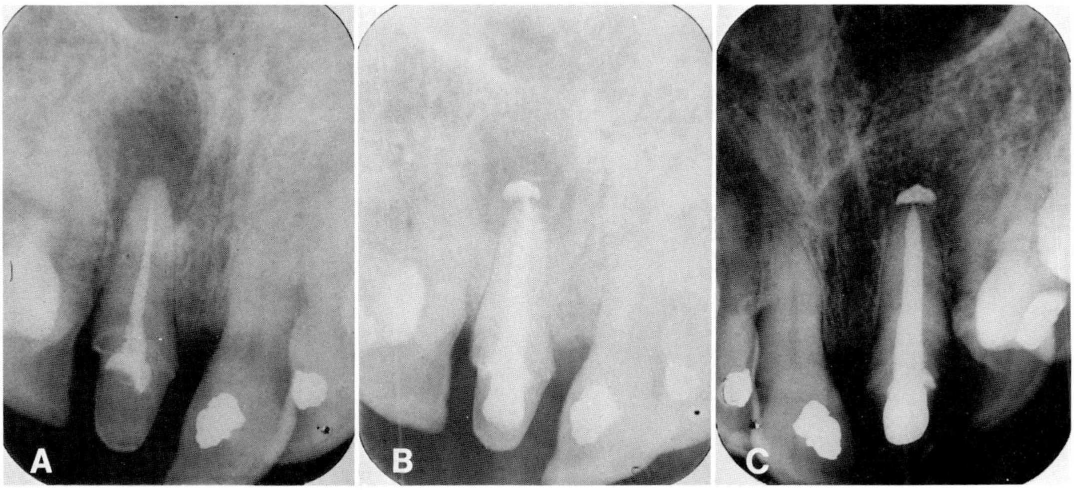

Fig. 11-3. Radiographs of another patient, showing the course of proper obturation of the root canal system. *(A)* Periapical pathology of a tooth with an inadequately filled root canal system (4/5/68). *(B)* Retreatment has been completed (4/19/68). *(C)* Complete resolution of periapical pathology (2/7/74). Note that foreign material in the periapical area does not interfere with healing if the root canal system has been properly obturated.

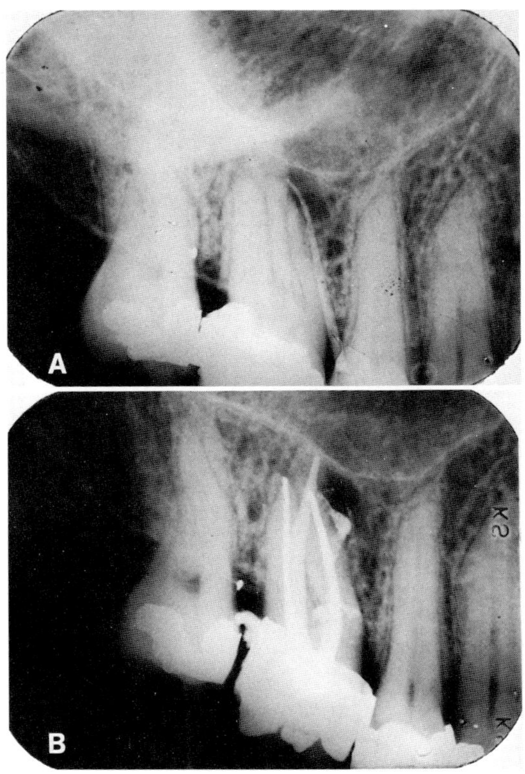

Fig. 11-4. Radiographs for another patient, showing the course of proper obturation of the root canal system. *(A)* Pre-operative radiograph, showing gutta-percha used as a marker in a fistula. *(B)* Postoperative radiograph showing proper filling of the root canal system. The fistula did not close after the canals were completely cleaned and shaped; it did close after obturation of the root canal system. The cause of the fistula was the necrotic pulp tissue in the lateral canal in the mesiobuccal root, which had never been cleaned out during instrumentation but which was obturated with root-canal sealer and warm gutta-percha as these materials were packed with pressure around the silver cones.

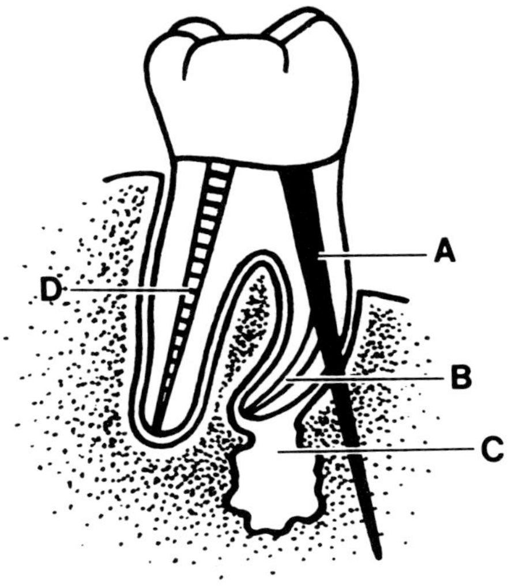

Fig. 11-5. Point A, Vitallium implant; Point B, unfilled root-canal space; Point C, resultant periapical pathology; Point D, root canal properly filled with gutta-percha.

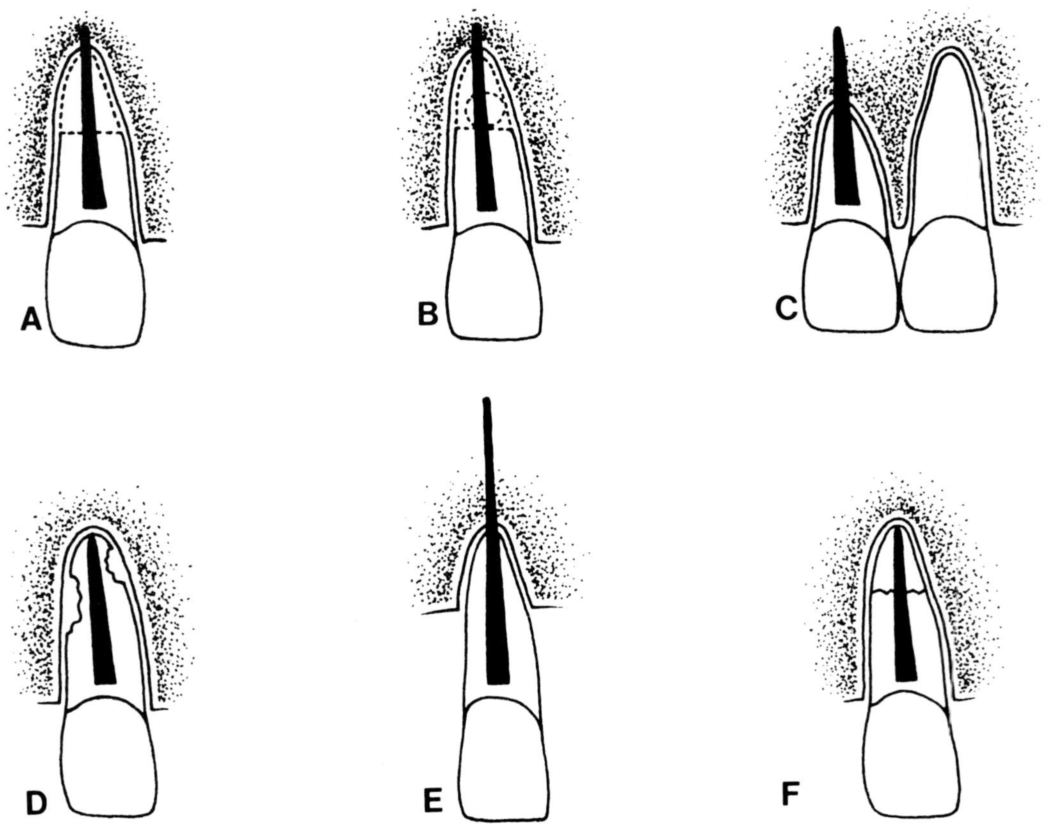

Fig. 11-6. Indications for endodontic implants. *(A)* Horizontal root fracture necessitating the removal of the apical portion of the root. *(B)* Internal resorption perforating to the outside, in an area that is inaccessible for repair. The apical portion of the root must be removed. *(C)* External resorption of the root, creating an unfavorable crown-root ratio. *(D)* External resorption along the lateral aspect of the root. *(E)* Horizontal periodontal bone loss, leading to an unfavorable crown-root ratio. *(F)* Horizontal root fracture wherein both portions of the fractured root can be retained.

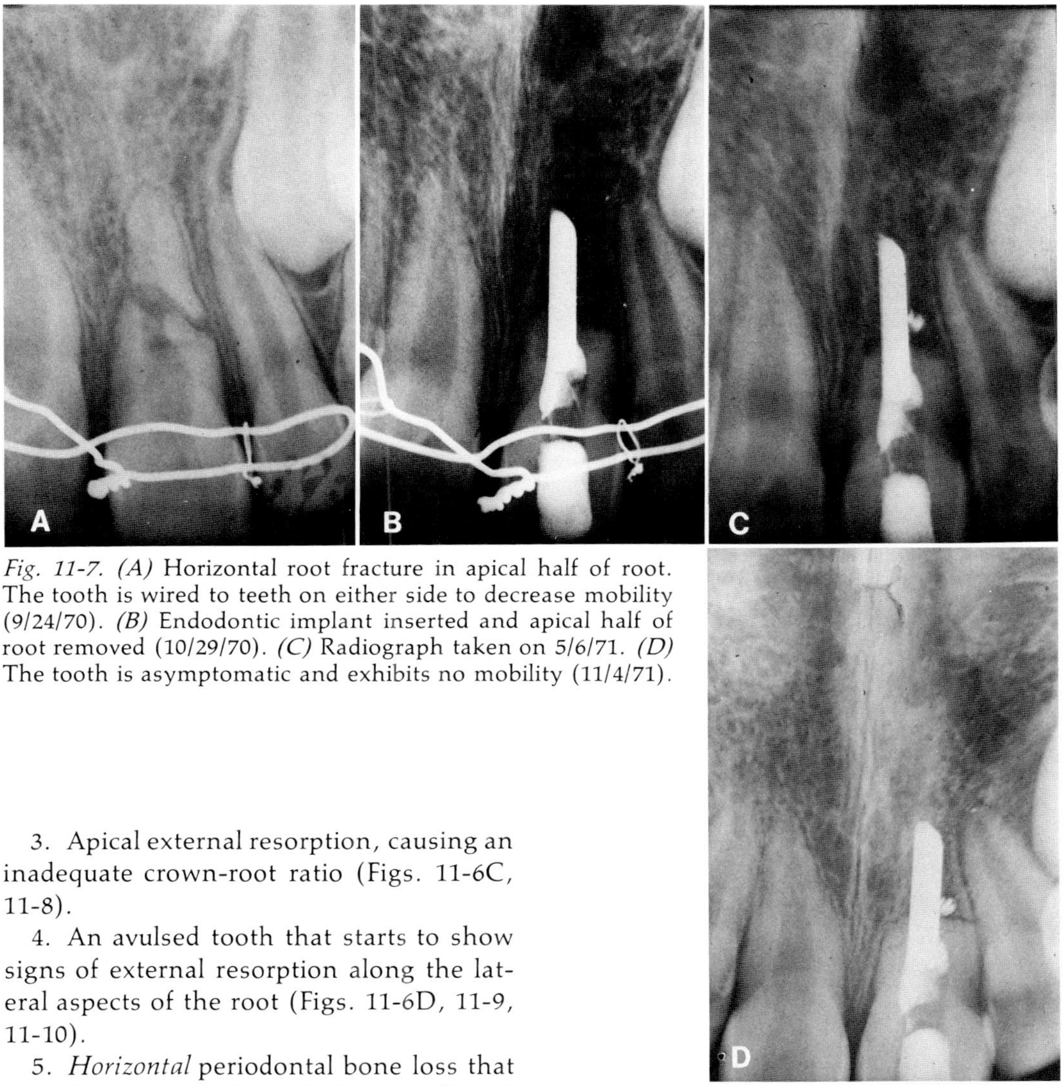

Fig. 11-7. *(A)* Horizontal root fracture in apical half of root. The tooth is wired to teeth on either side to decrease mobility (9/24/70). *(B)* Endodontic implant inserted and apical half of root removed (10/29/70). *(C)* Radiograph taken on 5/6/71. *(D)* The tooth is asymptomatic and exhibits no mobility (11/4/71).

3. Apical external resorption, causing an inadequate crown-root ratio (Figs. 11-6C, 11-8).
4. An avulsed tooth that starts to show signs of external resorption along the lateral aspects of the root (Figs. 11-6D, 11-9, 11-10).
5. *Horizontal* periodontal bone loss that extends between the apical one-half and one-third of the root. This tooth may be included in a fixed bridge; or it may be a tooth whose salvation eliminates the necessity of a bridge (Figs. 11-6E, 11-1C to F, 11-11).
6. A horizontal root fracture, where both portions of the root can be retained and stabilized with the implant (Figs. 11-6F, 11-12).

Ancillary Uses of Endodontic Implants

Both indications No. 4 and No. 6 above are not truly endodontic implants, because the Vitallium implant in these situations is not extended past the apex of the tooth into the bone. Because of its strength and rigidity, however, Vitallium is certainly the filling material of choice for the stabilization of fractured root portions, rather than silver or gutta-percha.

If problems develop due to irritants in the fracture line, the apical portion of the root may be split and removed surgically, and the coronal portion of the root and implant may be left in place. Amalgam can be placed around the implant, where the implant now exits from the root, to ensure

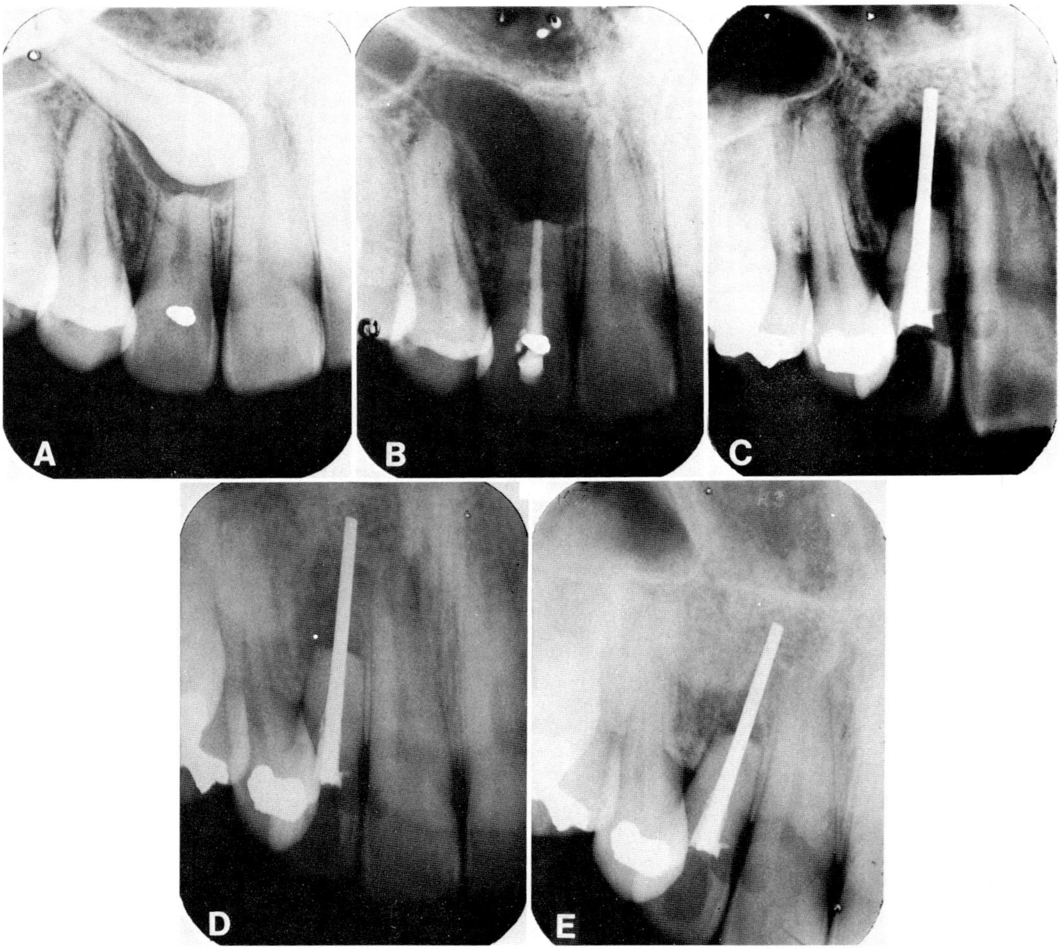

Fig. 11-8. (A) An impacted cuspid has caused external root resorption of the lateral incisor. Radiograph was taken on 12/30/65 immediately prior to removal of the cuspid. Root canal therapy was performed on the lateral incisor at the same time that the cuspid was removed. *(B)* Large periapical radiolucency is still present. The tooth exhibits Class 3 mobility (3/27/74). *(C)* Endodontic implant procedure performed on 4/3/74. *(D)* Radiograph taken on 12/20/74 shows bone filling in. The tooth exhibits no mobility. *(E)* Radiograph taken on 8/22/75 shows complete fill-in of bone and no mobility.

the seal. An endodontic implant would have then been created (Fig. 11-13).

Likewise, with the avulsed tooth showing lateral resorptions, if the root continues to resorb until the Vitallium is no longer within the tooth structure, an endodontic implant would have been created. This tooth has more of a chance of retention than would one filled with either silver or gutta-percha. If the endodontic seal of the Vitallium implant fails during the course of root resorption, the operator can try to improve the seal by using an apicoectomy type of approach and by inserting amalgam around the implant (Fig. 11-14).

Because a permanent bridge is contraindicated until a patient is approximately 17 to 18 years old, and because loss of a tooth

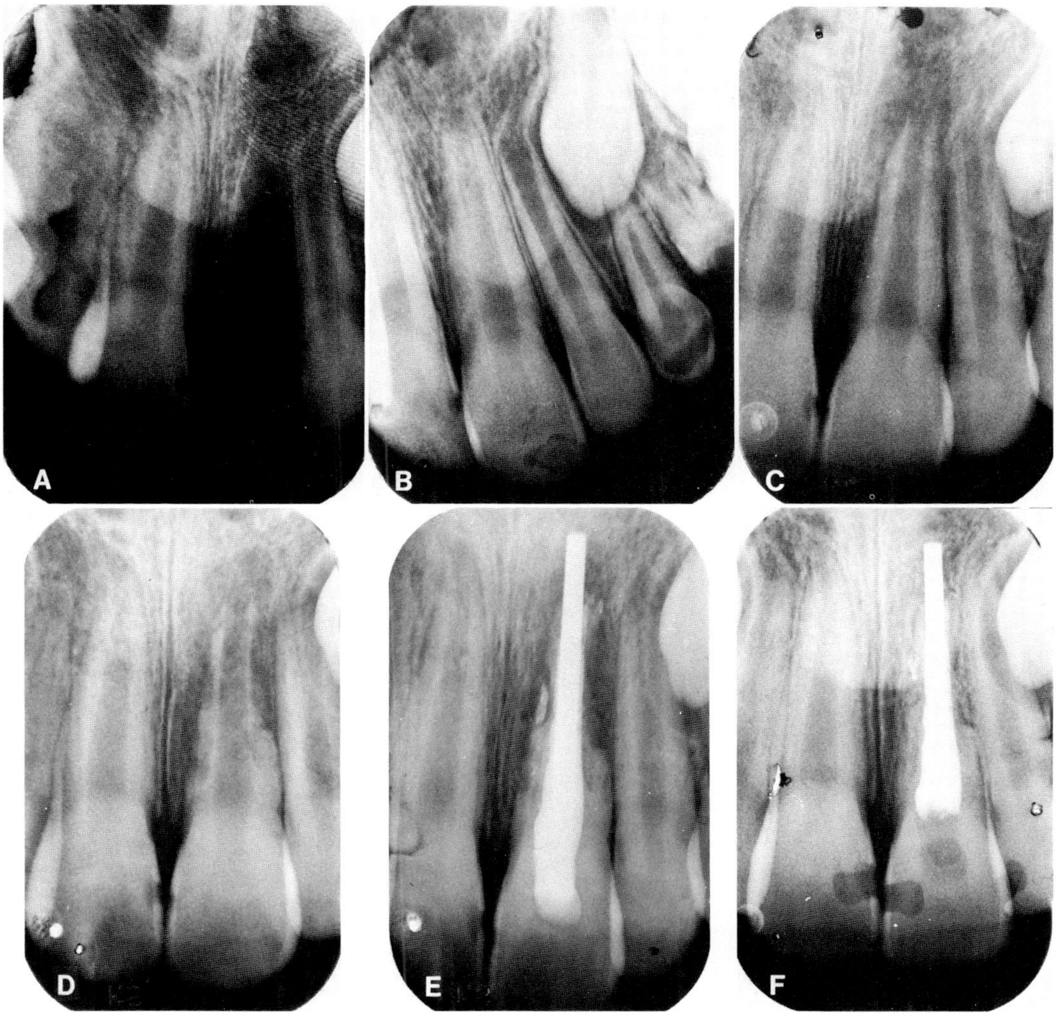

Fig. 11-9. (A) The above radiograph, although imperfectly processed, shows an upper left central incisor totally avulsed (8/23/73). *(B)* Tooth replaced into alveolus (8/28/73). *(C)* No external resorption evident. The tooth exhibits Class 1 mobility (9/24/73). *(D)* Lateral and apical external resorption evident. The tooth now exhibits 2 plus mobility (11/15/73). *(E)* Endodontic implant inserted. Implant is the same length as the original root (11/30/73). *(F)* Normal periapical bone. The tooth exhibits no mobility clinically (10/3/74).

prior to this age necessitates its replacement with a temporary removable appliance, retention of the tooth in either of the aforementioned situations until the patient reaches this age, thereby avoiding the necessity of a temporary removable appliance, is indisputably a recommended procedure.

CONTRAINDICATIONS FOR ENDODONTIC IMPLANTS

The contraindications for endodontic implants include the following situations:

1. The periodontal bone loss is so extensive that there is direct communication between the gingival sulcus and the apex of

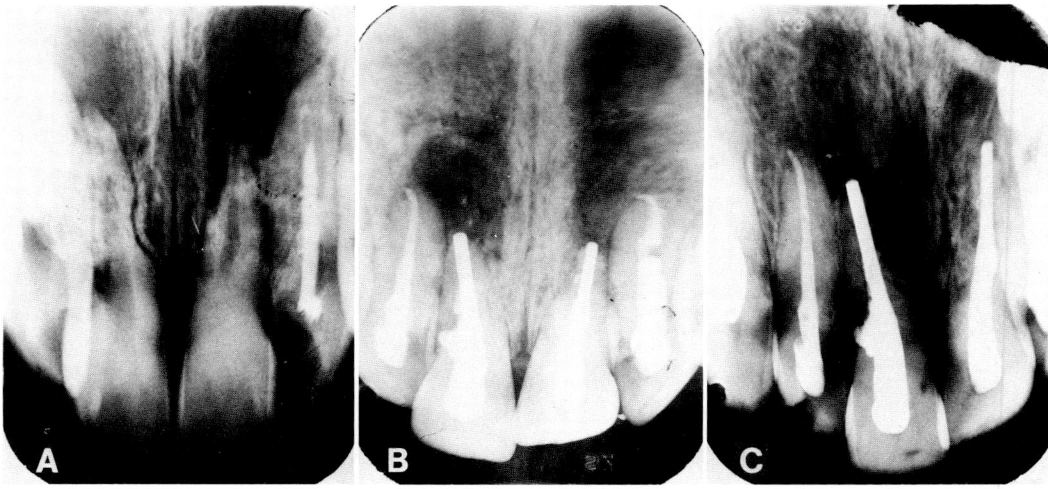

Fig. 11-10. (A) Pre-operative radiograph shows external root resorption along the lateral aspects of the roots. This condition is of unknown etiology. The teeth exhibit no mobility. *(B)* Endodontic treatment has been performed, with Vitallium implants used to fill the canals to the radiographic apices only. *(C)* One year later, no more resorption seems to have taken place. The teeth are asymptomatic and still exhibit no mobility.

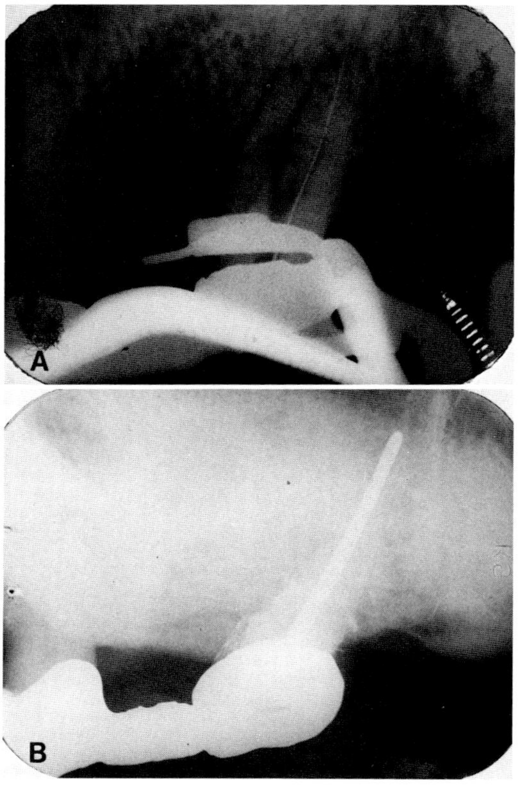

Fig. 11-11. Pre-operative radiograph of the upper left second molar, showing through and through trifurcation involvement, with extensive bone loss around both buccal roots. The tooth exhibited 2 plus mobility. Clinical examination revealed adequate attachment apparatus around the palatal root. *(A)* Endodontic treatment performed on the palatal root. An endodontic implant was inserted that extended 8 mm. beyond the apex, distal to the posterior wall of the maxillary sinus. Both buccal roots were amputated, and the occlusal table was reduced so that forces were directed along the long axis of the remaining palatal root. Mobility was immediately reduced from 2 plus to plus. A temporary splint was fabricated. *(B)* Three months later, the tooth was stable (immobile), and a permanent bridge was placed from the upper left cuspid to the upper left second molar. (Courtesy of Dr. Fredrick I. Muroff)

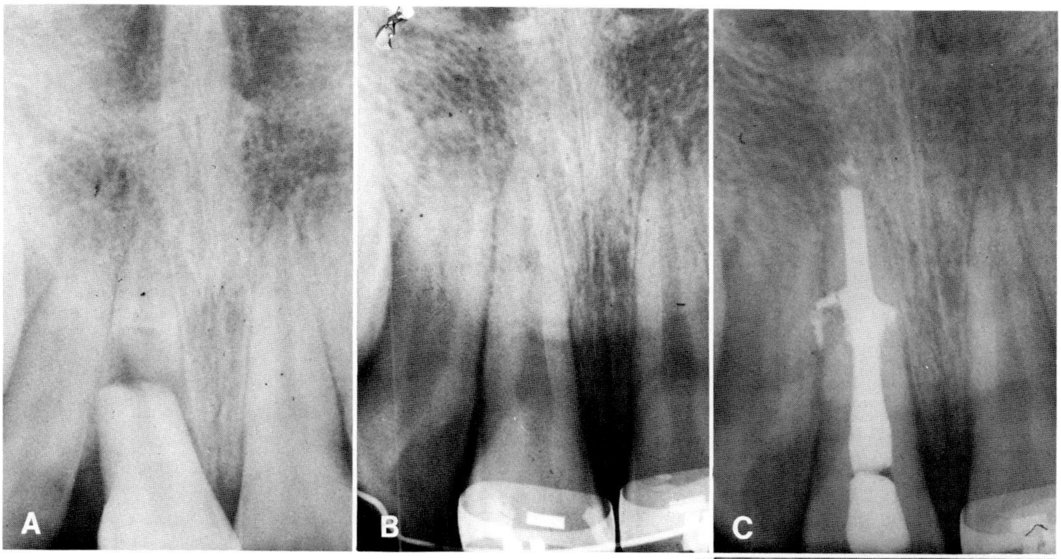

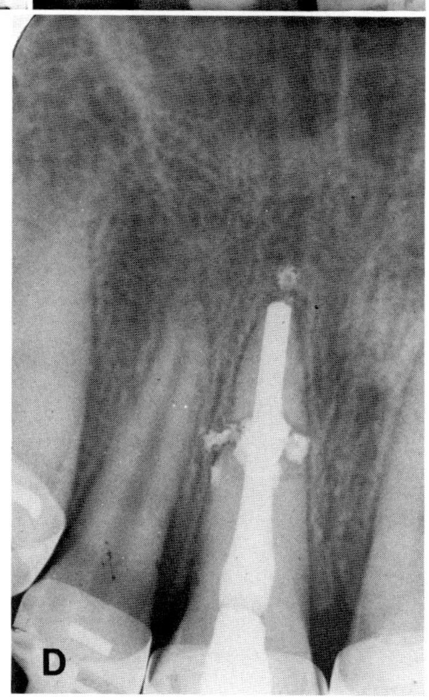

Fig. 11-12. (A) This patient presented on 5/4/71 with a horizontal root fracture of the upper right central incisor and a badly displaced coronal portion. Although told that the prognosis was extremely poor, the patient pleaded that something be attempted. The coronal portion of the tooth was repositioned, and orthodontic bands were inserted to help reduce mobility. *(B)* Perfect repositioning of the coronal and apical portions of the tooth (6/11/71). *(C)* An endodontic implant was placed from the coronal to the apical portions of the root in an attempt to stablize and retain both halves of the tooth. *(D)* The tooth is completely asymptomatic and exhibits no mobility (8/10/73).

the root. This would mean that the implant would have contact with the oral epithelium and would no longer follow the definition of an endodontic implant (Figs. 11-15A, 11-16).

2. The inclination of the root of the tooth is such that the extension of the implant would perforate through the facial plate of bone and into the soft tissues (Figs. 11-15B, 11-17).

3. The implant would impinge on an anatomic landmark, such as the mental foramen, inferior alveolar canal, or maxillary sinus (Fig. 11-15C).

4. The patient has a clotting problem (i.e., he is receiving anticoagulant therapy) or has a blood dyscrasia.

5. The patient is an uncontrolled diabetic.

PRE-IMPLANT CONSIDERATIONS

Naturally, before the insertion of an endodontic implant can be considered, a complete medical history of the patient must be taken in order to eliminate the medical contraindications for the use of the implant. Multiple radiographs should be taken from various angles to try to determine the relationship of the involved anatomic structures to the root of the tooth,

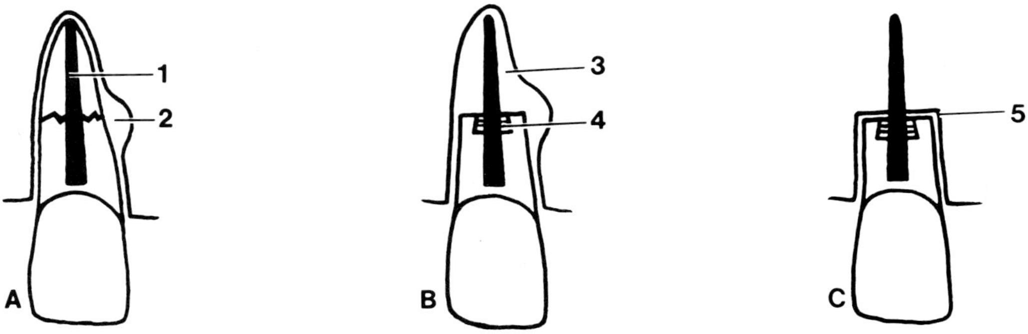

Fig. 11-13. *(A)* Point 1, an endodontic implant stabilizing both portions of a horizontally fractured root. Point 2, pathology developing along the fracture line. *(B)* Point 3, the apical portion of the root has been removed. Point 4, amalgam inserted to ensure seal. *(C)* Point 5, fill-in of bone; a true endodontic implant has been created.

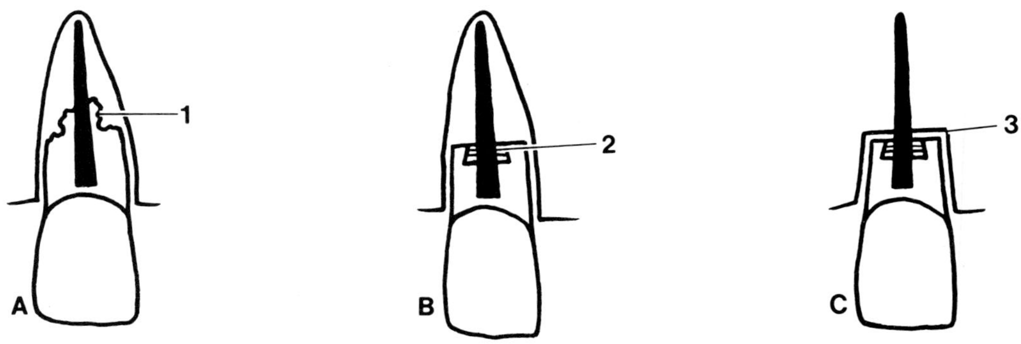

Fig. 11-14. *(A)* Point 1, root resorption has continued after an endodontic implant was inserted. The resorption has led to an incomplete endodontic seal and resultant pathology. *(B)* Point 2, resorptive area of the root has been removed, and amalgam has been placed to ensure seal. *(C)* Point 3, healing has taken place, and a true endodontic implant has been created.

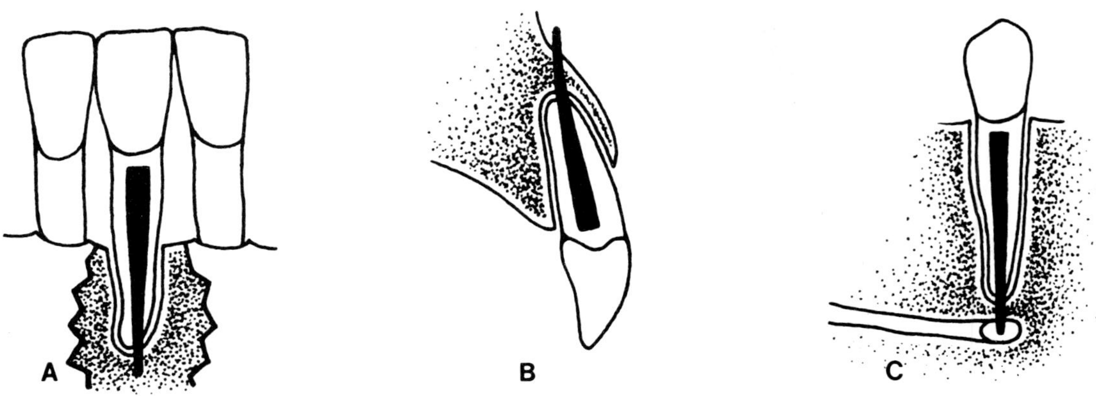

Fig. 11-15. Contraindications for endodontic implants. *(A)* Periodontal bone loss so extensive that the implant has contact with the oral epithelium. *(B)* The path of insertion of the implant has caused fenestration of the labial plate of bone. *(C)* The implant impinges on an anatomic landmark, the mental foramen.

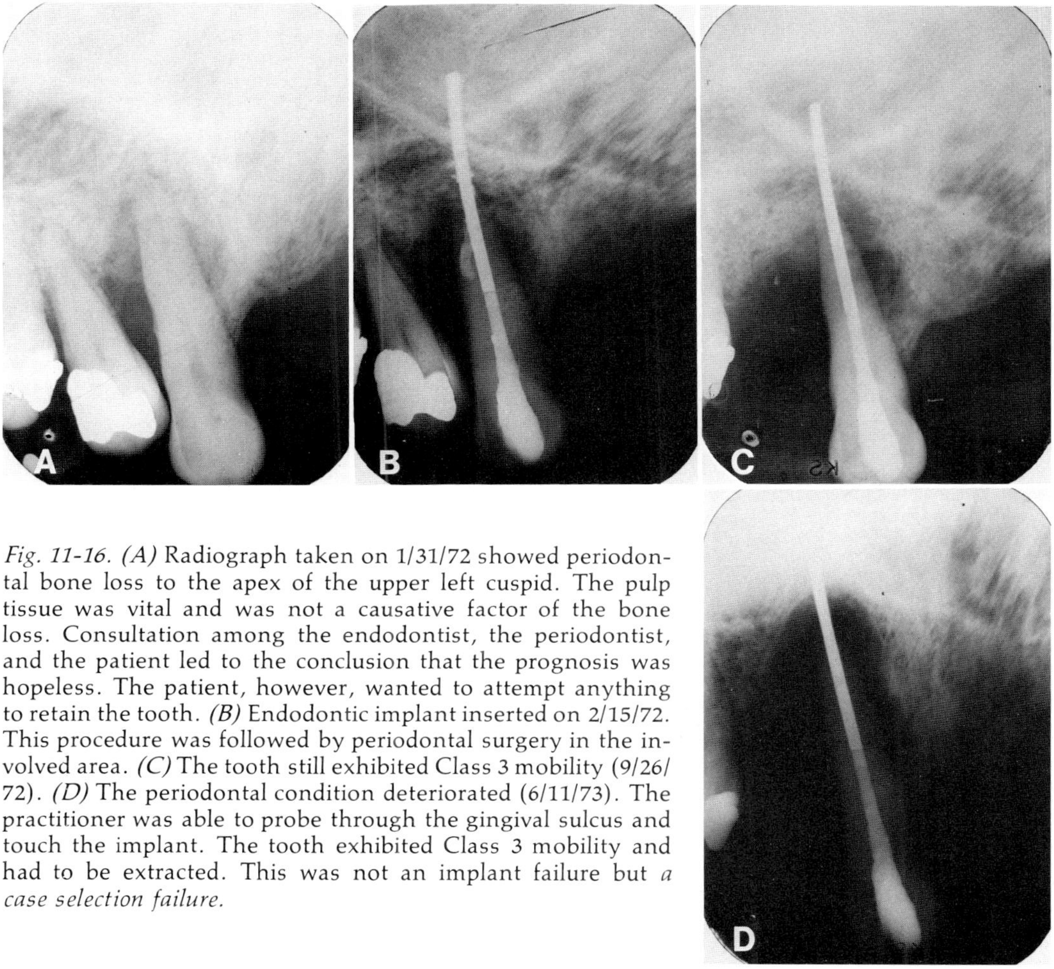

Fig. 11-16. (A) Radiograph taken on 1/31/72 showed periodontal bone loss to the apex of the upper left cuspid. The pulp tissue was vital and was not a causative factor of the bone loss. Consultation among the endodontist, the periodontist, and the patient led to the conclusion that the prognosis was hopeless. The patient, however, wanted to attempt anything to retain the tooth. *(B)* Endodontic implant inserted on 2/15/72. This procedure was followed by periodontal surgery in the involved area. *(C)* The tooth still exhibited Class 3 mobility (9/26/72). *(D)* The periodontal condition deteriorated (6/11/73). The practitioner was able to probe through the gingival sulcus and touch the implant. The tooth exhibited Class 3 mobility and had to be extracted. This was not an implant failure but *a case selection failure.*

and, if possible, to try to get some idea of the root inclination in relation to the labial or buccal plate of bone.

A periodontal probe should be a part of the basic examination-tray setup for every general dentist and dental specialist, as well as for the periodontist. The tooth being considered for an implant or for any endodontic procedure should be carefully examined with the periodontal probe before initiating any treatment. Probing often reveals conditions that are not evident on radiographs. For example, a radiograph may show that a lower anterior tooth has interproximal alveolar bone; however, the periodontal probe may reveal that the labial or lingual plate of bone has resorbed down to the apex of the root (Fig. 11-18). This would contraindicate the use of an endodontic implant.

ENDODONTIC IMPLANT TECHNIQUE

Stage 1

1. Only after the medical history and the dental examination indicate a favorable prognosis is the patient anesthetized and the tooth isolated under the rubber dam (Fig. 11-19). Strict endodontic principles of asepsis must be followed. The tooth and the surrounding rubber dam must be vigor-

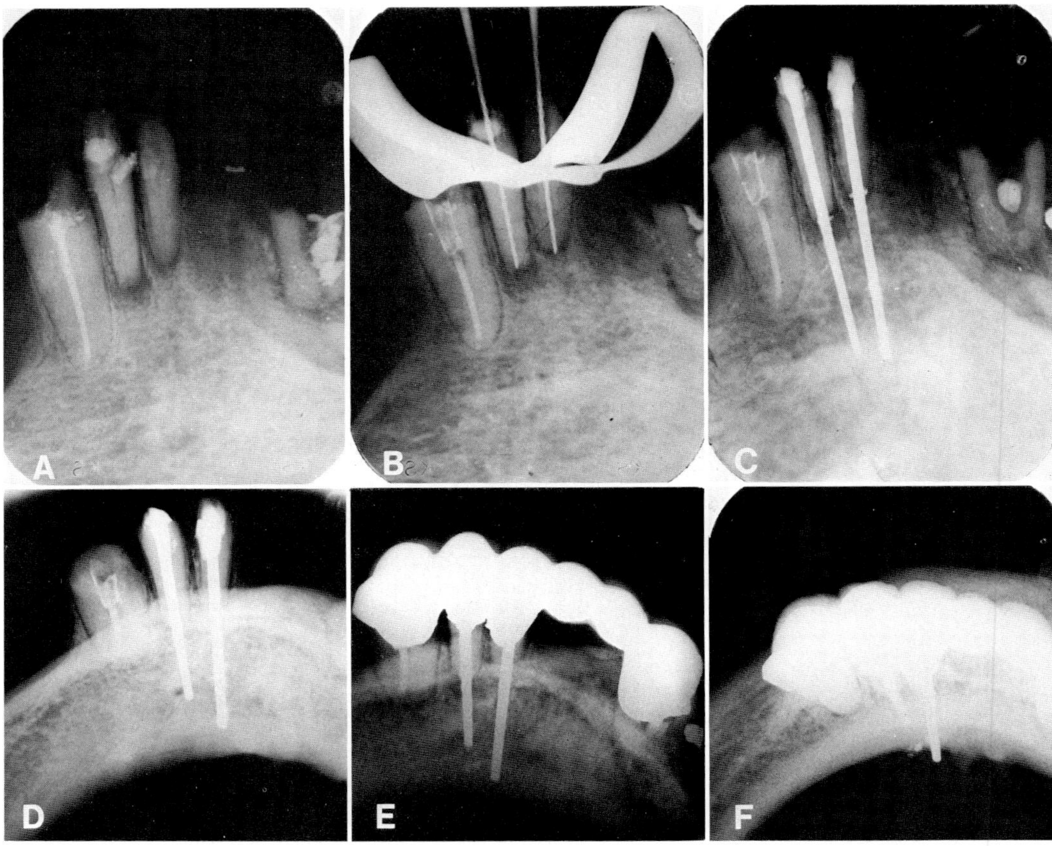

Fig. 11-17. (A) Pre-operative radiograph. The lower right central and lateral incisors exhibited 2 plus mobility. It was decided to retain these teeth so that a coping denture could be constructed over these two teeth and the lower right cuspid, which were to be the only remaining teeth in this arch. It was decided to extract the lower left cuspid. *(B)* Endodontic therapy performed on both incisors. *(C)* Endodontic implants inserted. Hours after the implants were inserted, the patient developed a swelling under the inferior border of the mandible and on the floor of the mouth. Antibiotic therapy was instituted. The next day the swelling was larger, and the patient exhibited systemic symptoms. *(D)* Another view of the implants taken in an effort to determine the cause of the problem. Everything appeared to be normal. *(E)* Still another view of the implants. Everything still appeared to be normal. *(F)* One week after insertion of the implants, the systemic symptoms had disappeared, but the patient still exhibited hard swelling. Occlusal view showed that the implant of the lower right central incisor perforated the lingual plate of bone through to the soft tissue. This tooth was extracted, and all symptoms disappeared. This was not an implant failure, but *a procedural failure* on the part of the operator.

ously swabbed with alcohol in an attempt to rid the area of bacteria.

2. Using a small round bur, access is then gained into the pulp chamber of the tooth (Fig. 11-20A).

3. The root canal is completely cleaned and shaped to the radiographic apex with at least a No. 50 reamer. Then the canal is flared by using Hedstrom files on the walls or by serial reaming. All reamers and files are kept sterile by a chair-side salt or bead sterilizer, at a temperature of between 425° F. and 475° F. for 5 seconds.

4. The canal is thoroughly irrigated and

dried, a culture is taken, and a medicament such as cresatin or camphorated para-monochlorophenol is placed into the pulp chamber on a cotton pellet. The access cavity is then sealed with a temporary filling such as Cavit.*

Stage 2

1. At the second visit, if the tooth fulfills the criteria for obturation of any root canal, the endodontic implant procedure may be completed. The criteria are: the tooth is asymptomatic, the culture is negative, and the canal is dry.

2. Local anesthesia is administered to the patient. The tooth is isolated under a rubber dam. Then both the tooth and the surrounding rubber dam are swabbed with alcohol.

3. The temporary filling is removed in order to gain access to the pulp chamber.

4. At this point, it is usually necessary to modify the access cavity and enlarge it in a more incisal direction (Fig. 11-20B). This must be done because the rigidity of the Vitallium implant requires more straight-line access than do either silver cones or gutta-percha.

5. The final instrument that reached the apex of the root at the last visit (at least a No. 50 reamer) is reinserted to make sure that no blockage has developed in the canal.

6. At this point, it is necessary to switch to reamers that are 40 mm. in length and are specially designed for endodontic implant procedures (Fig. 11-21). The operator must start with a reamer that is two to three sizes smaller than the last instrument that reached the apex of the root. A rubber band marker is set on the 40-mm. reamer at a level that includes the length of the canal *plus* the length that the implant is to extend into the bone (Fig. 11-22); this is usually the length of the canal plus ap-

*Premier Dental Products Co., Philadelphia, Pennsylvania.

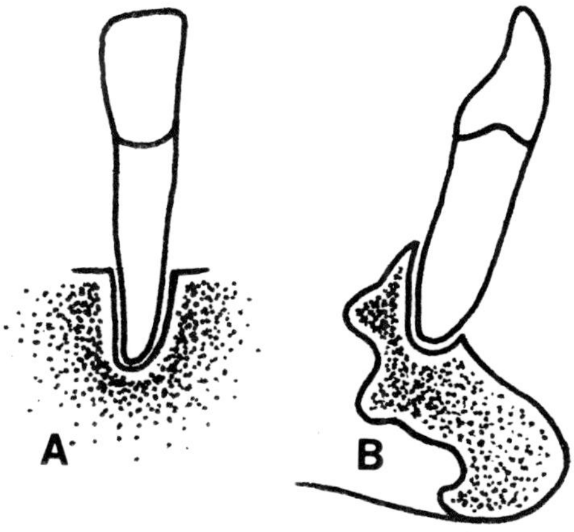

Fig. 11-18. Radiographic view of tooth may appear as if one-third of the root is supported by alveolar bone *(A)*. Side view would show that this is not the case *(B)*. Only a periodontal probe can show that there is no labial plate of bone present.

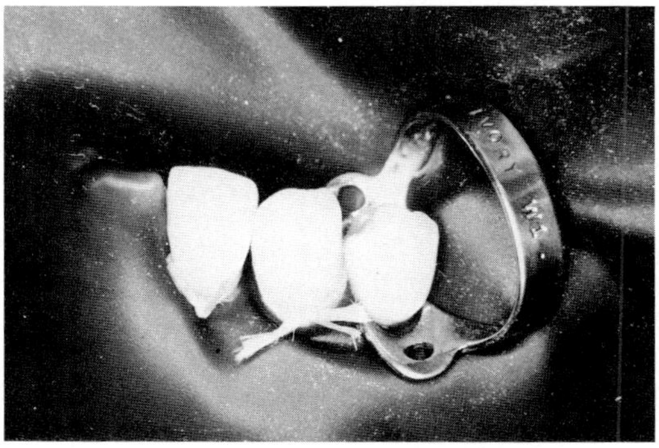

Fig. 11-19. Rubber dam in place.

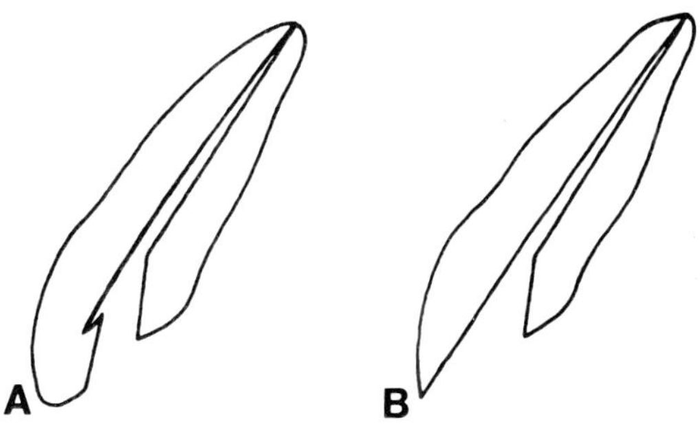

Fig. 11-20. (A) Normal access cavity for maxillary anterior tooth. *(B)* Access cavity enlarged in a more incisal direction to accommodate the rigidity of the implant.

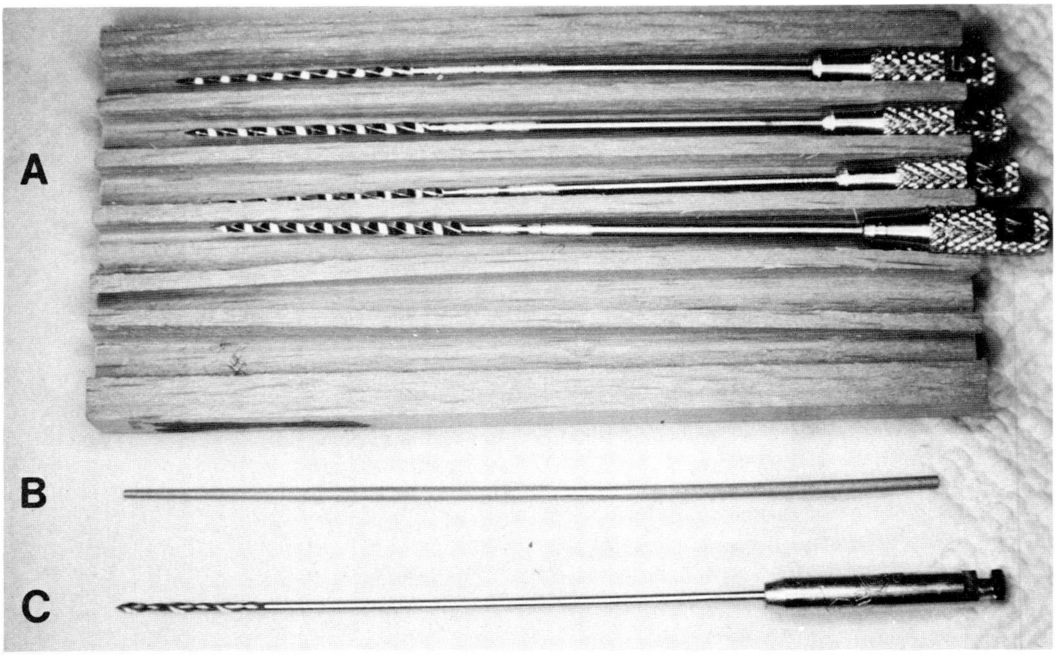

Fig. 11-21. Point *A,* 40-mm. reamers designed specifically for endodontic implant procedures. Point B, Vitallium implant. Point C, Bone drill.

proximately 10 mm. The bone is then reamed to the desired length. Sometimes it is very difficult to begin the reaming of the intra-osseous preparation; in these cases, a bone drill should be used. A rubber band stop should also be set on the bone drill at the proper length. Rotation of the bone drill should be started *prior* to placing it into the canal and *should be continued* until *after* the drill is removed from the canal. The bone drill is a fragile instrument. If it is allowed to stop rotating while it is still in the bone, the drill will be difficult to remove and may break off in the bone (Fig. 11-23).

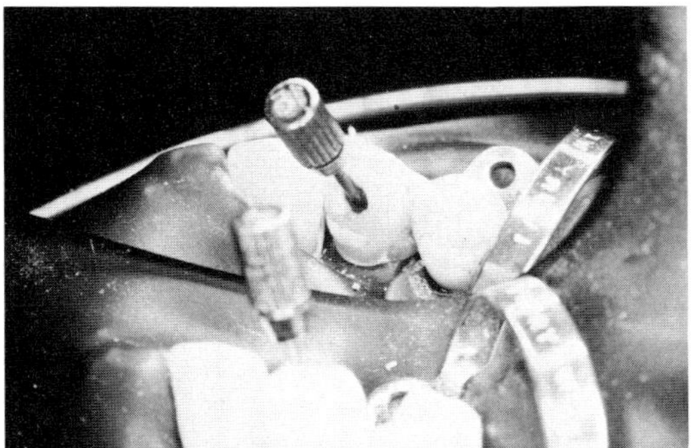

Fig. 11-22. A 40-mm. reamer inserted through the access cavity and root canal and into the bone.

The preparation in the bone proceeds very easily after it has been started. Instruments at least one or two sizes larger than the last reamer that reached the radiographic apex should be used at the new length. The canal must be constantly irrigated with saline, sterile water, or local anesthetic during the bone preparation.

7. A Vitallium implant is then chosen that corresponds in size to the last instrument used in the intra-osseous preparation. The implant is gripped by a heavy-beaked forceps at the desired length. The implant is kept sterile in the same manner by which the reamers and files were kept

sterile, i.e., by chair-side salt or bead sterilizer. The implant is then placed into both the canal and the prepared bone. If the implant fits loosely at the desired length, it should be removed, and 1 mm. should be removed from the apical end of the implant with a carborundum disc. This procedure should be continued until the implant fits tightly and is seated 1 mm. *short* of the intra-osseous preparation. This seating is one of the keys to a successful implant. If the implant fits tightly at the full length of the bone preparation, it may be binding (wedged tightly) in the bone, but it may be loose in the canal. Thus, the case may fail because of an endodontic failure. If, however, (a) the implant binds tightly, (b) it is 1 mm. short of the full intra-alveolar preparation, and (c) the root canal itself has been flared properly at the first visit, then the implant must bind at the apical foramen, and the case should be endodontically successful.

8. The implant is then disced at a level that is even with the incisal edge of the tooth. This disc mark will serve as a reference point when the implant is cemented into place. The implant is then removed from the tooth, and the canal is irrigated and dried with paper points that are confined to the root canal space. After cessation of hemorrhage in the root canal, a sealer such as AH-26* is placed into the canal with a spiral paste filler (Fig. 11-24). The implant is sterilized, and the portion of the implant that is to remain in the canal is coated with the sealer (Fig. 11-25). The implant is then gently inserted into the canal and apically into the bone preparation until the disc mark on the implant is again even with the incisal edge of the tooth and the implant fits tightly (Figs. 11-26, 11-27). Slow easing is necessary in inserting the implant, so that the sealer is not displaced from the canal into the periapical area, with the implant acting as a plunger.

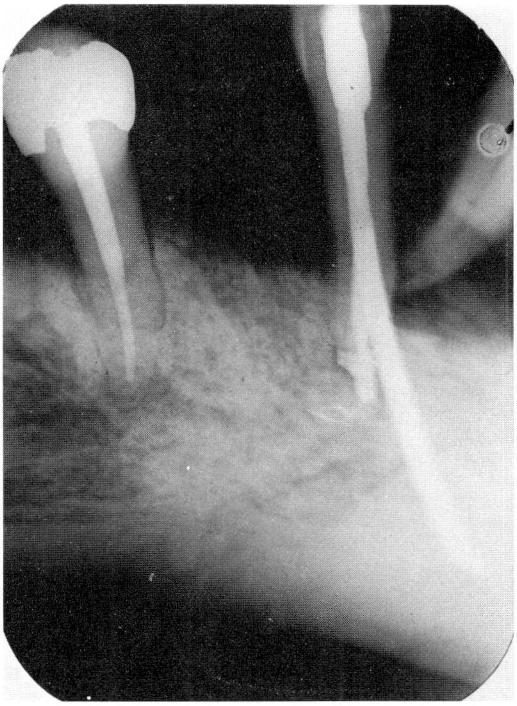

Fig. 11-23. The bone drill broke off in the tooth and extended into the alveolar bone. The canal was successfully obturated by packing sealer and warm gutta-percha around the drill. The root was then intentionally perforated, and the endodontic implant was inserted through the perforation. The implant has been successful for more than 1 year.

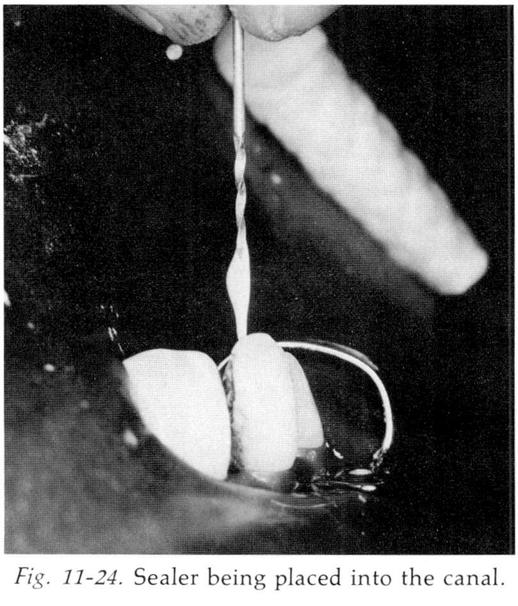

Fig. 11-24. Sealer being placed into the canal.

*Claudius Ash, Inc., Niagara Falls, New York.

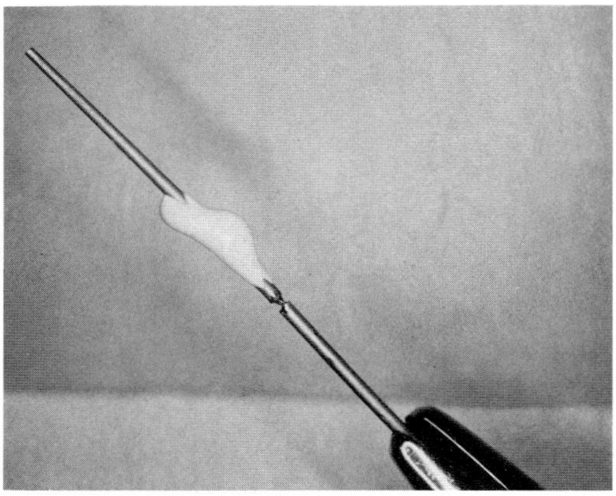

Fig. 11-25. The portion of the implant that will remain in the canal is coated with sealer.

9. Gutta-percha is then condensed around the Vitallium implant by using either warm vertical condensation or the lateral condensation technique. It is important to fill all the voids in the canal around the implant and to attempt to push the sealer into any large lateral canals that may be present or into any voids around the implant in the apical area of the root canal. Sealer that is pushed into the periapical area of the tooth during this part of the operation aids in the formation of an apical seal. As diligent as the endodontist may be, most canals are not reamed to a perfectly round shape. The Vitallium implant is machine-made and is perfectly round. Thus, the condensation of gutta-percha around the implant, and the excess sealer that is expressed periapically help ensure the formation of an apical seal, which undoubtedly leads to a greater success rate (Figs. 11-28, 11-29).

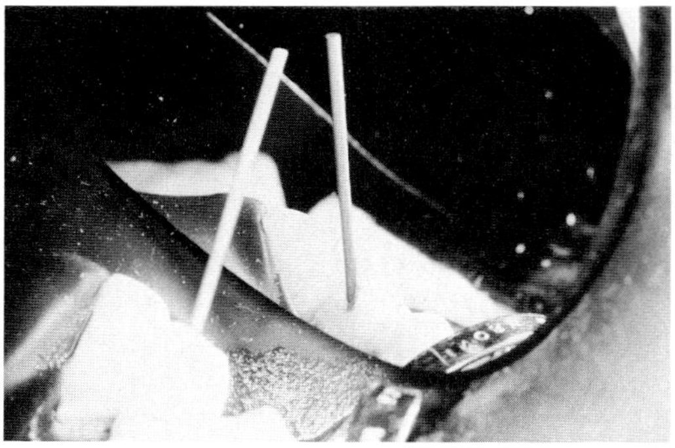

Fig. 11-26. Implant inserted into the canal, and apically into the bone preparation.

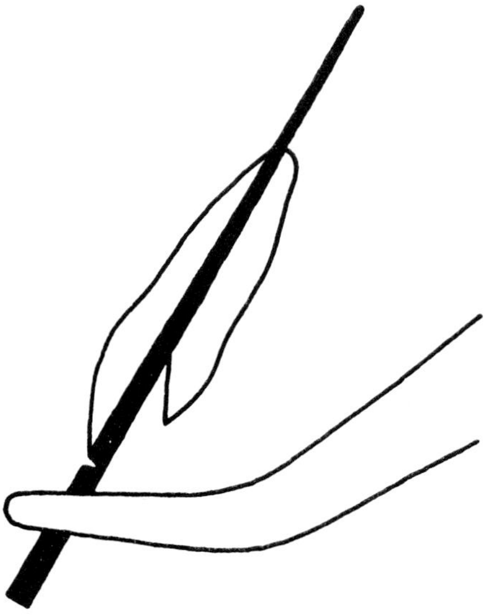

Fig. 11-27. With heavy beaked forceps, the implant is inserted until it fits tightly and the incisal mark is reached.

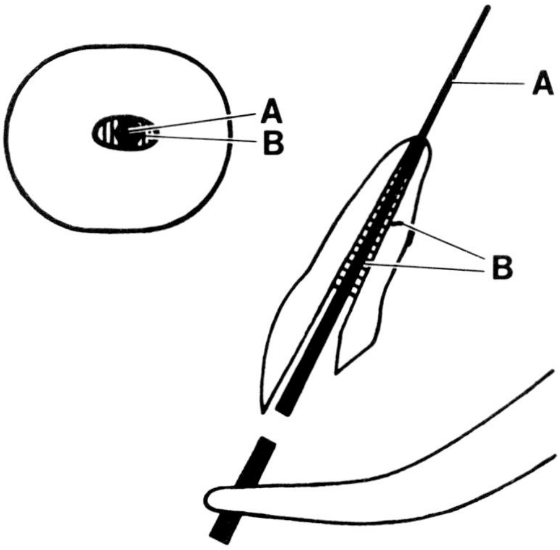

Fig. 11-28. Cross section *(left)* and longitudinal section *(right)* of the apex of a tooth root with an endodontic implant. Point A, Vitallium implant. Point B, Gutta-percha and sealer. The gutta-percha and sealer are condensed around the implant to help ensure the formation of an apical seal.

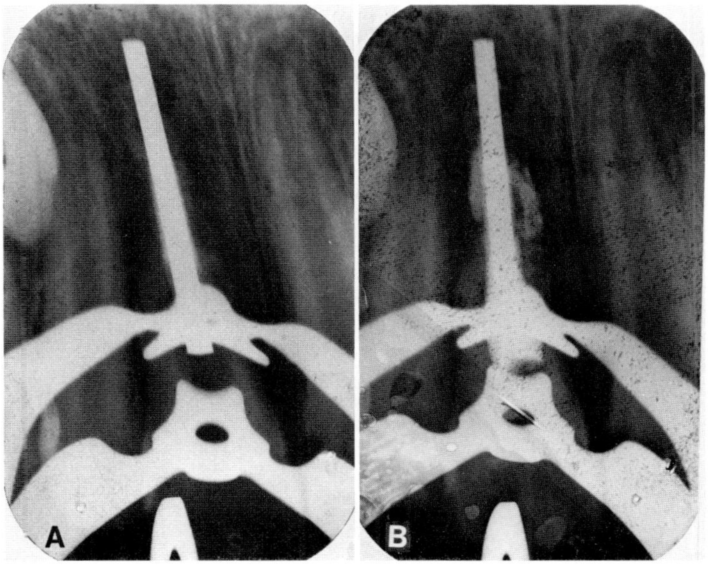

Fig. 11-29. (A) Endodontic implant seated into the intraosseous preparation. The implant fits very tightly. *(B)* The above radiograph, although imperfectly processed, shows gutta-percha condensed around the Vitallium implant, pushing the sealer into the periapical area. The perfectly round implant did not seal the nonround root-canal space. We have helped to create an apical seal by pushing gutta-percha and sealer into the voids.

10. The portion of the implant that extends beyond the enamel of the tooth is then removed with water-cooled, high-speed rotary instruments. Zinc oxyphosphate, Durelon,* amalgam, or Adaptic† is then used to fill the access cavity (Fig. 11-30).

Modification of Insertion

1. A modification of this insertion technique may be used if the tooth needs a post and core type of restoration, or if the operator feels that the tooth is likely to need such a restoration at any time in the future. Before the sealer is placed in the canal, the Vitallium implant is cut through with a carborundum disc at a level approximately two-thirds of the length from the incisal or occlusal reference point in relation to the radiographic apex of the tooth. Sealer is then placed into the canal and on the portion of the implant that is to remain in the canal. The implant is placed into the tooth and is pushed into place, with the coronal portion of the implant used as a plunger. In discing through the implant, about 1 mm. of the Vitallium is lost, so the incisal disc marking on the plunger end should come to rest about 1 mm. apical to the ref-

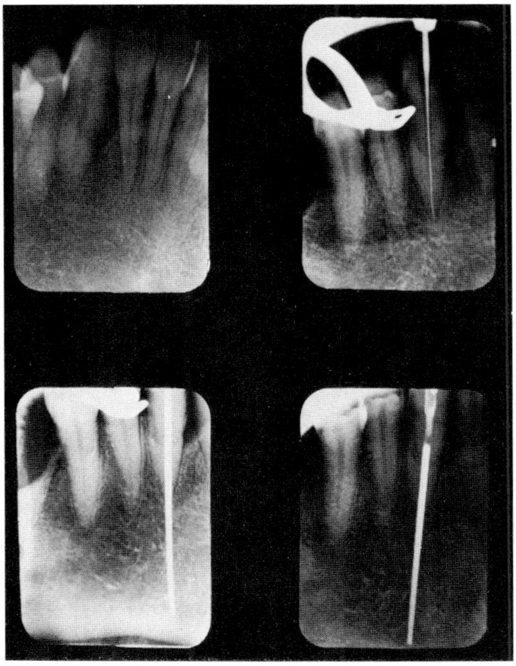

Fig. 11-30. Radiographs of case shown in Figures 11-19, 11-21, 11-22, and 11-24 to 11-26. (Courtesy of Dr. Jeffrey Shapiro)

*Premier Dental Products Co., Philadelphia, Pennsylvania.

†Johnson & Johnson, New Brunswick, New Jersey.

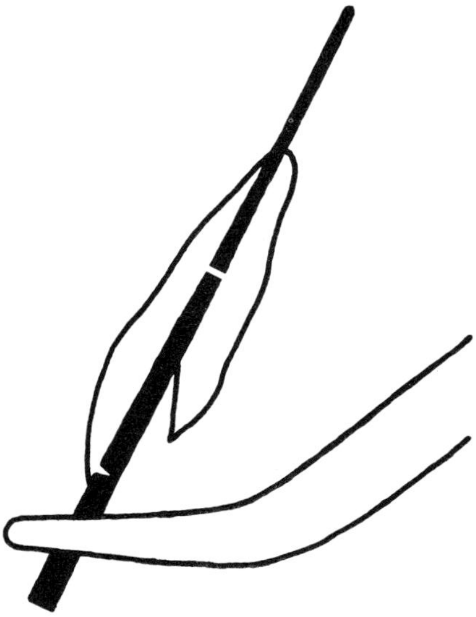

Fig. 11-31. Technique used if a tooth is to be restored with a post and core. The severance of the Vitallium should be at a point within the tooth, so as to ensure adequate post length.

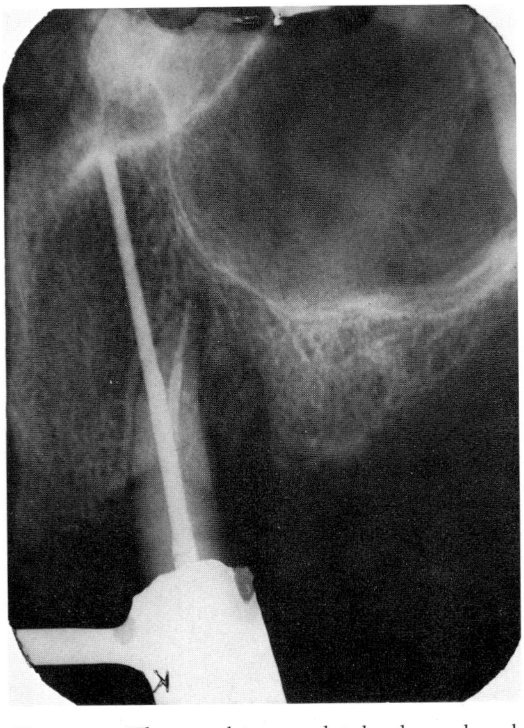

Fig. 11-32. The canal is completely cleaned and shaped, and filled with gutta-percha. The canal is then intentionally perforated, and the implant is inserted through the perforation. (Courtesy of Dr. Charles Weitzner)

erence point (Fig. 11-31). Again, the coronal aspect of the canal should be filled with gutta-percha in an attempt to seal large lateral canals and apical discrepancies.

2. Other modifications of the insertion technique include: (a) one-visit treatment for patients who have vital, uninfected pulp tissue in the tooth to be treated; (b) one-visit treatment when surgery is indicated (in this case, the surgical flap is raised, and —at the same time—coronal access is gained, the root canal is cleaned, and the implant is inserted); (c) a tooth whose canal is extremely curved and cannot be negotiated by a stiff Vitallium implant. In this type of case, the canal should be completely cleaned and shaped, and filled with gutta-percha, using conventional endodontic techniques. The canal is then *intentionally* perforated, and the implant procedure is performed in the normal manner, except through the perforation instead of the apex of the tooth (Figs. 11-32, 11-33).

SUCCESS IN ENDODONTIC IMPLANTOLOGY

Endodontic implants are not the ends, but rather the means; their proper utilization enables the practitioner to build prostheses on sound foundations. Proper case selection, periodontal preparation of the site, thorough endodontic techniques, and proper occlusion are all important factors for success.

Sometimes it is necessary to take heroic measures to maintain an important tooth in an arch. This approach is justified in order to make a fixed rather than a removable appliance for the patient or in order to prevent the necessity for *any* replacement. Such situations warrant the consideration of the endodontic implant.

Because of our present state of knowledge, all implants should be thought of as essentially experimental in nature, and they should be used only in very select cases. Success, however, is measured by the ability to maintain natural dentition.

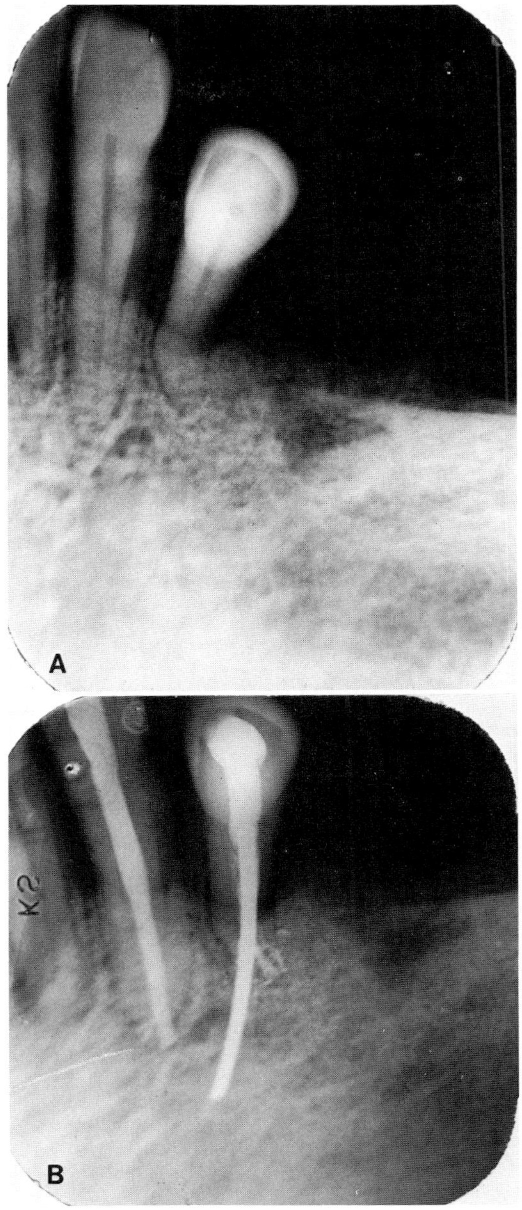

Fig. 11-33. (A) Pre-operative radiograph shows curvature of the root of the lower left first bicuspid. This curve cannot possibly be negotiated by the rigid Vitallium implant. *(B)* Routine endodontic treatment is performed, and the curved canal is filled with gutta-percha. The canal is then intentionally perforated, and the implant is inserted through the perforation.

Success is also measured by the ability to use a fixed rather than a removable prosthesis. To attain success, it is sometimes necessary to use an innovative procedure—but only if the patient understands the choices, and only if the operator applies the basic tenets of the many specialties of dentistry that are available to him today, in order to give the patient the best long-term prognosis.

BIBLIOGRAPHY

Andreasen, J. O.: Treatment of fractured and avulsed teeth. J. Dent. Children, *38:*29-31, 1971.

Baumhammers, A., Baumhammers, I., and Conway, J. C.: Periodontal considerations of endosseous implants. J. Periodont., *43:*135-140, 1972.

Berger, S. I., and Baskas, M. J.: Endodontic-endosseous implant root stabilizers. New York J. Dent., *41:*323-329, 1971.

Bernier, J. L., and Canby, C. P.: Histologic studies on the reaction of alveolar bone to Vitallium implants. J. A. D. A., *30:*188-197, 1943.

Dictrow, R.: Correction of endodontic endosseous implant existing supraperiosteally. New York State D. J., *35:*615-617, 1969.

Ehrmann, E. H.: Endodontic implants. Quintessence Internat., *4:*9-14(April); 13-20 (May); 11-14(June); 11-14(July); 1973.

Editorial: Endosseous implants. J. Brit. Endodontic Soc., *5:*1, 1971.

Feldman, G., Solomon, C., Notaro, P., and Moskowitz, E.: Endodontic implant stabilizers. New York J. Dent., *42:*259-260, 1972.

Flander, S.: Periodontic, orthodontic, and endodontic considerations in conjunction with implant dentistry. D. Clin. North America, *14:*137-143, 1970.

———: The endodontic implant. Quintessence Internat., *2:*9-14, 1971.

Frank, A. L.: Endodontic endosseous implants and treatment of the wide open apex. D. Clin. North America, *11:*675-700, 1967.

———: Improvement of the crown-root ratio by endodontic endosseous implants. J. A. D. A., *74:*451-462, 1967.

———: A standardized technique for the endodontic implant. *In* Grossman, L. I. (ed.): Transactions of the Fourth International Conference on Endodontics. pp. 112-121. Philadelphia, University of Pennsylvania Press, 1968.

Frank, A. L., and Abrams, A. M.: Histologic

evaluation of endodontic implants. J. A. D. A., *78:*520-524, 1969.

Giro, C. M.: Reclaiming the irretrievable tooth. New York J. Dent., *41:*97-100, 1971.

Gutentag, H., and Judy, K.: Endodontic-endosteal implants: biologic considerations. J. Oral Implantol. *4:*303-318, 1974.

Harris, R.: Use of chrome cobalt alloy and titanium endosseous implants. Australian Dent. J., *16:*94-108, 1971.

Hoyer, H., Holder, H., and Berggold, R.: Pin retention and stabilization of a transplanted tooth. Quintessence Internat., *1:*11-16, 1970.

Ingle, J. I.: Endodontics. Philadelphia, Lea & Febiger, 1965.

Johns, R. B.: The status of implants. J. Brit. Endodontic Soc., *5:*21-27, 1971.

Judy, K. W., Eilberg, R., Lew, I., and Greene, D.: Cement leakage and retention of threaded and non-threaded endodontic implants. J. Oral Implantol., *3:*28-43, 1972.

Judy, K. W., and Weiss, C. M.: A new coordinated system for the controlled placement of self-tapping, titanium endodontic stabilizers. Oral Implantol., *4:*567-579, 1974.

Kanth, L.: Late results in abutment implantation. Deutsche Zahn. Ztschr., *28:*561-565, 1973.

Lew, I.: The endosseous implant: evaluations and modifications. D. Clin. North America, *14:*201-213, 1970.

Lew, I., Greene, D., and Judy, K.: The endodontic implant. J. Acad. Gen. Dent., *20:*36-40, 1972.

Messinger, R.: Increasing the crown-root ratio with endodontic pin implants. J. Connecticut State D. A., *45:*140-144, 1971.

Morse, D. R.: Endodontic implants, a review and new approach. New York State D. J., *35:*5-12, 1969.

———: The significance of endodontics in implantation procedures. J. D. A. South Africa, *26:*263-277, 1971.

Morse, D. R., Barnett, A. M., and Maggio, J. M.: A scanning electron microscope examination of endodontic implants. Oral Implantol, *3:*139-167, 1972.

Morse, D. R., Nislow, F., and Busch, N.: The full arch splint using endodontic implants: report of a case, J. A. D. A., *85:*351-357, 1972.

Natiella, A. R.: Current evaluation of dental implants. J. A. D. A., *84:*1358-1372, 1972.

Orlay, H. G.: Endodontic splinting treatment in periodontal disease. Brit. D. J., *108:*118-121, 1960.

———: Non-prosthodontic oral implants. J. Oral Implantol. Transplant Surg. *11:*44-53, 1965.

———: Endodontic implants. *In* Grossman, L. I. (ed.): Transactions of the Fourth International Conference on Endodontics. pp. 97-109. Philadelphia, University of Pennsylvania Press, 1968.

Powell, W. D.: Endodontic implants for lower denture stabilization. J. Tennessee D. A. *53:*142-146, 1973.

Ritacco, A.: Endodontic implants for root fractures. Fauchard, *1:*428-431, 1970.

Scopp, I. W., Dictrow, R. L., and Lichtenstein, B. S.: Endodontic endosseous implants—a conservative method for stabilization in geriatric patients. J. Periodont., *40:*664-666, 1969.

Scopp, I. W., Dictrow, R. L., Lichtenstein, B. S., and Blechman, H.: Cellular response to endodontic endosseous implants. J. Periodont., *42:*717-720, 1971.

Seltzer, S., Greene, D., de la Guardia, R., and Barnett, A.: Vitallium endodontic implants: a scanning electron microscope, electronmicroprobe and histologic study. Oral Surg., *35:*828-860, 1973.

Shaykin, J. B.: Endodontic implants for fixed bridge support. Chron. Omaha Dist. D. Soc., *30:*56-58, 1956.

———: Endodontic implant. J. A. D. A., *68:*704-707, 1964.

Simring, M.: Discussion of a standardized technique for the endodontic implant. *In* Grossman, L. I. (ed.): Transactions of the Fourth International Conference on Endodontics. pp. 122-126. Philadelphia, University of Pennsylvania Press, 1968.

Skidmore, A. E.: Endodontic endosseous implants. West Virginia D. J., *46:*6-9, 1972.

Skidmore, A. E., and Sunshine, K. P.: Endodontic implants—a method of intraosseous stabilization. Iowa D. J., *56:*20-22, 1970.

Stacy, G. C.: Intra-alveolar root fracture treated by internal splinting. Brit. D. J., *118:*210-212, 1965.

Sterchi, A.: Histologic study of two endosseous implants. Schweiz. Monatschr. Zahnh. *82:*862-877, 1972.

Strock, A. E., and Strock, M. S.: Method of reinforcing pulpless anterior teeth—preliminary report. J. Oral Surg., *1:*252-255, 1943.

12 Potential Problems, Home Care, and Recalls

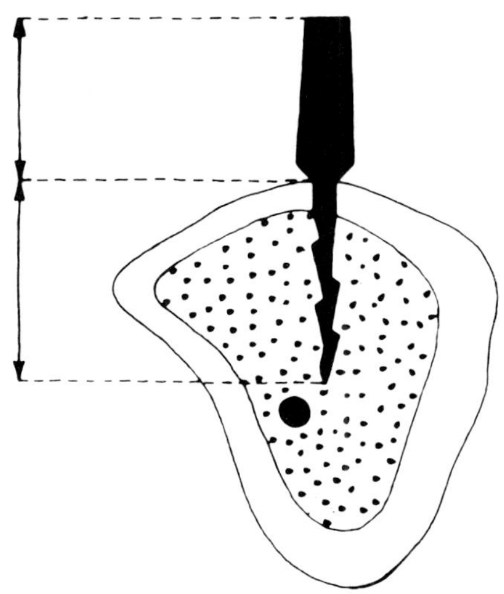

Fig. 12-1. Ideally, it would appear that any blade implant would have a favorable crown-root ratio. The added mesiodistal dimension of the blade implant frame, however, precludes such a direct measurement. Nevertheless, sound clinical judgment must be exercised so as not to abuse this basic crown and bridge principle.

POTENTIAL PROBLEMS WITH BLADE IMPLANTS

Blades with Inadequate Designs

Although the selection of the appropriate blade-vent implant to use for each patient is based on measurement of the depth, the mesiodistal length, and the buccolingual width of the bone, and on the relation to the topography of the bone, there are certain implant designs that are of questionable value. A direct crown-root ratio—which can be established with the natural abutment tooth—cannot be established with the blade-vent implant because of the added dimension of the broad mesiodistal expanse of the frame of blade-vent implants (Figs. 12-1, 12-2).

Despite the fact that no biomathematical formulas have yet been devised to facilitate the practitioner's selection of a blade-vent implant (other than the superimposition of the selection celluloid grid on a radiograph of the area), one fact is obvious. If the clinical crown that extends from the occlusal

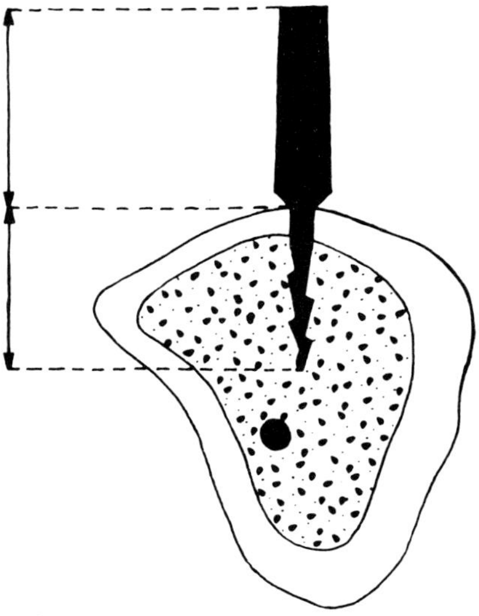

Fig. 12-2. Unless this blade implant has a frame that is long mesiodistally within the bone, its so-called crown-root ratio would be inadequate. The crown portion must not only consist of the implant post depicted herein, but must also include the projected additional occlusal height of the superimposed cast crown retainer.

surface of the retainer through the neck of the implant creates a top-heavy ratio, then such an implant may have a very limited longevity. Therefore, blade implant selection should be based not only on the bony topography of the implant site, but also on the projected height of the subsequently fabricated crown retainer.

Also, prefabricated blade-vent implants that are designed to circumvent sinus areas are of particularly questionable value, because one or more of the legs that extend from the frame into the bone around the sinuses are extremely short, thereby providing insufficient retention (Fig. 12-3). Therefore, in areas in the maxilla—such as the sinuses—that require a modification of the blade-vent implant, with a resultant inadequate depth of the blade-vent implant frame, it would be better to use the subperiosteal implant.

Realignment of the Implant Neck

The prefabricated blade-vent implant may, at times, present a problem in the alignment of the post for a path of insertion with adjacent abutment teeth. Although the metal can be physically bent into position by the use of two sets of hand-held pliers, this practice should be avoided. It is dangerous to bend any such appliance when it is in position in the mouth, because of the obvious possibility of osseous fracture. It is questionable whether the implant neck should ever be bent, because it is not known to what extent the metal would be weakened, even when the implant is reshaped out of the mouth. Therefore, by bending the implant neck, one risks creating a weak point,

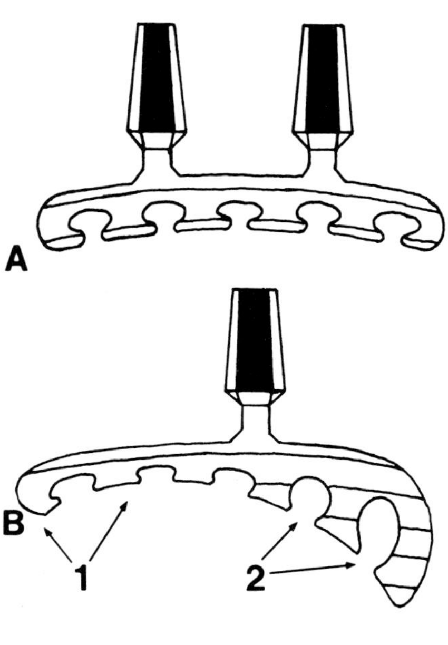

Fig. 12-3. Some blade implant designs, such as these, are of questionable value. *(A)* may have an inadequate amount of intra-osseous support, considering the top-heavy prosthesis that it is meant to support. *(B)* is designed to circumvent a maxillary sinus; although the depth of the legs of the frame may be adequate at one end *(2)*, the amount of bony retention at the other end *(1)* may be insufficient. The discretionary selection of intra-osseous implants should be based as much as possible on the principles expounded for "manmade attachment apparatus."

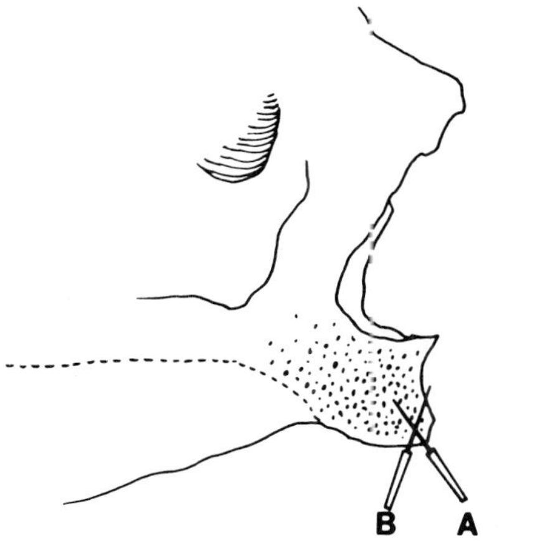

Fig. 12-4. Flaws in the placement of maxillary anterior blade implants. Although Position A appears to be proper in its intra-osseous support, it is obvious that the implant post would be useless because of its labial inclination. The implant neck would have to be mechanically bent, and the resultant severe angulation of the neck might produce a weakening of the neck. On the other hand, Position B may have a correct implant post alignment, but the potential for labial bone perforation by the implant frame would preclude its use. If neither of these pitfalls can be avoided, intra-osseous implants should not be used in this area.

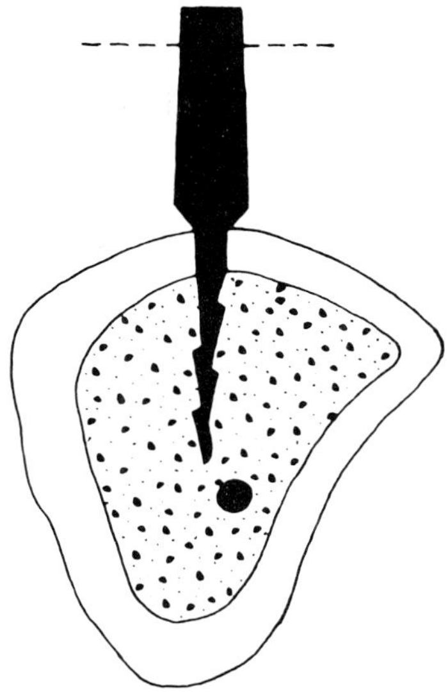

Fig. 12-5. The blade implant post should never be shortened while the frame is within the osseous channel. This pertains as much to the initial insertion appointment as to any subsequent session after healing. The amount of post structure that is to be removed should be determined before implant insertion, and any removal should be done chair-side, while the implant is out of the mouth, just prior to insertion.

which should be avoided particularly at the implant neck, because it is stress-bearing by virtue of its critical linkage of substructure to superstructure (Fig. 12-4). As has been previously mentioned (Chap. 9), the use of cast metal copings is the safest method of realigning the blade-vent implant post to a limited degree. Such a coping may also be used to lengthen the implant post, if necessary.

Shortening the Implant Post

The prefabricated blade-vent implant may at times be too long in occlusal height to enable a crown retainer to be superimposed. In such situations the implant post must be shortened (Fig. 12-5). The time to perform this simple procedure is prior to the insertion of the implant into its osseous channel. The post should never be shortened after healing has taken place, while the implant is in the osseous channel. Such intra-oral procedures may tend to overheat and to vibrate the implant, despite the use of intermittent pressure and copious amounts of water. The practice of shortening the post at the time of insertion of the implant *while the implant is in the osseous channel* should also be avoided because heat transmission and vibration may hamper the critical initial phase of healing. Therefore, if the implant is to be shortened, before the implant is finally seated with a hand mallet, occlusal clearance should be checked, and the implant should be removed before it is shortened. Once the amount of metal that should be removed has been calibrated intra-orally, an NM disc* should be used to cut the post

*Dental Development & Manufacturing Corp., Brooklyn, New York.

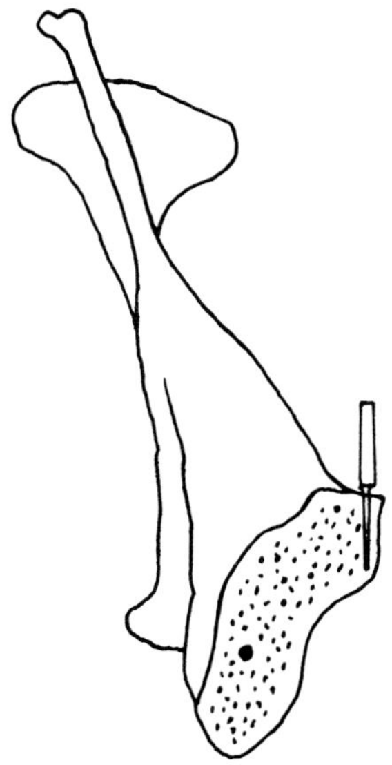

Fig. 12-6. Cross section through a mandible reveals the improper placement of an intra-osseous implant. Although a radiograph may reveal proper insertion, it is only by palpation that the angulation of the mylohyoid ridge area can be determined. In this case, the position of the blade lies precariously towards the lingual aspect. If an adequate amount of attached tissue were to lie buccal to this position, a blade implant could be safely inserted buccal to this position. Otherwise, such an implant is contraindicated.

chair-side. Polishing wheels may then be used to remove any metallic spurs at the occlusal aspect of the implant post. Before the blade-vent implant is reinserted into the prepared osseous channel for a final check, it should be placed in a bead sterilizer* for proper cleaning.

Angulation of the Implant Frame

The use of the radiograph to examine any implant site is of limited value. The critical third dimension must be observed by palpation and by visual examination (Fig. 12-6). There are two areas that are of prime concern for the intra-osseous insertion of an implant: (a) the lingual and sublingual aspects of the posterior mandibular region in the vicinity of the mylohyoid ridge; and (b) the labial aspect of the anterior maxillary region in the vicinity of the nasal spine (Fig. 12-4). In such areas, undercuts of varying degrees are usually present, so that the intra-osseous channel should not be made in an absolutely vertical plane. Instead of creating an angulation for the channel that is perpendicular to the occlusal surface of the residual ridge, the channel should parallel either the lingual aspect of the posterior mandibular region or the labial aspect of the anterior maxillary region. If only radiographic examination is relied upon, the lingual or labial plate of bone may be perforated, necessitating the cessation of the implant procedure.

Reshaping the Implant Frame

The blade-vent implant frame is straight, whereas the mandible and the maxilla have varying degrees of curvatures, which are especially noticeable in the cuspid areas. Therefore, it is necessary to accommodate the implant to the architecture of the bone, in order to avoid the creation of very thin surrounding osseous plates or even perforations. In such instances, the ability to bend the metal, form an arc, is indeed helpful; this does not create the same weakness of metal that has been mentioned before, especially because the blade-vent implant frame is completely confined *within* a supportive osseous framework. The thin wafer-like shape of the blade-vent implant makes it desirable for use in ridges that are especially narrow buccolingually. The ability to bend the metallic implant frame in order to accommodate osseous curvatures is not only of value, but is often necessary.

Resorption of Bone at the Implant

A minor amount of bone loss should be anticipated above the shoulder of the blade implant frame. The surgical procedures involved in both the creation of full-thickness mucoperiosteal flaps and the intra-osseous

*Buffalo Sterilizer Model 62 115V 200W, Buffalo Dental Manufacturing Co., Inc., Brooklyn, New York.

channel preparation involve enough manipulation of the hard and soft tissues to cause a slight amount of bone loss. Such loss is not critical, however, if (a) the implant was placed to its complete and proper depth within the bone, and b) the surgical procedures necessary for this insertion were executed expeditiously, with a minimum of tissue manipulation. Exposure of the occlusal portion of the shoulder of the implant should not be expected (Figs. 12-7, 12-8).

At times, a U-shaped area of bone resorption may appear at the neck of the implant. As long as this resorption is not accompanied by suppurative exudate or by a combination of exudate, pain, and a mobility greater than one on a scale of zero to three, the implant should not be removed. If there is no suppuration, pain, or hypermobility, then the presence of a radiolucent area around the implant frame that tends to look like a periodontal ligament space should not be considered to be a problem. This radiolucent area may just be a soft-tissue membrane (generally referred to as the peri-implant tissue) between the supporting bone and the implant frame; this tissue is not the same as the periodontal ligament that embraces the root of a natural tooth. If, during a recall visit, this radiolucency seems to have increased in size, or if it is accompanied by either pain, hypermobility, or purulent exudate, then the removal of the implant is indicated.

POTENTIAL PROBLEMS WITH SUBPERIOSTEAL IMPLANTS

Strut Exposure

At times, exposure of a primary or secondary strut or even of a portion of the peripheral border of a subperiosteal implant may occur (Fig. 12-9). This may be strictly a mechanical rupture of the superimposed friable mucosal tissue. The patient should be made aware of any such exposure at any recall visit so that he may brush this area with as much care as he would

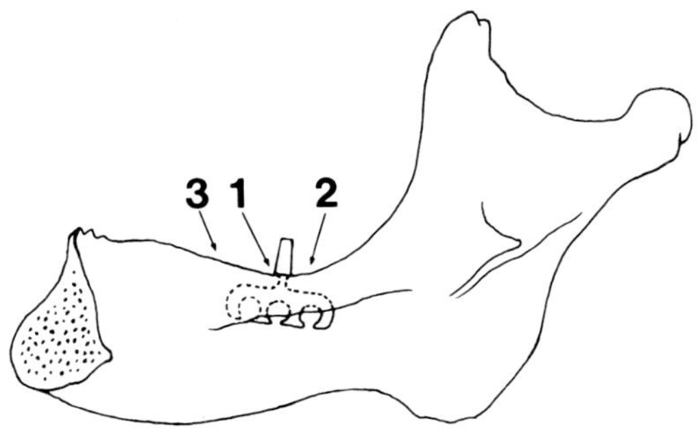

Fig. 12-7. A slight amount of post-insertion bone resorption is to be anticipated above the shoulder of any blade implant. This resorption occurs as a result of the manipulation of bone during the preparation of the intra-osseous channel. Although such resorption may be more extensive at the neck of the implant *(Point 1),* it is likely to occur at all points—both mesial *(Point 3)* and distal *(Point 2)*—at the crest of the residual ridge.

the implant neck. Usually, any inflammation accompanying such exposure can be readily resolved by good home-care practice.

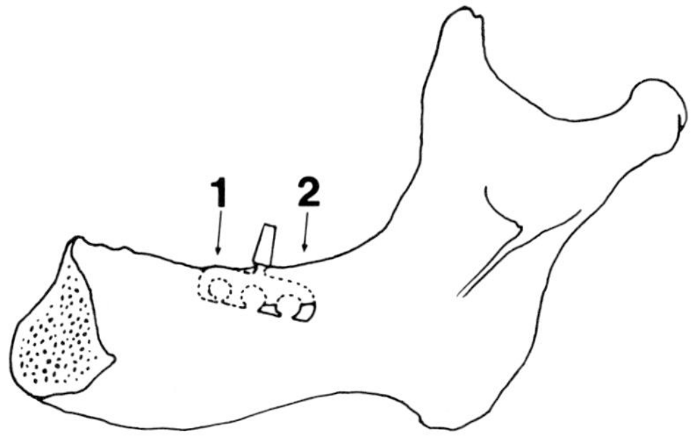

Fig. 12-8. This figure shows the improper placement of a blade implant; the mesial portion *(Point 1)* of the shoulder of the implant is exposed. The proper placement of the blade implant would usually make the shoulder of the implant parallel to the contours of the residual ridge. The shoulder of the implant should be evenly covered by bone at the time of insertion and should be seated to a sufficient depth so that postsurgical bone resorption would not cause exposure of any portion of the implant shoulder. In this figure, even though residual ridge resorption may have occurred at the distal portion *(Point 2)* of the implant shoulder, there is an adequate depth of remaining bone to prevent metal exposure.

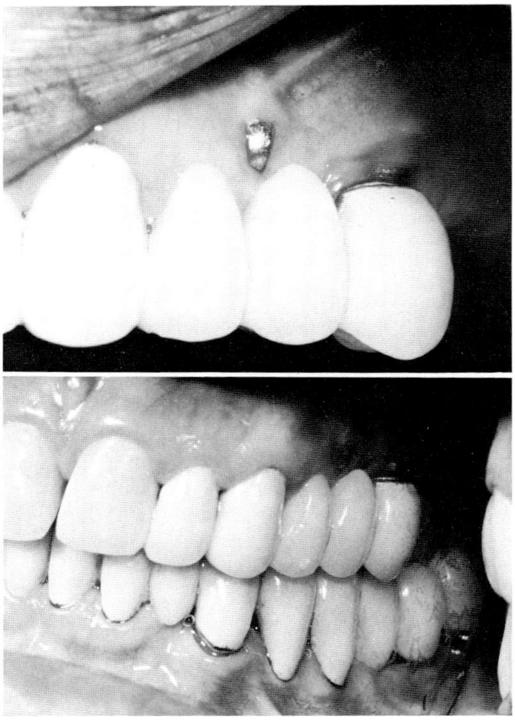

Fig. 12-9. Mirror images of the upper right posterior quadrant at 8-month intervals. Although a metal strut of a terminal subperiosteal implant has ruptured the labial mucosa, there are no positive signs or symptoms. Diligent home care has precluded the necessity of removing this strut, because no inflammation, suppuration, pain, or progressive deterioration has occurred.

If such exposure is accompanied by suppurative exudate, professional treatment is necessary. First, good oral hygiene combined with antibiotic therapy may suppress the infection, thereby preventing the necessity of any further surgery. Second, if such initial therapy does not suffice in eradicating the infection, then surgery is necessary. This surgery would involve full flap exposure of the area, so that the portion of the implant that is directly involved in this chronic situation can be removed. Subsequently, the full-thickness flaps are approximated and resutured to facilitate uneventful healing (Figs. 12-10, 12-11). Unless the portion of metal that is removed directly affects a primary supportive strut or implant neck, there should be no appreciable loss of retention of the subperiosteal implant frame. The frame should, by this time, have adequate connective tissue interwoven within the remaining portion (Fig. 12-12).

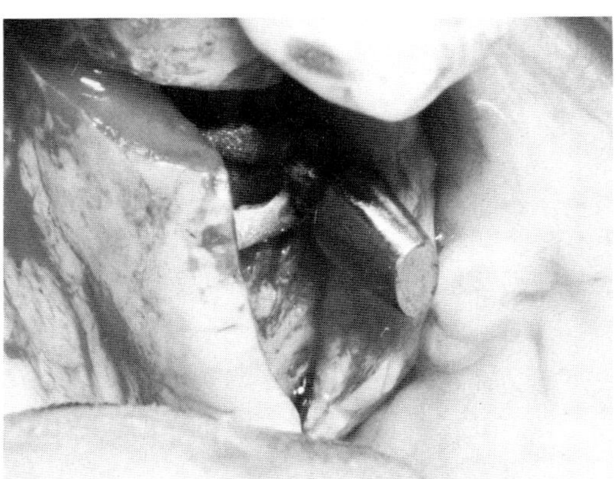

Fig. 12-10. Palatal view of a maxillary terminal subperiosteal implant. The inspection of any symptomatic implant requires procedures similar to those required for surgery for the insertion of the subperiosteal implant. Full-thickness flaps and blunt dissection make possible proper inspection, as well as curettage procedures where indicated.

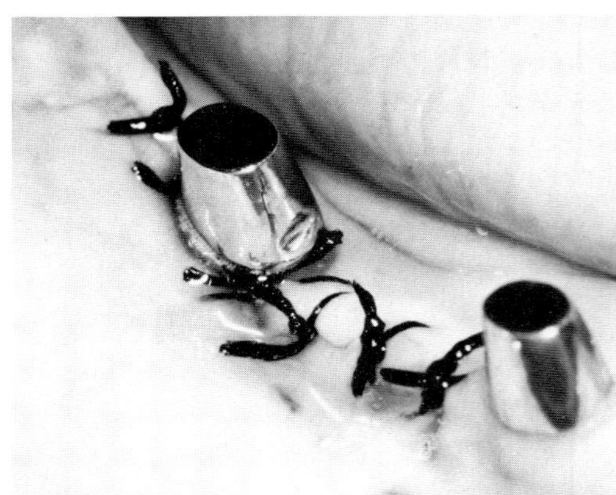

Fig. 12-11. Curettage surgical intervention at the distal portion of a complete subperiosteal implant has been followed by close suturing. The use of individual sutures to approximate the full-thickness flaps, with specific concentration around the implant neck, should facilitate uneventful healing. This is similar to the suturing that takes place after implant insertion.

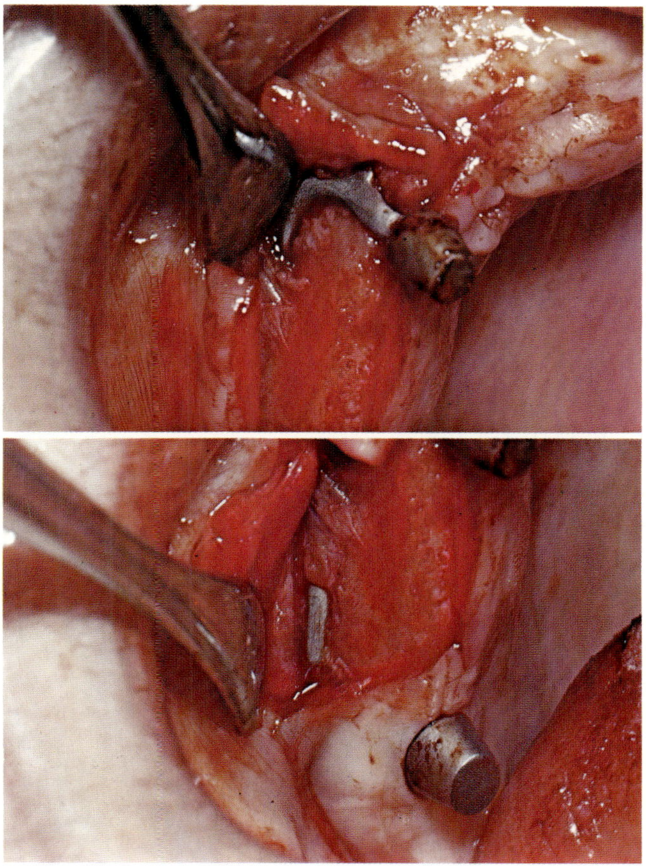

Plate 12–1. See Figure 12–12.

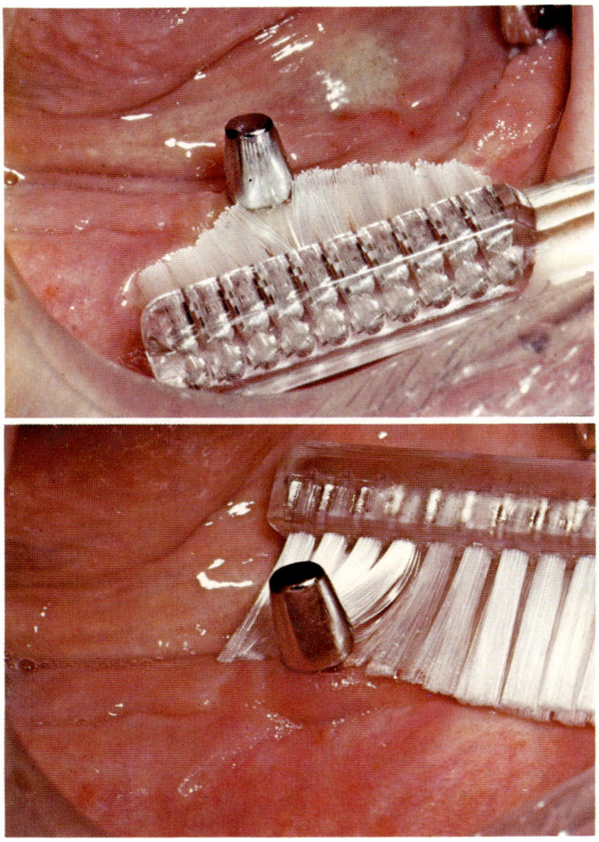

Plate 12–2. See Figure 12–19.

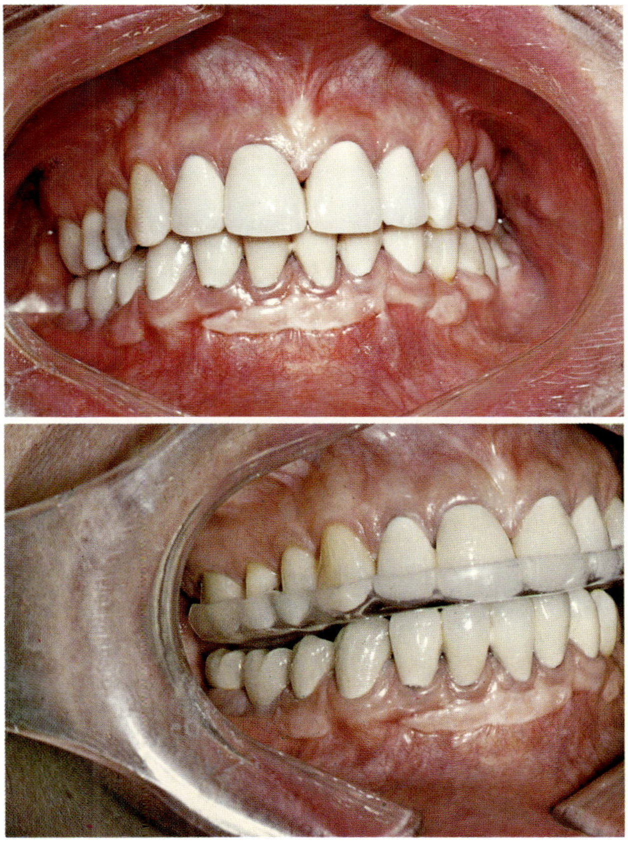

Plate 12–3. See Figure 12–21.

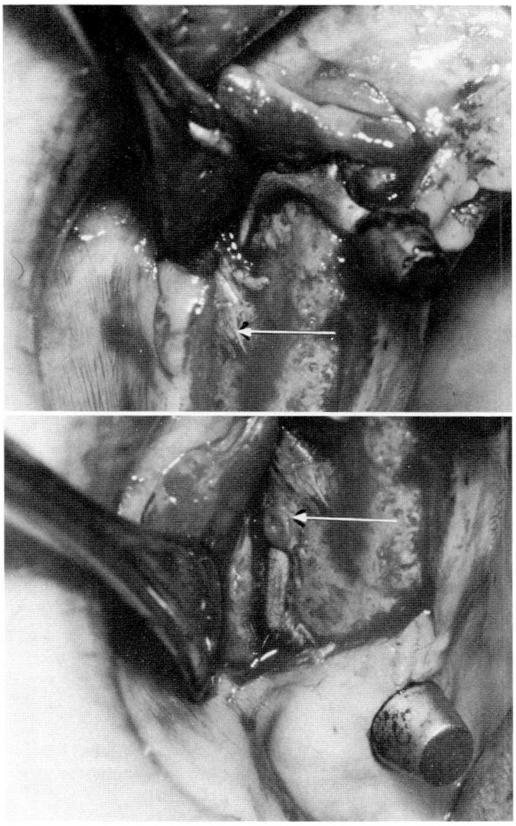

Fig. 12-12. Surgical reentry of subperiosteal implants normally reveals fibrous strands of connective tissue *(arrows)* engaging various parts of the implant frame. As long as there are no positive signs or symptoms, the subperiosteal implant frame would rest on bone, with the weaving ingrowth of a meshwork of such tenacious tissue.

Bone Resorption

An amount of bone resorption comparable to the thickness of any portion of the implant frame should be considered clinically inconsequential. It has been referred to by Dr. Roy Bodine and his fellow investigators as a "settling" of the implant (see Chap. 6), which may take place with any subperiosteal implant (Fig. 12-13). Each soft-tissue area surrounding each implant neck, however, should be milked with finger pressure, to check for any cumulative suppurative material. If such suppuration is milky in color and consistency, initial antibiotic therapy, accompanied by irrigation and diligent home care, may eradicate this positive sign. If exacerbations persist, or if this exudate is of a thick, coagulant nature, surgical intervention would be necessary. There are three different levels of such surgical intervention.

1. The most conservative surgical intervention is one that does not alter the implant itself. The area in question should receive a full-thickness incision at the height of the residual ridge (Fig. 12-14). This incision is similar to the one that was required for the insertion of the implant. Then, surgical curettes are used, in conjunction with blunt dissection of the overlying tissue, to remove any granulation tissue or what may appear to the naked eye to be a soft, nonsupportive tissue. Such tissue must be thoroughly and exactingly removed along every strut; this may necessitate further dissection in any given direction along any given strut in order to follow the path of such deterioration.

Usually, if recalls have been on a regular 6-month basis, such interceptive procedures may be instituted successfully with-

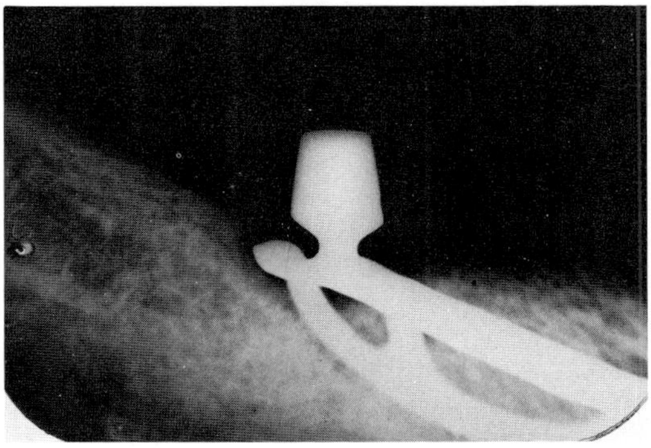

Fig. 12-13. At times, a radiograph may reveal bone resorption at the distal portion of a complete mandibular subperiosteal implant. This resorption may be due to a combination of masticatory force and *flexure of the mandible.* If there are no other positive signs, and if subsequent radiographic check-ups reveal no osseous change, then the implant may be left as is. If, however, uncontrolled suppuration occurs, or if the radiolucency becomes larger, then it may be necessary to remove that portion of the implant.

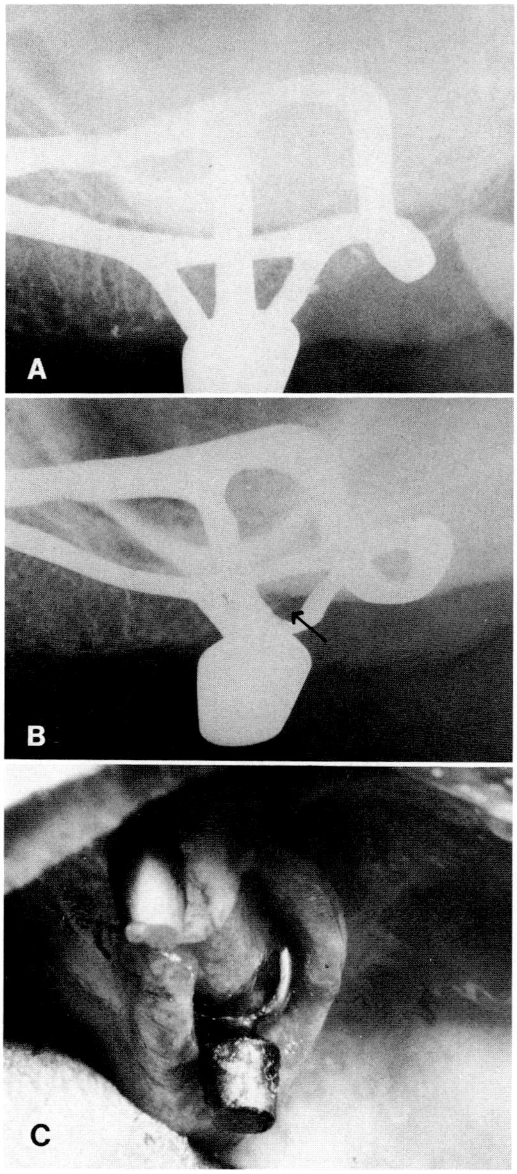

Fig. 12-14. The importance of several individual radiographs cannot be overemphasized. This series shows two apical radiographs *(A, B)* of an upper right posterior area, and the subsequent reflection of full-thickness flaps in that same area *(C)*. The only symptom was pain. A single apical radiograph *(A)* revealed no positive signs. Another apical radiograph *(B)*, taken at a different angle, revealed bone loss under the implant post *(arrow)*. The surgical opening of this segment *(C)* enabled the removal of the soft granulation tissue by curettage, which precluded any further deterioration that might have gone otherwise unnoticed.

out having to resort to anything more extensive. When performed properly, this curettage procedure is more time-consuming than the implant insertion procedure. This curettage procedure should be accompanied by antibiotic therapy in order to increase the chances of success.

2. There are times when the curettage procedure may not produce an effective positive long-term result. Also, the failure of the recall system—on the part of the patient or the clinician—with any patient may result in an area with advanced degenerative changes that may indicate, even radiographically, that the interceptive curettage procedure would not suffice. In such instances, if the area of concern is localized, then the removal of a strut or a portion of the border, or even of an entire post and its supportive frame (in the case of a complete-arch implant), may be necessary (Fig. 12-15). Such interception may result in the salvation of the remainder of the implant in a complete subperiosteal case. It should be remembered that when severing the implant frame with new high-speed carbide burs, intermittent pressure and copious amounts of water should be used, to minimize bone damage and to prevent disturbance of the sound portion of the implant frame. Because of the feasibility of such interceptive surgical procedures, it has been recommended that for fixed prostheses that are supported by either a partial or a complete subperiosteal implant, the superstructures should not be cemented with a permanent cementing agent (see Chap. 9). Accessibility for surgical intervention or for modification of portions of the fixed superstructure is best achieved by judicious cementation aided by Re Seté screw insertion.

3. If (a) antibiotic therapy accompanied by impeccable home care, or (b) curettage procedures, or (c) strut removal have not corrected a chronic purulent or increasingly radiolucent area, then removal of the entire implant would be necessary. There are times when suppuration may occur

around each neck of a complete implant, without accompanying pain. In such cases, the patient should be informed of the degeneration surrounding the implant, and the patient should be advised as to removal of the implant (Fig. 12-16). Sometimes, such suppuration is restricted to the implant neck area, and there may be no accompanying enlargement of the radiographic radiolucency. In these cases, sound clinical judgment may call for well-spaced intermittent antibiotic treatments, which may suffice in relieving such exacerbations, and the implant may not have to be removed.

The question always arises as to the feasibility of inserting an implant after a previous implant has been removed. Only after a 6- to 9-month healing period can such a decision be made. If healing has been uneventful, and if the accompanying bone loss has been minimal, then such implant procedures may be considered. Not only is a waiting period necessary, however, but the amount of bone loss must be assessed. The only alternative may be the use of a conventional removable complete or partial denture, if the bone loss is too extensive for another implant.

Screws in Subperiosteal Implants

The screws that accompany some mandibular implants are a potential source of soft-tissue inflammation. If inflammation occurs at any time after the initial healing that follows the insertion procedures, a small incision should be made above the screw area. Then the screw can be readily removed with the appropriate surgical screwdriver. At this stage, it should not be necessary to rely on the screw to hold the implant in place.

Sometimes, although inflammation may not occur, a radiographic radiolucency may be noticed during any of the recall appointments. This situation would also necessitate the removal of the screw. Any screw that has no accompanying inflammatory signs or radiographic anomalies, however, should be left in place indefinitely.

The Distal Aspects of the Complete Mandibular Subperiosteal Implant

The most frequent areas of change or pathosis with the complete mandibular implant are the distal-most areas around the molar implant posts. Inflammation in the buccal fold is the most innocuous of all possible situations and does not require surgical treatment. If there is a slight swelling *without* accompanying pain, bone resorption, or purulent exudate, then it is best not to intervene. If any of the aforementioned symptoms accompany this fullness, then a complete surgical curettage reentry is indicated.

Also, a radiograph may reveal slight bone resorption, without any accompanying inflammation, suppuration, or pain. If this resorption falls within the realm of what has been described as a settling of the implant, then no surgical intervention would be indicated. Here again, however, if this resorption is accompanied by suppuration upon milking, pain, or a large fistula in the vicinity, then surgical entry and intervention would be necessary. Radiographic examination alone (unless the results are gross) may not be sufficient for determining whether to intervene. Only (a) when radiolucencies are accompanied by other signs, or (b) if the area of radiolucency or resorption is larger than the norms anticipated in settling, or (c) if the area of radiolucency is of an active nature that differs from previous recall radiographic examinations, does the radiograph take on an added significance.

The more frequent occurrence of such radiographic signs in the distal aspects of the mandible *may relate to the flexibility of the mandible through opening and closing.* This is strictly conjecture; but it may call attention to the necessity for flexibility of the implant frame rather than more rigid materials and designs.

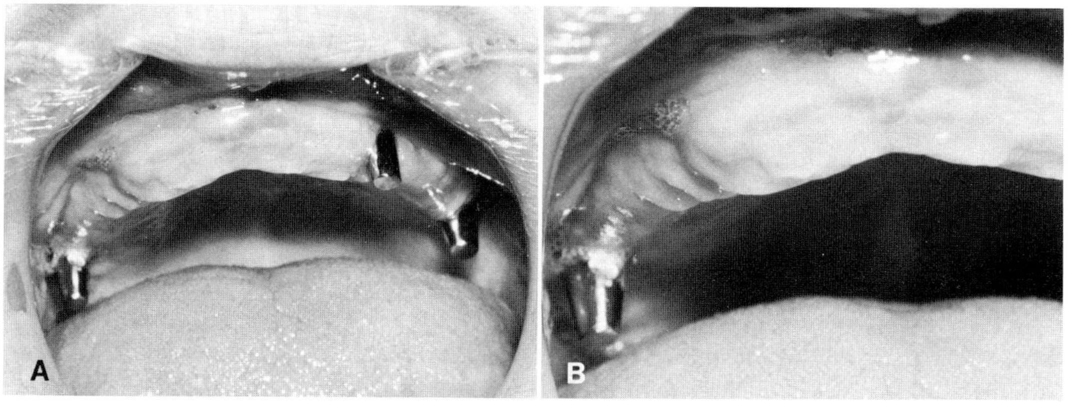

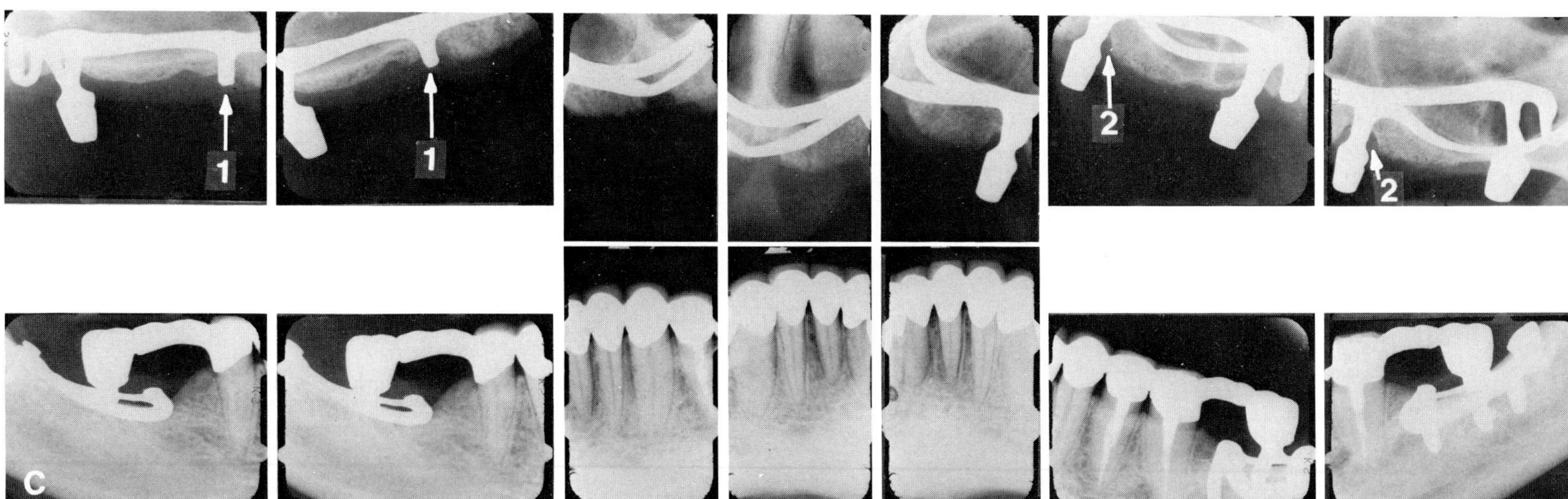

Fig. 12-15. Suppuration and inflammation developed in the upper right cuspid post area of an otherwise sound complete maxillary subperiosteal implant. Because of these symptoms, the post and the labial primary strut were removed, and the tissues were reapproximated. These photographs *(A, B)* and radiographs *(C)* were taken more than 1 year after surgical removal of the strut. (*B* is a close-up view of the upper right cuspid area after removal of the post and the labial primary strut.) The complete upper denture was relined to accommodate the new ridge topography. The surgical intervention *(C, Arrow 1)* prevented the possible loss of the entire implant. The saucering of bone *(C, Arrow 2)* at any post site should be observed during various check-ups. Usually, such resorption does not progress beyond the noted point. (The surgical intervention and post removal were done by Dr. Edward Listengart.)

HOME CARE INSTRUCTION

Upon insertion of the implant, or during the 7-day postoperative session for the removal of sutures, the patient should be thoroughly informed of the responsibilities of home care. Plaque control is as important in implantology as it is in any other aspect of dentistry (Figs. 12-17, 12-18). Home care is especially important in implantology because the area of soft tissue that surrounds each implant neck is a weak link. Regardless of the proximity and tightness of the tissue that surrounds an implant neck, such tissue is in no way a barrier to the ingress of oral fluids or debris, as is the intact epithelial attachment of the gingival unit of the natural tooth. Even though certain implant materials allow for the ingrowth or adhesion of soft tissue to the implant neck, *there is no barrier in implantology that is as complete as the sound base of the gingival sulcus of the natural tooth.*

The patient must both eliminate plaque and stimulate the tissues; this should be explained to the patient so that he understands what is to be accomplished. The use of the brush, dental tape, and soft pipe cleaners is encouraged. Because implant necks are usually located in highly resorbed areas to which it is difficult to gain access, the brush head should be small and the bristles soft (Fig. 12-19). The Oral B Sulcus Brush* is particularly appropriate. The brush should be used in a sweeping

*Division of Cooper Laboratories, Inc., Wayne, New Jersey.

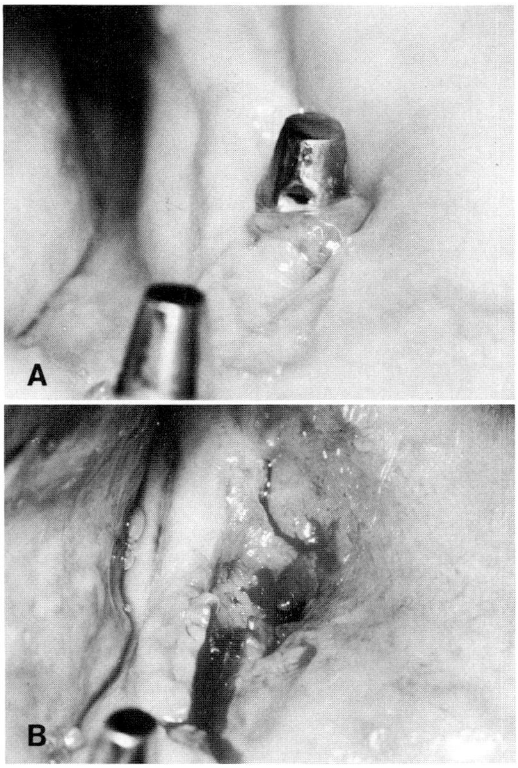

Fig. 12-16. The importance of recalls cannot be overemphasized. In this case, the patient presented *only* because of discomfort in the lower left posterior region of a complete subperiosteal implant *(A)*. Bone loss, together with discomfort, suppuration, and tissue hypertrophy, necessitated the removal of the distal post of this implant *(B)*. Fortunately, this unhealthy state did not progress along the path of least resistance to the progress and movement of suppurative exudate (along the implant frame), so that retention of the remainder of the implant was achieved.

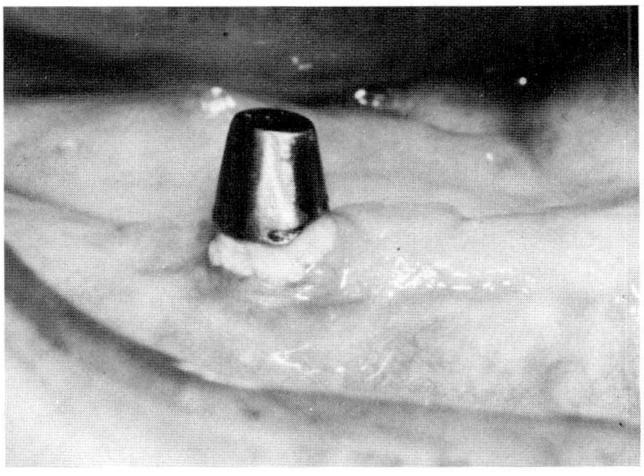

Fig. 12-17. The lack of proper home care can lead to the accumulation of varying amounts of plaque, which may lead to the deterioration of the soft tissues around the neck of the implant. Fortunately, the removal of this debris and the reinforcement of the home-care procedures during a recall visit prevented any detrimental effects on this implant.

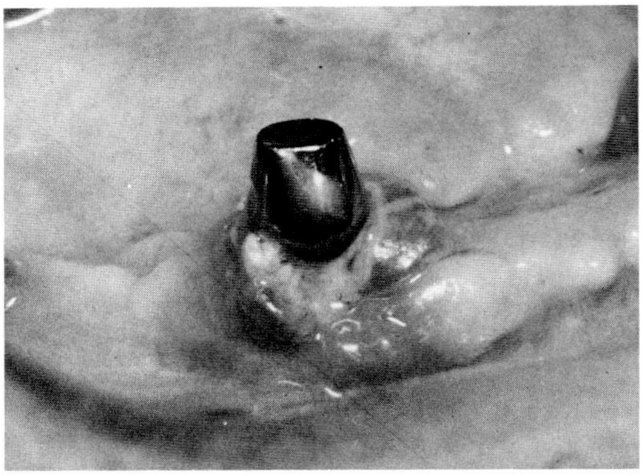

Fig. 12-18. Complete neglect of an implant by the patient can lead to failure—as in any case of any natural dentition. Not only is it important to screen patients prior to implant insertion, but home care instruction must be taught and reinforced during recalls. In all phases of dentistry, including implantology, however, patient neglect is sometimes unforeseeable. As this figure illustrates, complete lack of home care by the patient and failure to appear for routine recall appointments has resulted in gross pathosis around an implant post.

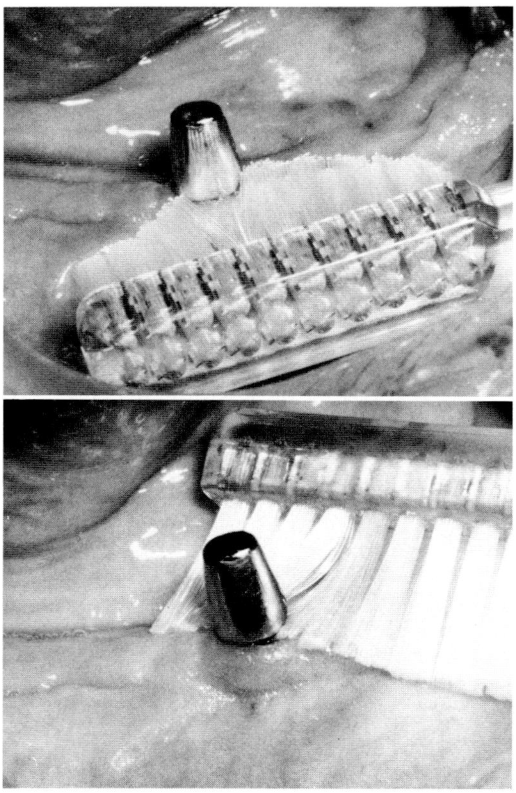

Fig. 12-19. Circumferential brushing of the necks and posts of all implants should be taught to all implant patients. The head of the brush should be small enough to provide access to all exposed metallic parts. The bristles are placed perpendicular to the implant post, and the brushing strokes are in short horizontal movements. The bristles should actually fit beneath the post base, in order to maintain a lustrous polish of the implant neck. (The Oral B Sulcus Brush is recommended.)

horizontal motion along both the buccal and lingual surfaces. The bristles should actually depress the soft tissues so that they fit below the base of the post along the implant neck. The proximal (mesial and distal) surfaces of the implant necks are best cleaned with soft pipe cleaners, which can be twisted into a convenient, manageable shape (Fig. 12-20). The pipe cleaners are placed along the neck of the implant, in the so-called sulcular area, and are used back and forth, in a shoeshine motion, to clean the implant neck and the surrounding tissues and to stimulate these tissues. Dental tape may be used instead of pipe cleaners. Although it is advised that pipe cleaners take precedence over dental tape, it is a matter of patient preference as to the ease of manipulation.

For the most part, the use of water irrigation devices is discouraged. These devices do not afford the same direct control of plaque removal as a brush or other hand-held cleaner. Also, with a water irrigation device, there is always a danger of lifting the tissue away from its osseous base, and the tissue may be lacerated, thus inducing a pathologic state (see Chap. 6). Only when gross debris is present can a water irrigation device be safely used at very low pressures, and only *in conjunction with* the other forms of plaque control.

At this same instructive appointment session, the patient should be made aware of the possibilities of abusing any implant. Because an implant is a prosthetic appliance, its abuse may tend to destroy the supportive tissues over a period of time. The patient should be made aware that sustained forces and adverse pressures are detrimental to the retention of any implant. Sustained forces relate to such habits as clenching or bruxism. Although a patient who exhibits clenching and bruxism would have been eliminated as an implant candidate, such sustained forces may be caused by holding a pipe or a cigar between the teeth. This would tend to place unrelieved stress on the implant and its supportive structures. Adverse pressures may relate to the manner of eating or to the consistency of foods that are ingested. Specifically, eating corn on the cob and biting into whole, fresh apples should be discouraged because of the adverse pressures and torque that would be sustained by the implant. The patient should be encouraged to still eat such foods but he should cut them into small pieces. Similarly, the constant chewing of gum, the cracking of nutshells by the teeth, the crunching of hard candies, and other similar oral habits should be discouraged, and their resultant detrimental effects should be explained to the patient.

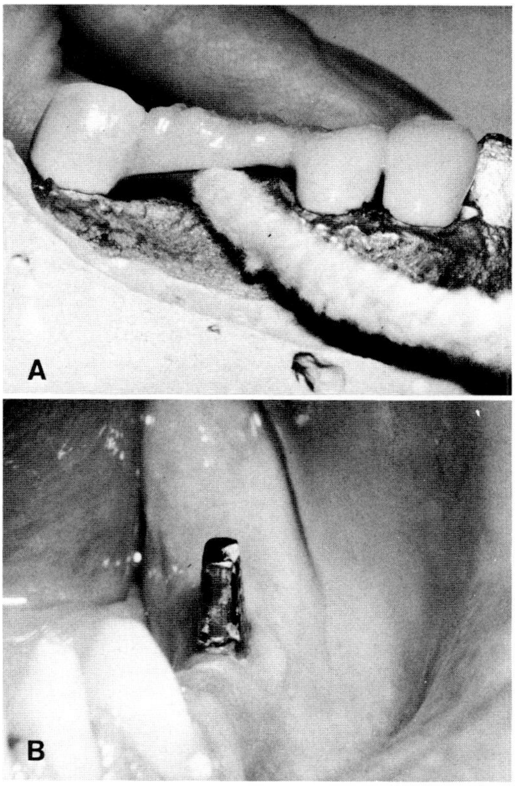

Fig. 12-20. Soft pipe cleaners are used by the patients as part of their home-care armamentarium. These pipe cleaners can be shaped to the patients' convenience. Thus, the distal and mesial portions of implant necks can be shoeshined, and the soft tissues that are beneath modified sanitary pontics can be massaged and maintained clean *(A)*. It is through the use of such devices that the mechanical removal of plaque and of food debris can be readily achieved with fixed implant prostheses *(B)*.

RECALL OF THE IMPLANT PATIENT

An important part of the entire implant service is the system of recalls. Even though a patient may not have discomfort, such recalls are necessary. Radiographic hints and visual signs may indicate potential problems. Usually, it is a good practice to observe the patient three to four times within the first year of implant insertion. Then, if no adverse conditions have been present, the patient may be observed during semiannual checkups.

The recall of any implant patient should take the form of a step-by-step routine:

1. Visual Examination: The patient's oral hygiene should be checked, and any deficiencies on his part should be brought to his attention prior to debris removal. The patient must see what he had not attended to. Usually, an inflammation can be seen by visual examination. Other important signs to look for are wear facets, which may indicate a need for either occlusal adjustment or the notation of a possible detrimental nonfunctional occlusal habit on the part of the patient. For example, the patient may have developed the habit of bruxism at any time since the insertion of the implant and the prosthesis that it supports. In such situations, severe wear

patterns may be noted on the occlusal surfaces of the prosthetic appliance. Of course, there is no definitive treatment for nocturnal bruxism, other than the interceptive use of a processed acrylic-resin night guard in some cases. If the bruxism is brought to the patient's attention, and if the patient can consciously refrain from bruxism during the day, then the detrimental effects of this habit may at least be partially removed. It is important to inform the patient, however, that clenching or bruxism ultimately results in the failure of a complete implant.

2. Palpation: Palpation consists of an actual milking procedure of the soft tissues towards the implant neck. Thus, any suppuration may be noted and attended to as previously described. If inflammation is present, the sublingual glandular area should be palpated extra-orally to ascertain the degree of any possible infectious process.

3. Periapical Radiographs: Individual periapical radiographs most accurately reveal any potential problems of the bone. Those radiographic changes that may accompany the strut thickness of implant settling or indicate the presence of an implant membrane are of no concern. Other radiolucencies, however, should be carefully related to signs and symptoms for possible interceptive surgical procedures.

4. Mobility Testing: Every aspect of the fixed superstructure should be checked for any possible cement washout. This is done by a gentle push and pull technique. First, every portion of the occlusal aspects of the fixed prosthesis is depressed with the index finger, and the examiner looks for either percolation at the crown margins or any rocking movement of the superstructure itself. Then, an explorer is hooked under the major embrasures at the abutment sites and pulled gently in each area. Here too, if any movement or percolation occurs, a washout of the prosthesis is evident. On the other hand, such procedures may reveal a stable fixed superstructure, but a mobility in a buccolingual direction. If such mobility is greater than 1, on a 0 to 3 scale, then the possibility of implant failure or occlusal traumatism should be explored. The same stabilities that should be expected for any fixed periodontal prosthesis should be expected for any implant prosthesis.

5. Occlusion: The even distribution of occlusal forces should be rechecked at each recall appointment. Articulating paper, or waxes, or a Joffe Marker* in conjunction with a thin cellophane paper are useful for examining occlusion. The newly acquired stability of occlusal surfaces of any complete arch through the use of implants may allow the patient to assume a much more relaxed muscular tone. Because of this, further occlusal adjustments and even remounts may be required in those cases wherein a highly resorbed edentulous ridge had failed to support and retain a comfortable removable complete denture over a period of years. In cases that have a terminal or intermediary implant abutment, the occlusal surfaces related to these specific areas should never be relieved of occlusal contacts except when bite guards are used (Fig. 12-21). Such relief of the fabricated dentition would not only preclude the even distribution of occlusal forces, but a resultant torque may occur that would tend to lift the implant in an occlusal direction.

6. A Reminder: It is advisable to remind the patient, during any recall appointment, of the nature of the implant prosthesis. Just as a patient must be made aware that surgery may leave him with a scar, or a hip implant may leave him with a slight limp, so must he be made aware of the fact that the dental implant is man-made and cannot endure the abuses that a natural intact dentition can endure. Not only should foodstuffs be cut into small pieces in order to avoid as much as possible incising on the anterior teeth, but sustained forces on any portion of the man-made dentition

*The Hygienic Dental Manufacturing Co., Akron, Ohio.

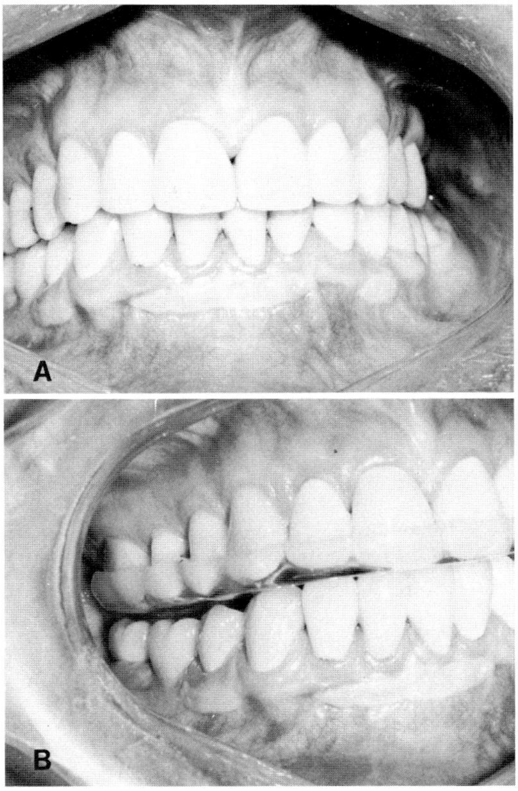

Fig. 12-21. An implant abutment supports a lower right four-unit fixed prosthesis *(A)*. Only *after* the completion of this case was it learned that the patient had become a night-time clencher. In order to alleviate such undue stresses upon the implant, a night guard was fabricated for the upper arch, with specific occlusal relief of the night guard for the lower right posterior segment *(B, after 4 years of using the night guard)*. Naturally, had it been known before treatment that this patient was a clencher or a bruxer, an implant would not have been indicated. Moderate mechanical interceptive procedures during check-ups, however, can prevent implant deterioration, just as check-ups may prevent deterioration of natural dentition and periodontium. (Periodontal treatment by Dr. Jeffrey Shapiro)

should be avoided. From time to time an occasional ache or soreness may occur without any other positive signs that would otherwise indicate degeneration of the implant and its surrounding structures. With proper home care, regular maintenance visits, and a modification and moderation of masticatory habits, the prostheses and their supporting implants can provide years of comfort and function for the stomatognathic systems of many edentulous and partially edentulous individuals.

BIBLIOGRAPHY

Bassett, C. A. L., and Becker, R. O.: Generation of electrical potentials by bone in response to mechanical stress. Science, *137:*1063-1064, 1962.

Bhaskar, S. N., *et al.*: Biodegradable ceramic implants in bone. Oral Surg., *32:*336-346, 1971.

De Angelis, V.: Observations on the response of alveolar bone to orthodontic force. Am. J. Orthodontics, *58:*284-294, 1970.

Fraunhofer, J. A. von, L'Estrange, P. R., and Mack, A. O.: Materials science in dental implantation and a promising new material: vitreous carbon. Biomed. Engin., *6:*114-118, 1971.

Grenoble, D. E., and Kim, R. L.: Progress in the evaluation of a vitreous carbon endosteal implant. Oral Implantol., *4:*216-235, 1973.

Lee, T. C.: The vitreous endosteal implant: a single tooth replacement system. J. California D. A., *1:*42-43, 1973.

Mandel, I. D.: Dental plaque: nature, formation, and effects. J. Periodont., *37:*537-567, 1966.

Polisar, R. S., and Cook, A. W.: Use of polyethylene in cranial implants. J. Pros. Dent., *29:*310-316, 1973.

Powell, R. N.: Oral hygiene and the dental plaque. J. Irish D. A., *16:*167-171, 1970.

Ringqvist, M.: Fibre sizes of human masseter muscle in relation to bite force. J. Neurol. Sci., *19:*297-305, 1973.

Ross, S. R.: What is plaque control? J. California D. A., *47:*8-13, 1971.

Sumner, C. F.: What is the value of water spray devices in maintaining adequate oral hygiene. Periodont. Abst., *14:*150, 1966.

Thomas, J. C.: The load factor in complete denture intolerance. J. Pros. Dent., *25:*4-11, 1971.

Toto, P. D., Evans, C. L., and Sawinski, V. J.: Effects of water jet rinse and toothbrushing on oral hygiene. J. Periodont., *40:*296-298, 1969.

Waerhaug, J.: Effect of rough surfaces upon gingival tissue. J. D. Res., *35:*323-325, 1956.

Index

Numbers in *italics* indicate an illustration.